Revised Third Edition

THE

"COMPLETE"

NATURAL

HEALTH

ENCYCLOPEDIA

NATURAL TREATMENTS

for the Worlds 400 Most Common Ailments

Plus a Complete Directory on
VITAMINS & MINERALS
WESTERN & ORIENTAL HERBS
HOMEOPATHIC MEDICINES
PROTEINS & AMINO ACIDS
THERAPEUTIC & TOXIC FOODS

By David H. Nyholt

THIS ENCYCLOPEDIA CONTAINS
REFERENCE INFORMATION ONLY
IT IS IN NO WAY INTENDED TO BE PRESCRIPTIVE OR DIAGNOSTIC.

This book is a reference work based on extensive research. The intent is to offer natural alternatives for complex solutions to treat the breakdown of the immunity system. In the event you use this information without your doctor's approval, you are prescribing for yourself, which is your constitutional right, but the publisher and author assume no responsibility.

Genesis 1: 29-30

"And God said, behold, I have given you every herb bearing seed, which is upon the face of all the earth, and every tree, in the which is the fruit of a tree yielding seed; to you it shall be for meat."

"And to every beast of the earth, and to every fowl of the air, and to everything that creepeth upon the earth, wherein there is life, I have given every green herb for meat: and it was so."

Canadian Cataloging in Publication Data
Nyholt, David H.
The Complete Natural Health Encyclopedia
Includes Bibliographical References and Index
1. Health. 2. Nutrition. 3. Herbs - Therapeutic use. 4. Homeopathy
I. Title
RA776.N94 1993   613   C93-091265-9
ISBN 0-921202-07-5

Printed in United States of America

DEDICATION

This book is dedicated to my parents Henry and Kelly Nyholt who gave direction, meaning, and cohesion to my life. My children Doren, Dixie, Darrell, Dwayne, and Lorne. My mother in-law Clara Davidson and to my loving wife Sandra whose vision sparked mine.

ACKNOWLEDGMENTS

I wish to express my sincere thanks to the Global Health's research staff for their time, energy, dedication, and support in the preparation of this book.

FOREWORD

This encyclopedia was assembled to provide the general public with the latest breakthroughs in natural health science and to keep you in touch with the proper natural treatments and remedies for the world's most common ailments. We are united in cause, to help you restore health, prevent premature aging, and prolong life. The Complete Natural Health Encyclopedia is the most comprehensive, concise, and straight forward natural health guide on the market today. Simplified, allowing you to skim through and find what you want and need to know when you're at your busiest, or digest at your leisure. Using the quick scan index, clearly designed charts on vitamins, minerals, therapeutic foods, herbs, homeopathic remedies, amino acids, and tissue salts. Giving you more information in less reading time.

The author has also included, quick reference R.D.A. charts. Effects and side effects of the common vitamins, minerals, and herbs and in which foods they can be found. Nutrition should be looked upon as a means of preventing as well as treating disease. This can be accomplished through appropriate supplementation, proper selection of foods, and lifestyle changes. This guide will expand your awareness of treating yourself as naturally as possible, and discover a comfortable relationship with the latest natural alternatives for your busy lifestyle.

It is our privilege and honor to participate in Mr. Nyholts efforts. He has put his experience, knowledge, and heart into his studies, for the continuing happiness and health of people around the world.

Gordon Jones

Director, Global Health Research Foundation.

QUICK REFERENCE INDEX

INDEX

TREATMENTS
FOR OVER 400
COMMON AILMENTS

INDEX

AILMENTS - Continued

INDEX

AILMENTS - Continued

INDEX

AILMENTS - Continued

INDEX

INDEX

WESTERN HERBS -
 Continued

INDEX

WESTERN HERBS -
Continued

INDEX

ORIENTAL HERBS

INDEX

HERBAL GLOSSARY

SPICE RACK REMEDIES

AMINO ACIDS

INDEX

AMINO ACIDS - Continued

HOMEOPATHY

HOMEOPATHIC

COMBINATION REMEDIES

HOMEOPATHIC

SINGULAR REMEDIES

INDEX

INDEX

HEALING FOODS

INDEX

GLOSSARY

BIBLIOGRAPHY

GLOBAL HEALTH BOOKS

NATURAL TREATMENTS FOR 400 OF THE WORLD'S MOST COMMON AILMENTS

ABSCESS

SPECIFICS: An abscess forms when pus accumulates externally or internally in a particular part of the body due to infection. Most abscesses are treated with antibiotics which destroy the B vitamins as well as the friendly bacteria.

(BeneficialRemedies,Treatments,andNutrients)

SINGLE HERBS: Burdock root, Cayenne, Chaparral, Dandelion root, Echinacea, Red Clover, Yellow Dock root.

VITAMINS: A, B complex, E, C, plus a Multivitamin.

MINERALS: Zinc, plus Mineral complex.

ALSO: Acidophilus, Garlic capsules, Pau d'arco, Raw Thymus, and Proteolytic enzymes.

HELPFUL FOODS: Beef, broccoli, carrots, fish liver oils, fruits, green leafy vegetables, herring, nuts, soybeans, spinach, pumpkin seeds, and whole wheat.

ACNE

SPECIFICS: A disorder of the oil(sebaceous) glands in the skin. It is believed that stress is a significant factor in acne. Other factors that contribute to acne are allergies, heredity, oral contraceptives, overindulgence in carbohydrates, and foods with high fat or sugar content and androgens(male hormones) produced in increased amounts when the girl or boy reaches puberty.

(BeneficialRemedies,Treatments,andNutrients)

HERBAL COMBINATION: (AKN).

PHYSIOLOGIC ACTION: Acne is nearly always the product of blood impurities. AKN helps cleanse toxins and mucus. Enhances overall good health and well-being, and helps eliminate skin blemishes and acne.

SINGLE HERBS: Burdock, Chaparral, Chlorophyll, Echinacea, Garlic, Gotu Kola, Red Clover, Yellow Dock, and Yucca.

VITAMINS: A, B complex, B3, B6, C, E, and F.

MINERALS: Potassium, Sulfur, and Zinc.

ALSO: Primadophilus

HELPFUL FOODS: Avocados, bananas, broccoli, lean beef, carrots, celery, fruits (citrus and other), green leafy vegetables, pumpkin, radish, and vegetable oils.

ADRENAL EXHAUSTION

SPECIFICS: The adrenal glands are organs resting on top of each kidney. They are responsible for the production of the hormone epinephrine that speeds up the rate of metabolism in order to cope with stress and are involved in the metabolism of carbohydrates and the regulation of blood sugar. Adrenal exhaustion is most often caused by the long term use of cortisone drugs. Other causes are continuous stress, smoking, poor nutritional habits, and alcohol and drug abuse.

(Beneficial Remedies, Treatments, and Nutrients)

SINGLE HERBS: Astragalus, Echinacea, Milk Thistle, and Siberian Ginseng.

VITAMINS: B2, B12, B complex, Folic acid, Pantothenic acid, C, and E.

MINERALS: Copper, Potassium, Sodium, and Zinc.

ALSO: Coenzyme Q10, Germanium, L-Tyrosine, and Unsaturated fatty acids.

HELPFUL FOODS: Beef, broccoli, bananas, bacon, all fruits, herring, sea salt, raisins, soybeans, sweet potatoes, spinach, turnip greens, and whole wheat.

AGE SPOTS
(refer to Skin Problems)

AIDS
(Acquired Immune Deficiency Syndrome)

SPECIFICS: The virus that causes AIDS is called HIV, which stands for human immune deficiency virus. The virus is spread primarily through sexual contact or through the sharing of needles during intravenous drug use. Building up the immune system is the best defense for the potential AIDS victim. The following nutrients can help the AIDS victim and those at risk to contact AIDS.

(BeneficialRemedies,Treatments,andNutrients)

SINGLEHERBS: Cayenne, Chinese Ginseng, Garlic, Milk Thistle Weed, Shiitake mushroom, Sheep Sorrel, Suma, and Yucca.

VITAMINS: A, B6, B12, B complex, and E.

MINERALS: High potency multi-mineral formula, Copper, and Zinc.

ALSO: Canaid herbal drink, Acidophilus, Coenzyme Q10, Germanium, Gluconic from DaVinci Labs, Proteolytic enzymes, Quercetin plus bromelin, Raw thymus, and Multiglandulars.

AIR SICKNESS

SPECIFICS: Air sickness can indicate the presence of many diseases including inner ear infection, low blood sugar, food poisoning, and nutrient deficiency. The most common cause is a deficiency of the vitamin "B6", and the mineral "magnesium". Ginkgo is excellent for chronic dizziness and light headedness.

(BeneficialRemedies,Treatments,andNutrients)

HERBAL COMBINATION: (Motion Mate).

PHYSIOLOGIC ACTION: In a recent university study ginger root caps proved more effective than either a drug or placebo at controlling motion induced nausea, also queasy travelers have found taking B complex at night and just before the trip is most effective.

SINGLEHERBS: Ginger Root Caps, and Ginkgo.

VITAMINS: B complex plus B6.

MINERALS: Magnesium.

HELPFUL FOODS: Fruits, lean beef, nuts, unpolished rice, whole grains, and yellow corn.

ALCOHOLISM

SPECIFICS:A chronic physiological or psychological condition marked by a dependence on alcohol. Deficiencies of many nutrients occur when alcohol itself satisfies the body's caloric needs.

Some effects of alcohol are a depressed immune system, damage to the central nervous system, brain, duodenum, pancreas, liver, and a loss of inhibition.

Note: Tobacco, alcohol, caffeine and other drug "cravings" are brought about by a physiological body dependence on the poison which develops during prolonged use. The addicts blood poison level must remain at a certain level at all times. As the poison level drops, there is a "desire" to take in more of the drug, to bring the level back again.

(Beneficial Remedies, Treatments, and Nutrients)

HERBAL COMBINATIONS: (Thisilyn) (Milk Thistle) (PC) (Liveron) (AdrenAid).

PHYSIOLOGIC ACTION: The above herbal formulas support and rebuild the liver, pancreas, and adrenal glands. By supporting these systems, the taste for alcohol will eventually subside. The vitamin and mineral supplements strengthen the body's nutritional integrity to a state where the need for a "lift" will be eliminated.

SINGLE HERBS: Cayenne, Dandelion, Siberian Ginseng, Golden Seal, Licorice Root, Lobelia, Nettle, Skullcap, and Valerian.

VITAMINS: A, B complex, B1, B2, B6, B12, Choline, Folic acid, Niacin, Pangamic acid, Pantothenic acid, C, D, E, and K.

MINERALS: Calcium, Chromium, Iron, Magnesium, Manganese, Selenium, and Zinc.

ALSO: Acidophilus, Brewers Yeast, Glutamine, Liver, L-Cysteine, L-Glutamine, L-Methionine, Proteolytic enzymes, Tryptophan, Unsaturated fatty acids, and avoid meat and all refined and processed foods, especially white sugar and white flour.

HELPFUL FOODS: Butter, bran, broccoli, carrots, cheese, all fruits, green leafy vegetables, milk, peas, shellfish, spinach, and whole grains.

ALLERGIC RHINITIS
(refer to Hay Fever)

ALLERGIES

SPECIFICS: The inappropriate response by the body's immune system to some particular substance known as an allergen. The immune system wrongly identifies a non toxic allergen causing the white blood cells to overreact creating more damage to the body than the allergen itself.

The allergic reaction may cause asthma, dizziness, eczema, fever, hay fever, high blood pressure, hives, hypoglycemia, mental disorders, and stomach ulcers.

(BeneficialRemedies,Treatments,andNutrients)

HERBAL COMBINATION: (HAS: Original and Fast Acting Formulas) (Allergy Care).

PHYSIOLOGIC ACTION: HAS is an excellent formula which contains herbs that help relieve symptoms of hay fever, sinus congestion, and respiratory allergies. Helps drain nasal passages, relieve swollen membranes, eliminate mucus, and cleanse the body. The Fast Acting Formula adds Pseudoephedra, a natural plant extract from the Ephedra plant. This substance quickly opens nasal passages allowing free breathing. While HAS Fast Acting is not for prolonged use, HAS Original can be taken for as long as needed.

Caution: Both formulas are not to be used during pregnancy, nor by small children.

Allergy Care: Maximum-strength natural allergy medicine that will not cause drowsiness. It contains 60mg of the active ingredient Pseudoephedrine Hcl.

SINGLE HERBS: Burdock Root, Cayenne, Chaparral, Elderberry, Eyebright, Lobelia, Golden Rod, Golden Seal, and Nettles

HOMEOPATHIC COMBINATION: Allergy Formula

VITAMINS: A, B complex, B3, B5, B6, B12, C, E, and F.

MINERALS: A multi-mineral complex plus Calcium, Magnesium, Manganese, and Potassium.

ALSO: Acidophilus, Bee Pollen, Coenzyme Q10, Germanium, L-Tyrosine, L-Cysteine, Digestive Enzymes, Propolis, Raw adrenal, Raw thymus, and Unsaturated fatty acids.

HELPFUL FOODS: Almonds, apples, beef, beets, broccoli, carrots, cheese, bananas, fruits, safflower and linseed oil, spinach, and sweet potatoes.

ALOPECIA
(refer to Baldness)

ALZHEIMER'S DISEASE

SPECIFICS: Alzheimer's disease affects fifteen percent of Americans over the age of sixty five. This disease is characterized by tangled nerve fibers surrounding the brains memory center(hippocampus).

This entanglement does not destroy the information stored, but it can no longer be transferred to and from the brain. Science does not yet know what can be done to stop the mental deterioration, however autopsies of the victims of Alzheimer's disease show excess amounts of aluminum, bromine, calcium, silicon, and sulfur in the brain, and a deficiency of boron, potassium, selenium, zinc, and B12. in the brain. The excesses and deficiencies could be the key to the prevention or cure of Alzheimer's disease.

(BeneficialRemedies,Treatments,andNutrients)

SINGLE HERBS: Butcher's Broom, Kelp, and Ginkgo Biloba.

VITAMINS: B complex, plus B6, B12, C, and E.

MINERALS: Boron, Potassium, Selenium, Vanadium, and Zinc.

ALSO: Coenzyme Q10, consume steam distilled water only, Germanium, Lecithin, Protein, and Superoxide dismutase.

HELPFUL FOODS: Beef, broccoli, bananas, bran, fish, green leafy vegetables, raisins, sweet potatoes, turnip greens, whole wheat, and all fruits.

ANCYLOSTOMIASIS
(refertoHookworms)

ANEMIA
(Iron deficiency anemia)

SPECIFICS: The component of the blood that carries oxygen is hemoglobin, Iron is an important factor because this mineral makes hemoglobin, and the formation of red blood cells will be impaired by the lack of iron. Causes of iron deficiency anemia include heavy menstrual bleeding, hormonal disorders, liver damage, peptic ulcers, dierticular disease, thyroid disorders, and dietary disorders.

(BeneficialRemedies,Treatments,andNutrients)

SINGLE HERBS: Barley Grass, Beet Powder, Black Current, Chlorophyll, Chorella, Comfrey, Dandelion, Fenugreek, Kelp, and Yellowdock.

VITAMINS: A complete multi-vitamin and additional C.

MINERALS: Complete multi-mineral.

HELPFUL FOODS: Broccoli, citrus fruits, sweet potatoes, turnip greens, red meat, whole rye, and black molasses.

JUICES: Parsley and blackberry juice; parsley and grape juice.

ANGINA
(refer to Myocardial infraction)

ANKYLOSING SPONDYLITIS

SPECIFICS: This condition is caused by inflammation affecting the joints between the vertebrae of the spine and the sacroiliac joints (the joints between the spine and the pelvis). Symptoms include stiffness and pain in the lower back, chest, and hips.

(Beneficial Remedies, Treatments, and Nutrients)

SINGLE HERBS: Devils Claw, Tumeric, and White Willow.

VITAMINS: B6, B12, C, and E.

MINERALS: Calcium and Magnesium.

ALSO: Bioflavonoids, Omega-3, Omega-6, Bromelain, and Digestive Enzymes.

HELPFUL FOODS: Broccoli, citrus fruits, kale, all green leafy vegetables, and whole grains.

ANOREXIA NERVOSA

SPECIFICS: In this disorder the individuals have an intense fear of becoming obese, and refuse to eat to the point of starvation. Symptoms include taking large doses of laxatives, deliberate vomiting, and self starvation. Recent studies show that some cases of anorexia nervosa may be caused by a severe zinc deficiency. When trying to stimulate the anorexic, consider the aroma and appearance of foods, as well as the nutritional value.

(Beneficial Remedies, Treatments, and Nutrients)

SINGLE HERBS: Catnip, Fennel, Ginger, Ginseng, Gotu Kola, Kelp, Papaya, Peppermint, and Saw Palmetto.

VITAMINS: Multi-vitamins plus A, B12, B complex, D, and E.

MINERALS: Multi-minerals plus Potassium, Selenium, and Zinc.

ALSO: Acidophilus, Bio-Strath, Brewer's yeast, Liver, Protein, and Proteolytic enzymes.

HELPFUL FOODS: Butter, bran, beef, bananas, herring, sunflower seeds, soybeans, spinach, tuna, and nuts.

ANURIA
(refer to Prostate and Kidney Disorders)

ANXIETY

SPECIFICS: Anxiety disorders affect roughly 4 percent of the population, mainly young adults. These disorders are generally a direct result of stress. The body can handle some stress but long term stress causes the body to break down. Long term stress occurs when the situation that causes anxiety is not relieved. Find the cause and handle it constructively. People experiencing anxiety should maintain a well-balanced diet and replace the nutrients depleted during stress.

(Beneficial Remedies, Treatments, and Nutrients)

HERBAL COMBINATIONS: (Calm-aid) or (Ex stress comb).

PHYSIOLOGIC ACTION: A proven formula that is soothing, strengthening, and healing to the whole nervous system to relieve nervous tension and rebuild the nerve sheaths. Excellent aid for insomnia, chronic nervousness, and stress-related conditions.

SINGLE HERBS: Evening Primrose Oil, Hops, Mistletoe, Skullcap, Valerian, and Yucca.

VITAMINS: B complex, B1, B2, B3, B5, B6, and C.

MINERALS: Calcium, Iodine, Iron, Magnesium, Phosphorus, Potassium, Silicon, and Sodium.

HELPFUL FOODS: Dulse, flax seed, sea salt, fruit(citrus and other), bacon, beef, chicken, all dairy products, all vegetables, and whole rye.

JUICES: Radish and prune juice.

APTHOUS ULCERS

SPECIFICS: An apthous ulcer is a contagious and painful mouth ulceration that can appear on the lips, gums, tongue, and on the inside cheeks. The sores have white centers and are surrounded by a red border. Canker sores may be caused from eating to many sweets, poor dental hygiene or stress. They are identified by a tingling sensation and a slight swelling of the mucous membrane.

(Beneficial Remedies, Treatments, and Nutrients)

SINGLE HERBS: Goldenseal, Pau d'Arco, and Burdock Root tea, Red Clover, or Red Raspberry tea is very helpful.

VITAMINS: A, B5, B12, B complex, and large doses of C.

MINERALS: Iron.

ALSO: Acidophilus and L-Lysine.

Note: Avoid chewing gum, sugar, processed or refined foods, coffee, and citrus fruits.

HELPFUL FOODS: Black molasses, carrots, lean red meat, fish, leafy green vegetables, turnips, onions, potatoes, vegetable oils, and unpolished rice.

ARTERIOSCLEROSIS
(Hardening of arteries)

SPECIFICS: Arteriosclerosis is the thickening and hardening of the walls of the arteries. This condition is due to the gradual build-up of calcium and fatty deposits on the inside of the artery walls. This buildup will slow or restrict the circulation of the blood causing high blood pressure. Symptoms of arteriosclerosis are cramping of muscles, chest pains and pressure, and hypertension. Causes for arteriosclerosis are poor diet, drug abuse, alcoholism, smoking, heredity, obesity, and stress.

(Beneficial Remedies, Treatments, and Nutrients)

HERBAL COMBINATION: (Garlicin HC).

PHYSIOLOGIC ACTION: A combination of herbs which supports the cardiovascular system. Helps to strengthen the heart, while building and cleansing the arteries and veins.

SPECIFICS: Recent animal studies suggest that vitamin C deficiency could be involved in the causation of arteriosclerosis. E.F.A.s (essential fatty acids) play a fundamental role in keeping cell membranes fluid and flexible.

SINGLE HERBS: Cayenne, Comfrey, Evening Primrose Oil, Fish Oil, Garlic, Golden Seal, and Rose Hips.

VITAMINS: B complex, C, E, Niacin, Inositol, and choline.

MINERALS: Calcium and magnesium.

ALSO: (E.F.A.s) — Fish oils and cold pressed vegetable oils.

HELPFUL FOODS: Apples, lean beef, broccoli, fruits(citrus and other), sprouted seeds, sunflower seeds, sweet potatoes, sardines, tuna, turnip greens, and yellow corn.

ARTHRITIS

SPECIFICS: The most common forms of arthritis are osteoasthritis, and rheumatoid arthritis.

Rheumatoidarthritis is inflammatory in nature and attacks and destroys the synovial membranes surrounding the lubricating fluid in the joints. This damaged tissue is replaced with scar tissue, causing the space between the joints to narrow and to fuse together.

Osteoarthritis is a degenerative joint disease involving the deterioration of the cartilage at the ends of the bones, causing the cartilage to become rough resulting in friction.

(BeneficialRemedies,Treatments,andNutrients)

HERBAL COMBINATION: (Rheum-Aid) or (Yucca -AR).

PHYSIOLOGIC ACTION: Relieves symptoms associated with bursitis, calcification, gout, rheumatoid arthritis, rheumatism, and osteoarthritis. Helps the body reduce or eliminate swelling and inflammation in the joints and connective tissue and helps to relieve stiffness and pain.

SINGLEHERBS: Alfalfa, Black Cohosh, Burdock, Cayenne, Celery seed, Chaparral, Devil's Claw, Valerian root, and Yucca.

HOMEOPATHIC COMBINATION: Arthritis Pain Formula.

VITAMINS: Niacin, B5, B6, B12, B complex, C, D, E, F, and P.

MINERALS: A strong Multi-mineral complex, plus Calcium, and Magnesium.

ALSO: Cod liver oil, Yu-ccan herbal drink, Green Magma, Aqua life, Seatone, and Bromelain.

HELPFUL FOODS: Almonds, apricots, beef, butter, broccoli, buckwheat, all fruits, cheese, sardines, soybeans, spinach, safflower, goats milk, and mung beans.

JUICES: Parsley and celery juice; cherry and pineapple juice.

ASCARIASIS
(refer to Worms)

ASTHMA

SPECIFICS: A chronic respiratory condition caused by spasms in the muscles surrounding the small airways in the lungs called bronchi. Typical symptoms of asthma are coughing, difficulty in breathing usually accompanied by a wheezing sound, and a feeling of suffocation. The main causes of asthma are air pollution, respiratory infections, disorders of the adrenal glands, specific allergies, and physical or emotional stress.

(BeneficialRemedies,Treatments,andNutrients)

HERBAL COMBINATIONS: (B R E) or (Breathe-Aid) and (ANTS Liquid Extract).

PHYSIOLOGIC ACTION: BRE or Breath-Aid effectively relieve symptoms associated with asthma, chest congestion, and inflammation. Promotes free breathing, eliminates mucus, and cleanses the body. ANTS Liquid Extract helps to relax bronchial spasms. It helps to cut mucus, and is helpful for chronic coughs.

SINGLE HERBS: Lobelia, Comfrey, Chlorophyll, Fenugreek, Mullein, and Nettle

VITAMINS: A, B complex, B2, B3, B5, B6, B12, C, E, F, and Paba.

MINERALS: Manganese.

ALSO: Bee pollen, honey (which will aid in clearing mucus out of the lungs), garlic, juice fast, and a vegetarian diet.

USEFUL FOODS: Almonds, beets, broccoli, carrots, celery, all fruits, green leafy vegetables, nuts, peas, soybeans, spinach, and whole wheat.

JUICES: Celery and papaya juice; carrot, celery, and endive juice.

ATHLETES FOOT

SPECIFICS: A highly contagious yeast like fungal infection, that lives off dead skin cells, and calluses of the feet. Athlete's foot victims should eat a well-balanced diet, supplemented by megadoses of vitamins A, B, and C.

(Beneficial Remedies, Treatments, and Nutrients)

HERBAL COMBINATION: (Black Walnut extract).

PHYSIOLOGIC ACTION: High in organic iodine, this herb has proven effective against fungal infections such as ringworm and athlete's foot.

SINGLE HERBS: Pau d'Arco and Tea Tree oil.

VITAMINS: A, B complex, and C.

MINERALS: Zinc.

ALSO: Acidophilus, Caprinex (caprylic acid), Germanium, and Unsaturated fatty acids. Vitamin C powder (crystals) applied directly to affected area helps destroy fungus infestation. Keep dry and out of shoes until infection clears.

HELPFUL FOODS: Red meats, all fruits, green leafy vegetables, herring, nuts, whole grains, and unpolished rice.

ATHLETIC INJURIES

SPECIFICS: Using the muscles for prolonged periods without rest can create muscle strain. If an athlete stresses a muscle beyond its capability the ligament connecting the bone to the muscle may tear causing a sprain. A well-balanced diet that is high in protein and the following supplement program will help these injuries heal.

(BeneficialRemedies,Treatments,andNutrients)

HERBAL COMBINATION: (B F + C)

PHYSIOLOGIC ACTION: A special formula to aid in healing processes for torn cartilage's, sprained limbs, and broken bones. (Multiple athletic injuries and associated swelling and inflammation).

SINGLE HERBS: White Oak Bark, Comfrey Root, Black Walnut Hulls, Lobelia, Scullcap and Yucca.

HOMEOPATHIC COMBINATION: Injury and Backache Formula.

VITAMINS: B complex, B5, B6, B12, C, and E.

MINERALS: A complete multi-mineral one a day, (time released).

ALSO: Bee pollen, Coenzyme Q10, Germanium, L-Arginine, L-Carnitine, L-Lysine, Green-Lipped Mussel, Liver, Protein, Proteolytic enzymes, Silica, and Unsaturated fatty acids.

HELPFUL FOODS: Beef, fruits, nuts, unpolished rice, soybeans, spinach, vegetable oils, liver, and whole wheat.

JUICES: Aloe Vera juice.

ATOPIC DERMATITIS

SPECIFICS:A type of skin eruption characterized by tiny blisters that weep and crust. Chronic forms produce flaking, scaling, itching, and eventual thickening and color changes of the skin.

(BeneficialRemedies,Treatments,andNutrients)

HERBAL COMBINATION: (AKN).

PHYSIOLOGIC ACTION: When toxins are not properly eliminated from the body, they may surface through the skin creating atopic dermatitis. This formula has been created to support liver and gall bladder function, to ensure toxins are filtered from the blood.

SINGLE HERBS: Aloe Vera, Chickweed, Evening Primrose Oil, Pau d'Arco, Red Clover, Thisilyn (Milk Thistle), and Yellow Dock.

VITAMINS: A, B complex, C, D, Paba, Biotin, Choline, and Inositol.

MINERALS: Magnesium, Sulfur Ointment, and Zinc ointment.

HELPFUL FOODS: Apples, apricots, cherries, citrus fruits, all sea foods, lean red meat, chicken, broccoli, carrots, celery, vegetable oils, and grain sprouts.

JUICES: Carrot, Celery, and Lemon juice.

ALSO: This condition is aggravated by food allergens such as dairy and wheat. These foods should be avoided. Powders and pastes should not be applied during acute or weeping stages. After acute stage passes, ointments and salves may be applied. Herbal ointments which contain Chickweed and Calendula are particularly helpful.

AUTISM

SPECIFICS: An illness that involves personalities of children who do not react to their environment. Children with autism are withdrawn, do not learn to talk or have learning disabilities, and exhibit marked unresponsiveness to affection and love. Scientific studies have shown that the combination of vitamin B6, and magnesium produces good results in children and adults with autism.

(BeneficialRemedies,Treatments,andNutrients)

HERBAL COMBINATION: (Wild Lettuce and Valerian Extract).

PHYSIOLOGIC ACTION: This excellent formula is a natural sedative. Promotes overall calming of the nerves and restores a sense of control and balance without causing drowsiness.

ALSO: Ginkgo or Ginkgold. Although this herb is often used to promote circulation, it also has a positive effect on the nervous system. Used in conjunction with the following single herbs and with a balanced, chemical free diet, good results can be expected.

SINGLE HERBS: Evening Primrose Oil, Ginkgo, Lobelia, Oat Extract, Skullcap, St. Johns Wort, Valerian and Wild Lettuce.

VITAMINS: High potency B vitamins, B3, B5, B6, and C.

NOTE: Yeast free B vitamins may be required if yeast intolerance is present.

MINERALS: High doses of all minerals.

NOTE: Avoid all foods with artificial flavoring and coloring. Processed foods should be eliminated from the diet. Foods which contain natural salicylates such as apples, tomatoes, and oranges need to be avoided. Carbonated drinks will worsen the condition.

HELPFUL FOODS: Beets, broccoli, fruits, nuts, sweet potatoes, turnip greens, peas, and unpolished rice.

AUTOIMMUNE DISORDERS

SPECIFICS: When the immune system weakens and is unable to respond to invading microorganisms you become more susceptible to infections and viruses. The key factors in the treatment and prevention of autoimmune disorders are proper nutrition and good supplementation.

(BeneficialRemedies,Treatments,andNutrients)

HERBAL COMBINATION: (EchinaGuard).

PHYSIOLOGIC ACTION: Stimulates the immune response systems. Especially helpful in rebuilding the body during convalescence and as a preventative.

SINGLE HERBS: Echinacea root, Chaparral, Evening Primrose, Korean White Ginseng, Goldenseal root, Pau d'Arco, and Rosemary.

VITAMINS: A multi-vitamin plus B6, B12, C, and E.

MINERALS: A strong mineral complex.

ALSO: Canaid herbal drink, L-Cysteine, L-Methionine, L-Lysine, L-Ornithine, Omega-3, Omega-6, Propolis, Proteolytic enzymes, and Primadophilus.

HELPFUL FOODS: Beef, broccoli, fruit(citrus and other), nuts, soybeans, spinach, sweet potatoes, turnip greens, unpolished rice, and whole grains.

BACK PAIN

SPECIFICS: Most back problems are associated with long term habits. Chronic pain in the lower back is usually caused by improper footwear, sleeping on a mattress that is too soft, poor posture, and walking habits.

(BeneficialRemedies,Treatments,andNutrients)

HERBAL COMBINATIONS: (Extress) (Kalmin Extract)

PHYSIOLOGIC ACTION: The herbs in these combinations help to relax muscles and reduce muscle tension. The Kalmin Extract has anti-spasmodic and anti-inflammatory qualities which are helpful in back pain caused by muscle strain.

SINGLE HERBS: Burdock, Horsetail, Licorice, Valerian, and White Willow Bark.

VITAMINS: B12, C D, and E,

MINERALS: Calcium, Magnesium, Manganese, Silicon, and Zinc.

ALSO: Cod liver oil, Enzymes with bromelin, DL-Phenylalanine, L-Tryptophan, and Protein.

HELPFUL FOODS: All dairy products, beef, cod liver oil, tuna, beets, broccoli, peanuts, sunflower seeds, soybeans, and sprouted seeds.

BAD BREATH

SPECIFICS: Bad breath is generally attributed to putrefactive bacteria living on undigested food. Nutrients necessary for efficient digestion are essential. Other causes are poor dental hygiene (gum or tooth decay), nose or throat infection, excessive smoking, liver malfunction, and constipation.

(BeneficialRemedies,Treatments,andNutrients)

SINGLE HERBS: Chlorophyll, Myrrh, Parsley, Peppermint, Rosemary, Sage, and Yucca.

VITAMINS: A, B complex, B3, B6, C, and Paba.

MINERALS: Magnesium, and Zinc.

ALSO: Primadophilus, Digestive enzymes, and Yu-ccan herbal drink.

HELPFUL FOODS: Apples, carrots, citrus fruits, and parsley.

BALDNESS

SPECIFICS: There is no known cure to hair loss in males due to heredity. If one is a victim of hair loss due to acute illness, pregnancy, surgery, poor circulation, or stress, the following nutrients can be helpful.

(BeneficialRemedies,Treatments,andNutrients)

SINGLE HERBS: Aloe Vera, Horsetail, Kelp, Rosemary, Sage, Nettle, Yarrow, and Yucca.

VITAMINS: A, B complex, B3, B5, B6. C, Biotin, Folic Acid, and Inositol.

MINERALS: Copper, Iodine, Magnesium.

ALSO: Coenzyme Q10, L-Cysteine, L-Methionine, Primadophilus, Protein, Raw thymus glandular, and Unsaturated fatty acids.

HELPFUL FOODS: Asparagus, broccoli, cabbage, beef, seafood, fish liver oils, all fruit, green leafy vegetables, turnip greens, and unpolished rice.

BEDSORES

SPECIFICS: Bedsores are deep skin ulcers that are the result of continuous pressure exerted over bony areas restricting circulation and leading to the death of skin tissue. Massaging the affected area daily is very helpful. Frequent sponge baths with warm water and a mild herbal soap or a soap containing vitamin E are recommended.

(Beneficial Remedies, Treatments, and Nutrients)

HERBAL COMBINATION: (X-Itch ointment)(Derm-Aid ointment)

PHYSIOLOGIC ACTION: X-Itch, and Derm-Aid are used for the relief and prevention of minor skin irritations. Black ointment has a drawing and healing effect for those tough to heal sores.

SINGLE HERBS: Goldenseal, Myrrh gum, and Pau d' Arco.

VITAMINS: A, B complex, C, D, and E.

MINERALS: Copper, Calcium, Magnesium, and Zinc.

HELPFUL FOODS: Beef, butter, cheese, all fruits, tuna, fish liver oils, nuts, and sunflower seeds.

BED-WETTING

SPECIFICS: The exact cause of bed-wetting (nocturnal enuresis) is still unknown, however it is believed that nervous or hyperactive children, and children having a faster heart beat and higher respiration rate during the sleep cycle are more likely to be bed-wetters. The most common theories speculate that the causes may be heredity, behavioral disturbances, stress, weak bladders, urinary tract infections, and nutritional deficiencies.

(Beneficial Remedies, Treatments, and Nutrients)

SINGLE HERBS: Buchu, Corn silk, Oat straw, Parsley, and Plantain.

VITAMINS: A multi-vitamin plus A, B complex, and E.

MINERALS: A mineral complex plus Potassium, and Zinc.

ALSO: Cod liver oil, and Protein.

HELPFUL JUICES: Celery and parsley juice.

BEE STINGS

SPECIFICS: If stung, a very severe reaction can occur to people that are allergic to bee venom. Symptoms include severe swelling, labored breathing, hoarseness, confusion, difficulty in swallowing, and weakness. If you have a known allergy to bee stings, have your doctor prescribe an emergency treatment kit.

(BeneficialRemedies,Treatments,andNutrients)

SINGLE HERBS: Echinacea, Pau d'Arco, and Yellow Dock tea.

VITAMINS: B1 is a good insect repellent, and it creates a smell at the level of the skin that insects do not like. Already stung, use vitamin C to ease allergic reaction (acts as a natural anti-histamine).

MINERALS: Calcium.

HELPFUL FOODS: Citrus fruits, turnip greens, all dairy products, and sardines.

BELCHING
(refer to Gas "Intestinal")

BERIBERI

SPECIFICS: A disease caused by a deficiency of B vitamins, particularly thiamine. The disease seldom occurs outside the Far East, where the principal diet of polished rice does not supply sufficient thiamine. Beriberi cases that do occur in America are associated with chronic alcoholism, hypothyroidism, infections, pregnancy, and stress.

(BeneficialRemedies,Treatments,andNutrients)

VITAMINS: B1, B complex, and C.

MINERALS: A complete mineral complex.

ALSO: Brewers yeast.

HELPFUL FOODS: Beef, broccoli, fruits(citrus and other), nuts, sweet potatoes, and turnip greens,

BIPOLAR DISORDER

SPECIFICS:A mental disorder characterized by swings in mood between opposite extremes. Mood swings may be accompanied by extreme negative delusions or by grandiose ideas. The main causes of this ailment are drugs, inherited tendency, and malnutrition.

(BeneficialRemedies,Treatments,andNutrients)

VITAMINS: B complex, B12, and Folic Acid.

MINERALS: Lithium.

ALSO: Omega-6 oils, L-phenylalanine, and L-tryptophan.

HELPFUL FOODS: Liver, red meat, eggs, asparagus, citrus fruits, turnip greens, sprouted seeds, cheese and other dairy products, sunflower seeds, wheat germ, and whole grains.

BLADDER INFECTION
(refer to Kidney and Bladder Disorders)

BLEEDING GUMS

SPECIFICS: Bleeding gums are nearly always caused by a nutrient deficiency. The recommended prevention and treatment is a well-balanced diet that is rich in all nutrients.

(BeneficialRemedies,Treatments,andNutrients)

SINGLE HERBS: Chamomile, Echinacea, Lobelia, Myrrh Gum, and White Oak Bark.

VITAMINS: A, B complex, C, D, P, and Folic Acid.

MINERALS: Calcium, Magnesium, Phosphorus, and Silicon.

HELPFUL FOODS: Apple, apricots, corn, carrots, butter, cheese, tuna, fish liver oils, green leafy vegetables, peanuts, sunflower seeds, and sprouted seeds.

BLOOD CLEANSER

SPECIFICS: If you are run down and full of toxins, watch out! A person should cleanse his or her blood at least once every six months, to eliminate the germs that live on the mucus, toxins, and poisons in the body.

(BeneficialRemedies,Treatments,andNutrients)

HERBAL COMBINATION: (Red Clover combination)

PHYSIOLOGIC ACTION: Helps cleanse the blood of toxins, mucus, and infections thus helps improve and sustain overall good health; used for many years with very good results.

SINGLE HERBS: Red Clover, Chaparral, Dandelion, Garlic, and Burdock.

MINERALS: Iron.

ALSO: Chlorophyll and Diulaxa tea.

HELPFUL FOODS: Black molasses, carrots, celery, parsley, red meat, tomatoes, and whole rye.

JUICES: Blackberry, blackcherry, carrot, celery, dandelion, parsley, and tomato juice.

BLOOD CLOTS

SPECIFICS: Blood clots are due to the gradual build-up of calcium and cholesterol-containing masses known as plaques on the inside of the artery walls. The clot will slow or restrict the circulation of the blood causing high blood pressure. Symptoms of this disease are cramping of muscles, chest pains and pressure, and hypertension. The main causes are poor diet, drug abuse, alcoholism, smoking, heredity, obesity, and stress.

(BeneficialRemedies,Treatments,andNutrients)

HERBAL COMBINATION: (Garlicin HC).

PHYSIOLOGIC ACTION: A combination of herbs which supports the cardiovascular system. Helps to strengthen the heart, while building and cleansing the arteries and veins.

SPECIFICS: Recent animal studies suggest that vitamin C deficiency could be involved in the causation of thrombosis. E.F.A.s

(essential fatty acids) play a fundamental role in keeping cell membranes fluid and flexible.

SINGLE HERBS: Cayenne, Comfrey, Evening Primrose Oil, Fish Oil, Garlic, Golden Seal, and Rose Hips.

VITAMINS: B complex, C, E, Niacin, Inositol, and Choline.

MINERALS: Calcium, Magnesium, and Selenium.

ALSO: (E.F.A.s) — Fish oils and cold pressed vegetable oils.

HELPFUL FOODS: Fish and fish liver oils, vegetable oils, oat bran, high fiber fruits, kelp, green tea, yogurt, and legumes.

JUICES: Alfalfa, beet, blackberry, grape, parsley, and pineapple juice.

BLOOD PRESSURE (High)

SPECIFICS: The main cause of high blood pressure is arteriosclerosis. This condition is due to the gradual build-up of calcium and fatty deposits on the inside of the artery walls. This buildup will slow or restrict the circulation of the blood causing high blood pressure. Symptoms of high blood pressure are cramping of muscles, chest pains and pressure, and hypertension. Causes for high blood pressure are poor diet, drug abuse, alcoholism, smoking, heredity, obesity, and stress.

(BeneficialRemedies,Treatments,andNutrients)

HERBAL COMBINATIONS: (Cayenne-Garlic) (Garlicin HC) (BP)

PHYSIOLOGIC ACTION: In addition to lowering the blood pressure, the above will help to relieve colds, influenza, and general infections, strengthen the heart and improves blood circulation.

SINGLE HERBS: Cayenne, Garlic, Kelp, Hawthorn, Mistletoe, Valerian Root, Yarrow, and Yucca.

VITAMINS: A, B complex (stress) B3, B5, B15, C, D, E, P, Inositol, Choline, and Lecithin

MINERALS: Calcium, Magnesium, and Potassium.

HELPFUL FOODS: Apples, apricots, bananas, cherries, broccoli, carrots, green leafy vegetables, soybeans, sunflower seeds, vegetable oils, and fish liver oils.

JUICES: Carrot, celery, grape, and lime juice.

BLOOD PRESSURE (LOW)

SPECIFICS: There are many disorders associated with circulatory problems. The most common disease for sluggish circulation is Raynaud's disease, characterized by constriction and spasm of the blood vessels in the limbs. Poor circulation can also result from varicose veins, caused by the loss of elasticity in the walls of the veins.

(BeneficialRemedies,Treatments,andNutrients)

HERBAL COMBINATION: (B/P).

PHYSIOLOGIC ACTION: A time proven formula that improves overall blood circulation and tends to normalize high or low pressure to the body's normal level. Also reduces cholesterol build-up in the blood vessels. Helps relieve symptoms of cold and flu.

SINGLE HERBS: Garlic, Hawthorn, Siberian Ginseng, Kelp, Golden Seal Root, Ginger Root, and Spirulina,

VITAMINS: A, B Complex, B5, C, E, and P.

ALSO: EPA. Salmon oil, and Lecithin.

HELPFUL FOODS: Fruits(citrus and other), carrots, broccoli, spinach, lean beef, and all seafood's.

BODY ODOR

SPECIFICS: Most body odors are related to the internal health of the body, caused by sluggish or infected bowel, kidney, or bladder. Certain nutrients such as the B vitamins, magnesium, and zinc appear to remove wastes in the body that cause odors.

(BeneficialRemedies,Treatments,andNutrients)

VITAMINS: B6, PABA, and B complex.

MINERALS: Magnesium, and Zinc.

ALSO: Chlorophyll and Yu-ccan herbal drink.

HELPFUL FOODS: Brewers yeast, nuts, fruits, unpolished rice, and whole grains.

BOILS

SPECIFICS: A painful localized infection producing pus filled areas in the deeper layers of the skin tissues. A boil forms when the skin tissue is weakened by chafing and there is inadequate nutrition to fight infection. Treatment for boils demands proper hygiene, frequent washing with soap and water, and application of an antiseptic.

(BeneficialRemedies,Treatments,andNutrients)

HERBAL COMBINATION: (AKN).

PHYSIOLOGIC ACTION: Many skin diseases such as boils are often related to liver dysfunction. This herbal formula combines herbs which support the liver, and clean the blood.

FOR PAIN: Make a paste of wheat flour and honey, spread over area, and cover with cotton dressing.

SINGLE HERBS: Chaparral, Dandelion, Echinacea, Lobelia, Mullein, and Red Clover.

VITAMINS: A, C, E. Vitamin A may be applied locally.

MINERALS: Zinc (preventative).

HELPFUL FOODS: Citrus fruits, herring, tuna, fish liver oils, soybeans, sunflower seeds, carrots, sweet potatoes, turnip greens, and melon.

BONE, FLESH AND CARTILAGE
(Disorders)

SPECIFICS: Using the muscles for prolonged periods without rest can create muscle strain. If an athlete stresses a muscle beyond its capability the ligament connecting the bone to the muscle may tear causing a sprain. A well-balanced diet that is high in protein and the following supplement program will help these injuries heal.

(BeneficialRemedies,Treatments,andNutrients)

HERBAL COMBINATION: (BF + C).

PHYSIOLOGIC ACTION: A special formula to aid the body's healing processes involved with broken bones, athletic injuries, sprained limbs, and related inflammation and swelling. A tonic used after acute and chronic diseases to help rebuild the body.

SINGLE HERBS: Comfrey Root, Black Walnut, Horsetail, Lobelia, Skullcap, White Oak Bark, and Yucca.

HOMEOPATHIC COMBINATION: Injury and Backache Formula.

VITAMINS: A, Pantothenic acid, C, and D.

MINERALS: Calcium, Magnesium, and Potassium.

NOTE: Protein and silicon accelerate bone healing.

HELPFUL FOODS: Beef, tuna, fish liver oils, all dairy products, citrus fruits, carrots, green and green leafy vegetables, nuts, seeds, and sprouted seeds.

BONE SPUR
(refer to Heel Spur)

BOWEL CLEANSER (Lower)

SPECIFICS: Constipation results when the waste material moves too slowly or there is decreased frequency of bowel movements. Constipation usually arises from insufficient amounts of fiber and fluids in the diet. Other causes include lack of exercise, nervousness, stress, infections, and poor diet.

(BeneficialRemedies,Treatments,andNutrients)

HERBAL COMBINATION: (Multilax #2) or (Naturalax #2).

PHYSIOLOGIC ACTION: Accelerates natural cleansing of the body and improves intestinal absorption by gentle evacuation of the bowels. It cleans out old, toxic fecal matter, mucus and encrustation's from the colon wall, and helps normalize the peristaltic action and rebuild the bowel structure. Use until the bowel is cleansed, healed, and functioning normally.

Warning: Do not take during pregnancy.

SINGLE HERBS: Cascara Sagrada, Golden Seal Root, Lobelia, Red Raspberry, Senna, and Yucca.

VITAMINS: B complex.

ALSO: Yogurt, soaked Prunes and Figs, and Yu-ccan herbal drink.

HELPFUL FOODS: Brewers yeast, flax seed, fruits, lean beef, nuts, prunes, unpolished rice, whey powder, and yogurt.

BREAST CANCER
(refer to Cancer)

BREAST FEEDING

SPECIFICS: The three main breast feeding problems are:

- **Engorgement;** which results in the swelling of the tissues in the breast causing the breasts to feel full, hard, and tender. Treatment and prevention of this disorder includes short frequent feedings and the non restriction of sucking time.

- **Sore nipples;** this is usually caused by improper nursing schedules and improper nursing positions.

- **Plugged duct;** this is usually caused by a tiny clot of dried milk plugging the nipple, or incomplete emptying of the milk ducts.
If the breast is infected refer to Mastitis in this manual.

(Beneficial Remedies, Treatments, and Nutrients)

SINGLE HERBS: Alfalfa, Blessed Thistle, Chlorophyll, Fennel, Red Raspberry, or Marshmallow (warm) will bring in good rich milk. Sage will help dry up the milk when the mother is ready to quit nursing.

VITAMINS: If the baby has a cold, the mother can take extra vitamin C.

CAUTION: A nursing mother should not take cleansing herbs as it may cause colic or diarrhea in the baby.

BREATHING DIFFICULTIES

SPECIFICS: The main causes of breathing difficulties are air pollution, respiratory infections, disorders of the adrenal glands, specific allergies, and physical or emotional stress. Also refer to asthma, and bronchitis in this manual.

(BeneficialRemedies,Treatments,andNutrients)

HERBAL COMBINATIONS: (B R E) or (Breathe-Aid) (Fenu-Comf)

PHYSIOLOGIC ACTION: Effectively relieves irritation and promotes healing throughout the respiratory tract. Eliminates mucus, inflammation of the lungs, and helps relieve symptoms of coughs, colds, and bronchitis.

SINGLE HERBS: Comfrey Leaves, Lobelia, Marshmallow Root, and Mullein.

VITAMINS: C.

ALSO: Respa-Herb, Bee Pollen.

HELPFUL FOODS: Broccoli, citrus fruits, and turnip greens.

BRIGHTS DISEASE

SPECIFICS: A chronic inflammation of the kidneys, characterized by blood in the urine with associated hypertension and edema which results in the kidney retaining salt and water. When the bloodstream becomes toxic with wastes due to kidney malfunction, uremia develops. The following nutrients will aid in controlling urinary tract infection.

(BeneficialRemedies,Treatments,andNutrients)

HERBAL COMBINATION: (KB).

PHYSIOLOGIC ACTION: Extremely valuable in healing and strengthening the kidneys, bladder, and genito-urinary area.

Useful to stop bed-wetting, but is a diuretic when congestion of the kidneys is indicated. Helps remove bladder, uterine, and urethral toxins.

Warning: Intended for occasional use only. May cause green-yellow discoloration of the urine.

VITAMINS: A, B complex, C, D, E, Choline.

SINGLE HERBS: Alfalfa, Barberry root, Catnip, Dandelion, Fennel, Ginger root, Horsetail, and Wild Yam.

ALSO: Cranberry juice, Propolis, Uratonic, 3-way herb teas, and other Diuretic tablets.

HELPFUL FOODS: Lean red meat, carrots, soybeans, tuna, fish liver oils, all fruits, and sprouted seeds.

BRONCHITIS

SPECIFICS: An inflammation of the tissues lining the air passage, or obstruction of the breathing tubes that lead to the lungs. The inflammation is usually followed by a mucus buildup, coughing, sore throat, fever, and back and chest pains. The main causes of bronchitis are air pollution, fatigue, malnutrition, and cigarette smoking. Treatment requires a well-balanced diet high in vitamins A and C.

(BeneficialRemedies,Treatments,andNutrients)

HERBAL COMBINATION: (Fenu-Comf).

PHYSIOLOGIC ACTION: Helps relieve symptoms of coughs, colds, bronchitis, and helps eliminate mucus, congestion, and inflammation from the lungs.

SINGLE HERBS: Comfrey, Eucalyptus, Lobelia, Chickweed Tea, Slippery Elm. Cayenne taken with Ginger cleans out the bronchial tubes.

VITAMINS: A, B12, C, and E.

MINERALS: A multi-mineral formula plus Zinc.

ALSO: Acidophilus, Coenzyme Q10, L-Arginine, L-Cysteine, L-Ornithine, Protein, Proteolytic enzymes, and Unsaturated fatty acids.

HELPFUL FOODS: Citrus fruits, fish liver oils, carrots, sweet potatoes, and turnip greens.

JUICES: Lemon juice with honey.

BRUISES

SPECIFICS: An injury that involves the rupture of small blood vessels resulting in swelling and black and blue marks due to the blood that has collected under the skin. The most common factors that make a person susceptible to bruises are anemia, time of menstrual period, and being overweight. The following nutrients can be helpful in the prevention and treatment of bruises.

(BeneficialRemedies,Treatments,andNutrients)

SINGLE HERBS: Alfalfa, Garlic, and Rosehips.

VITAMINS: B9, B complex, C, D, E, and K.

MINERALS: Calcium, Iron, and Magnesium.

ALSO: Germanium, Proteolytic enzymes, and Coenzyme Q10.

HELPFUL FOODS: Beef, butter cheese, all fruits, kelp, liver, soybeans, sunflower seeds, spinach, sprouted seeds, whole wheat, and yogurt.

BRUXISM
(refer to Teeth Grinding)

BURNING FEET

SPECIFICS: Burning feet are caused by a deficiency of B6, B12, and Iron.

(Beneficial Remedies, Treatments, and Nutrients)

VITAMINS: B6 and B12.

MINERALS: Iron.

HELPFUL FOODS: Black molasses, citrus fruit, nuts, and whole rye.

BURNING MOUTH AND TONGUE

SPECIFICS: Nearly all mouth and tongue disorders such as sore mouth, tongue, and gums are attributed to a deficiency of the B vitamins. The gums become puffy, tender, and the oral membranes become susceptible to canker sores with the deficiency of vitamin C and niacin.

(Beneficial Remedies, Treatments, and Nutrients)

SINGLE HERBS: Aloe Vera, Golden Seal, Myrrh, Red Raspberry, and White Oak Bark.

VITAMINS: A, B complex, B2, B3, B12, C, and E.

MINERALS: Iron, Magnesium, Phosphorus, and Zinc.

ALSO: Chlorophyll, Lysine, and Primadophilus.

HELPFUL FOODS: All fruits, carrots, corn, broccoli, herring, oysters, red meat, soybeans, and spinach.

BURNS

SPECIFICS: There are three degrees of burns. The first degree burn appears reddened, the second degree burn appears reddened and includes blisters, in the third degree burn the entire thickness of the skin is destroyed and possibly the underlying muscle. For third degree burns immediate treatment is required, see your doctor.

(BeneficialRemedies,Treatments,andNutrients)

SINGLEHERBS: Aloe Vera, and Comfrey.

PHYSIOLOGICACTION: Aloe Vera is very good for burns, it may be used internally and externally. Some Aloe Vera preparations contain lanolin, which will intensify burns. Use a preparation without lanolin. Aloe Vera is especially good for acid burns.

VITAMINS: A, C, E, Niacin, Paba. (Vit E applied directly to burn). Take vitamin C hourly-this will help prevent infection from occurring.

MINERALS: Calcium, Magnesium, Potassium, and Zinc.

ALSO: Ice, cold water, Paba cream, liquid honey, Comfrey poultice.

HELPFUL FOODS: Apples, bananas, broccoli, carrots, cheese, citrus fruits, herring, fish liver oils, green leafy vegetables, turnip greens, and vegetable oils.

BURSITIS

SPECIFICS: Bursitis is an inflammation of the bursae, liquid filled sacs found in the joints, tendons, muscles, and bones. This disorder is commonly found in the elbow, hip, and shoulder joints, causing swelling, tenderness, and extreme pain. During infection, elevated doses of A, C, and E are beneficial in the treatment of bursitis.

(BeneficialRemedies,Treatments,andNutrients)

HERBAL COMBINATIONS: (Rheum-Aid) (Cal-Silica) (Kalmin).

PHYSIOLOGIC ACTIONS: These herbal combinations contain herbs which exhibit anti-inflammatory and relaxing effects. Help to build nerve tissue and relieve stiffness and pain.

SINGLE HERBS: Alfalfa, Chaparral, Comfrey, and Yucca. Mullein is often used as a poultice to give relief externally.

VITAMINS: A, B12, B complex, C, E, and P.

MINERALS: Calcium and Magnesium.

ALSO: Alkaline diet, Coenzyme Q10, Germanium, Proteolytic enzymes, Yu-ccan herbal drink, and a protein supplement.

HELPFUL FOODS: Apples, apricots, cherries, citrus fruits, sardines, tuna, fish liver oils, spinach, and sweet potatoes.

CADMIUM TOXICITY

SPECIFICS: Cadmium is a tin like metal. Poisoning is usually due to breathing in cadmium dust and fumes by industrial workers. This problem may also arise when people consume foods that have been stored in cadmium lined containers. This metal has been linked to the development of high blood pressure and acute exposure can lead to kidney failure and permanent lung damage. Cadmium levels are much higher in smokers and non smokers may also accumulate higher levels from second hand smoke.

(BeneficialRemedies,Treatments,andNutrients)

SINGLE HERBS: Alfalfa and Garlic.

VITAMINS: E.

MINERALS: Calcium, Copper, Magnesium, and Zinc.

ALSO: L-Cysteiene, L-Lysine, and L-Methionine.

HELPFUL FOODS: Whole grains, fibrous fruits, pumpkin seeds, and other foods that have a high zinc content.

CALAMYDIA

SPECIFICS: Calamydia is the most common sexually transmitted disease. The microorganisms that cause this disease, can also be passed from the mother to the newborn infant, as it passes through the infected birth canal. Complications of calamydia may result in sterility in both sexes. Penicillin or another antibiotic is the usual treatment. In addition to medical treatment, an afflicted person should maintain a high nutrient diet to help repair the tissue damage that has occurred.

(BeneficialRemedies,Treatments,andNutrients)

SINGLE HERBS: Echinacea, Goldenseal, Kelp, Pau d'Arco, Red Clover, and Suma.

VITAMINS: A, B complex, C, E, and K.

MINERALS: Zinc.

ALSO: Acidophilus, Coenzyme Q10, Germanium, and Proteolytic Enzymes.

HELPFUL FOODS: All red meats, cabbage, fruits, aloe vera, kelp, herring, oysters, liver, nuts, and yogurt.

CALCIUM DEFICIENCY

SPECIFICS: Low levels of calcium in the blood may seriously disrupt cell function in muscles and nerves. Vitamin D will help control the overall amount of calcium in the body by regulating the amount of calcium removed from the body by the kidneys and the amount absorbed from food.

(BeneficialRemedies,Treatments,andNutrients)

HERBAL COMBINATION: (Ca -T).

PHYSIOLOGIC ACTION: This proven formula contains organic calcium, silica, and other tranquilizing minerals help prevent cramps. A natural way to calm nerves and aid sleep in addition to rebuilding the nerve sheath, vein, artery walls, teeth, and bones.

SINGLE HERBS: Comfrey Root, Horsetail, and Lobelia.

VITAMINS: D.

MINERALS: Calcium.

HELPFUL FOODS: Dark green leafy vegetables such as kale, mustard greens, collard greens, cabbage, broccoli are rich sources of easily assimilated calcium. Foods such as lentils, almonds, and sesame seeds are other good sources.

CALCULUS
(refer to Kidney and Bladder Stones)

CANCER

SPECIFICS: With cancer, cells begin to reproduce for no obvious reason. The cancer cells rob the normal cells of their essential nutrients causing the cancer patient to waste away quickly. The major causes of cancer are stress, environmental factors, and diet. Research indicates that pancreatic and other enzymes are a vital part of a cancer program. It has also been noted that potassium is vital. Along with all the supplements, coffee enemas are important to cleanse the system and stimulate liver function.

(BeneficialRemedies,Treatments,andNutrients)

HERBAL COMBINATION: (Red Clover Combination).

PHYSIOLOGIC ACTION: This herbal combination contains herbs that are very similar to the Hoxey formula used to treat cancer. It is unique in that it cleanses and feeds the body.

NOTE: Canaid herbal drink could be one of the cancer fighting breakthroughs that the world has so desperately been seeking. It's formula is similar, in nature and properties, to the famous Essiac treatment that has supposedly cured thousands of terminal cancer patients.

The herb Pau d' Arco possesses antibiotic, tumor inhibiting, virus killing, anti-fungal, and anti-malarial properties.

Red clover, burdock, and chaparral act as blood cleansers.

SINGLE HERBS: Bloodroot, Buckthorn Bark, Burdock, Chaparral, Cleavers, Garlic, Ginger, Ginseng, Golden Seal, Sheep Sorrel, Liquid Echinacea Extract, Pau d' Arco, Red Clover, Suma, Violet Leaves, and Yucca.

ALSO: There are various Chinese herbs which have been used successfully while treating cancer. Some of these herbs include: Reshi Mushroom, Astragalus, Ligustrum, Codonopsis, and Schizandra.

VITAMINS: A, B3, B complex, C, E, Beta Carotene, Digestive Enzymes

MINERALS: Germanium, Magnesium, Potassium, and Selenium.

ALSO: Almonds, Apricot Pits, Red Beet Juice, Liver Extract, Brewers Yeast, Raw Food, Low Animal Protein, Green Juices.

HELPFUL FOODS: Aloe Vera, apples, bananas, broccoli, bran, carrots, citrus fruits, green leafy vegetables, soybeans, sweet potatoes, turnip greens, vegetable oils, lean red meat, and fish liver oils.

CANDIDA ALBICANS (Candidiasis)

SPECIFICS: A yeast-like fungus that inhabits the genital tract, intestines, mouth, and throat. Candidiasis affects both men and women, when the fungus infects the vagina it results in vaginitis, when it infects the oral cavity, it is called thrush. Diabetics are at great risk of contracting the fungus, so if a person is diagnosed with yeast infection, he or she should be checked for diabetes.

(Beneficial Remedies, Treatments, and Nutrients)

HERBAL COMBINATION: (Cantrol).

PHYSIOLOGIC ACTION: An excellent well-balanced formula of herbs and supplements which balance the system while killing yeast. It includes caprylic acid and anti-oxidants for the control and eventual elimination of candida overgrowth.

SINGLE HERBS: Black Walnut, Caprinex, Garlicin, Pau d'Arco, and Yucca.

VITAMINS: Biotin and B complex.

ALSO: Candida Cleanse, Yu-ccan, Caprylic Acid, Coenzyme Q10, L-Cysteine, Primadophilus, Primrose oil, and Salmon oil.

HELPFUL FOODS: Egg yolk, apricot, citrus fruits, beef kidney, beef liver, and vegetable and fish liver oils.

CANKER SORES

SPECIFICS: A canker sore is a contagious and painful mouth ulceration that can appear on the lips, gums, tongue, and on the inside cheeks. They are identified by a tingling sensation and a slight swelling of the mucous membrane. The sores have white centers and are surrounded by a red border. Canker sores may be caused from eating to many sweets, poor dental hygiene or stress.

(BeneficialRemedies,Treatments,andNutrients)

SINGLE HERBS: Goldenseal, Pau d'Arco, and Burdock Root tea, or Red Raspberry tea is very helpful.

VITAMINS: A, B5, B12, B complex, and large doses of C.

MINERALS: Iron.

ALSO: Acidophilus and L-Lysine.

Note: Avoid chewing gum, sugar, processed or refined foods, and citrus fruits.

HELPFUL FOODS: Black molasses, carrots, lean red meat, fish, leafy green vegetables, turnips, potatoes, vegetable oils, and unpolished rice.

CARBUNCLES

SPECIFICS: A painful localized infection producing pus filled areas in the deeper layers of the skin tissues. Carbuncles are caused when bacteria enters lesions in the skin. They are deeper, slower healing and usually more painful than an ordinary boil.

(BeneficialRemedies,Treatments,andNutrients)

HERBAL COMBINATION: (AKN).

PHYSIOLOGIC ACTION: AKN helps cleanse the bloodstream. Pimples, blackheads, and other superficial skin eruptions, and more serious conditions such as boils, carbuncles, dermatitis, eczema, and pleuritis will be eliminated when the blood has been cleansed.

VITAMINS: A, B2, B3, B5, B6, C, F, P, Biotin, and Paba.

MINERALS: Iron, Silicon, and Sulfur.

ALSO: Canaid herbal drink, Whey Powder, and Brewers Yeast.

HELPFUL FOODS: Almonds, apricots, avocados, beef, broccoli, black molasses, carrots, celery, flax seed, all fruits, safflower and linseed oil.

CARDIOVASCULAR DISEASE
(refer to Arteriosclerosis and Circulation)

CARPAL TUNNEL SYNDROME

SPECIFICS: Carpal tunnel syndrome is a common nerve entrapment disorder caused by pressure on the median nerve at the point where it goes through the carpal tunnel of the wrist.

This disorder is common in individuals who perform repetitive movements with their hands and wrist at work. It is characterized by pain, tingling, and burning sensations in the hand and fingers.

(Beneficial Remedies, Treatments, and Nutrients)

SINGLE HERBS: Ginger Root Caps.

VITAMINS: B complex, plus B6, and C.

MINERAL: Calcium and Magnesium.

ALSO: Bromelain.

HELPFUL FOODS: Kale, broccoli, green peppers, turnip greens, spinach, and pineapple.

CAR SICKNESS

SPECIFICS: Car sickness can indicate the presence of many diseases including inner ear infection, low blood sugar, food poisoning, and nutrient deficiency.

The most common cause is a deficiency of the vitamin "B6" and the mineral "magnesium". Ginkgo is excellent for chronic dizziness and light headedness.

(Beneficial Remedies, Treatments, and Nutrients)

HERBAL COMBINATION: (Motion Mate).

PHYSIOLOGIC ACTION: In a recent university study, ginger root caps proved more effective than either a drug or placebo at controlling motion induced nausea. Also queasy travelers have found taking B complex at night and just before the trip is most effective.

SINGLEHERBS: Ginger Root Caps and Ginkgo.

VITAMINS: B complex, plus B6.

MINERAL: Magnesium.

HELPFUL FOODS: Fruits, lean beef, nuts, unpolished rice, whole grains, and yellow corn.

CATARACTS

SPECIFICS: A cataract is a condition in which the lens of the eye becomes clouded or opaque, and unable to focus on close or far objects. Most cataracts are caused by free radical damage (exposure to low level radiation from x-rays and ultraviolet rays). Free radicals attack the structural enzymes, proteins, and cell membranes of the lens.

(BeneficialRemedies,Treatments,andNutrients)

HERBCOMPLEX: Cineraria Maritima, D3.

PHYSIOLOGIC ACTION: This product is a Homeopathic medicine and only available through your Homeopathic Doctor. Used regularly, this product will dissolve cataracts completely, after cataracts have disappeared use gencydo for minor inflammation.

HERBAL COMBINATION: (Herbal Eyebright Formula).

PHYSIOLOGIC ACTION: This herbal product contains valuable nutrients for the eyes. If taken regularly, in conjunction with a proper diet, cataracts are likely to dissolve.

SINGLEHERBS: Standardized Bilberry Extract.

VITAMINS: A, B1, B2, B5, C, and E.

MINERALS: Copper, Manganese, Selenium, and Zinc.

ALSO: L-Lysine neutralizes viruses, and is important in collagen formation, which is necessary for lens repair.

HELPFUL FOODS: Bran, beets, broccoli, carrots, green leafy vegetables, raisins, soybeans, sweet potatoes, vegetable oils, herring, and fish liver oils.

CELIAC DISEASE

SPECIFICS: Celiac disease is an intestinal disorder caused by the intolerance to a protein in wheat, barley, and rye called gluten. Treatment includes eating a well-balanced gluten-free diet, high in proteins, calories, and normal in fats. Exclude all cereal grains except corn and rice.

(BeneficialRemedies,Treatments,andNutrients)

VITAMINS: A, B6, B12, B complex, C, D, E, and K.

MINERALS: Calcium, Iron, Magnesium, and Potassium.

HELPFUL FOODS: Apples, bananas, beets, black molasses, carrots, cheese, butter, goats milk, all fruit, kelp, and green leafy vegetables.

CERVICAL DYSPLASIA

SPECIFICS: A pre cancerous condition that occurs in the cervix of the female uterus. Cervical dysplasia is characterized by the presence of abnormal cells usually causing vaginal bleeding between menstrual periods and there may also be increased vaginal discharge. The (PAP) smear is most effective in diagnosing this condition.

(BeneficialRemedies,Treatments,andNutrients)

SINGLEHERBS: Bloodroot and Calendula.

VITAMINS: A, B complex, B6, B12, Folic acid, and C.

MINERALS: Selenium and Zinc.

ALSO: Bitter orange oil, Bromelain, and Escarotic treatment.

AVOID: Saturated fats from meat, white sugar, refined carbohydrates, and smoking.

HELPFUL FOODS: Greens, citrus fruits, strawberries, tomatoes, yellow fruits, and vegetables.

CHARLEY HORSE

SPECIFICS: A pulled or bruised muscle that results in soreness and stiffness caused by impaired blood circulation. It is usually caused by a forceful stretch of the leg during heavy exertion or athletic activity. Charley horse victims should have a protein rich diet to rebuild the damaged tissues.

(BeneficialRemedies,Treatments,andNutrients)

HERBAL COMBINATION: (B F + C).

PHYSIOLOGIC ACTION: A special formula to aid in healing processes for torn cartilage's, sprained limbs, broken bones, multiple athletic injuries, and associated swelling and inflammation.

SINGLE HERBS: Comfrey Herb, Horsetail Grass, Oat Straw, Skullcap, and Yucca.

HOMEOPATHIC COMBINATION: Injury and Backache Formula.

VITAMINS: B complex, B1, B2, B5, C, D, and E.

MINERALS: Calcium, Magnesium, and Phosphorous.

ALSO: #12 tissue salts, Green-Lipid Mussel, Silica, Protein, and Unsaturated fatty acids.

HELPFUL FOODS: Red meat, butter, cheese, citrus fruits, soybeans, rice, sunflower seeds, nuts, whole grains, and sweet potatoes.

CHEMICAL ALLERGIES

SPECIFICS: The inappropriate response by the body's immune system to some foreign chemicals or environmental contaminants. The immune system wrongly identifies a toxic allergen causing the white blood cells to overreact creating more damage to the body than the allergen itself. Chemical allergies may cause asthma, diarrhea, dizziness, eczema, fever, hay fever, high blood pressure, hives, hypoglycemia, mental disorders, ringing in the ears, and stomach ulcers.

(Beneficial Remedies, Treatments, and Nutrients)

HERBAL COMBINATION: (HAS: Original and Fast Acting Formulas) (Allergy Care).

PHYSIOLOGIC ACTION: HAS is an excellent formula which contains herbs that help relieve symptoms of hay fever, sinus congestion, and respiratory allergies caused by chemicals. Helps drain nasal passages, relieve swollen membranes, eliminate mucus, and cleanse the body. The Fast Acting Formula adds Pseudoephedra, a natural plant extract from the Ephedra plant. This substance quickly opens nasal passages allowing free breathing. While HAS Fast Acting is not for prolonged use, HAS Original can be taken for as long as needed.

Caution: Both formulas are not to be used during pregnancy, nor by small children.

Allergy Care: Maximum-strength natural allergy medicine that will not cause drowsiness. It contains 60mg of the active ingredient Pseudoephedrine Hcl.

SINGLE HERBS: Burdock Root, Cayenne, Chaparral, Elderberry, Eyebright, Lobelia, Golden Rod, Golden Seal, and Nettles

HOMEOPATHIC COMBINATION: Allergy Formula

VITAMINS: A, B complex plus extra B3, B6, C, and E.

MINERALS: A multi-mineral complex plus Calcium, Magnesium, Manganese, and Potassium.

ALSO: Acidophilus, Bee Pollen, Coenzyme Q10, Germanium, L-Tyrosine, L-Cysteine, Digestive Enzymes, Pancreatic Enzymes, Propolis, Raw adrenal, and Raw thymus.

HELPFUL FOODS: Almonds, apples, beef, beets, broccoli, carrots, cheese, bananas, fruits, oat bran, safflower, and linseed oil.

CHICKEN POX

SPECIFICS: A highly contagious viral disease that first manifests as a fever and a mild headache. After twenty-four to thirty-six hours, the chief symptom is generalized skin eruptions. It is most important to keep infected children away from the elderly as the virus that causes chickenpox in children (Varicella Zoster) also causes shingles in adults.

(Beneficial Remedies, Treatments, and Nutrients)

HERBAL COMBINATION: (Fenu-Thyme) (ANT-PLG Syrup) (EchinaGuard).

PHYSIOLOGIC ACTION: Helps the body to resist infectious diseases and reduce fever. Acts as a support to the system during such illnesses as chicken pox, mumps, and measles.

SINGLE HERBS: Cayenne, Chickweed, Cleavers, Echinacea, Lobelia, and Red Clover.

ALSO: Canaid herbal drink strengthens the immune system. A bath can be made from bulk chickweed to alleviate itching. Chickweed ointment is also excellent for itching.

VITAMINS: Complete multi-vitamin plus A, C, and E.

MINERALS: Multi-mineral, plus Potassium, and Zinc.

HELPFUL FOODS: Bananas, citrus fruits, melon, herring, fish liver oils, carrots, broccoli, green leafy vegetables, sweet potatoes, and turnip greens.

CHOLESTASIS

SPECIFICS: Cholestasis is not in itself a disease, but a sign of a liver, kidney, or blood disorder, which causes a build-up of bilirubin in the blood. Bilirubin is the presence of pigments from worn out blood cells that are deposited in the tissues, which leads to a characteristic type of jaundice, causing the skin and whites of the eyes to become abnormally yellow.

(Beneficial Remedies, Treatments, and Nutrients)

HERBAL COMBINATION: (LG).

PHYSIOLOGIC ACTION: This herbal combination helps to correct malfunctioning of the liver and gall bladder. It is a liver detoxifier, and a bile stimulant.

SINGLE HERBS: Birch Leaves, Dandelion, Fennel, Horse Tail, Irish Moss, Parsley, and Rose Hips.

VITAMINS: A, B6, C, D, and E.

MINERALS: Calcium, Magnesium, and Phosphorus.

ALSO: Lecithin, Protein, and Unsaturated fatty acids.

HELPFUL FOODS: Apples, bananas, broccoli, carrots, cheese and other dairy products, tuna, fish liver oils, red meat, vegetable oils, and sprouted seeds.

JUICES: Sauerkraut and tomato juice.

CHOLESTEROL LEVEL (high)

SPECIFICS: Cholesterol is a fatty substance manufactured by the liver and found only in animal fat. It is essential in building sex hormones, cell membranes, and also aids in digestion. High cholesterol levels are the primary cause of heart disease and is implicated in clogging of the arteries, gall stones, high blood pressure, impotence, and mental impairment. High cholesterol can only be reduced by lowering ones consumption of low-density lipoproteins (LDLs - animal fats), eating a balanced diet, and exercise.

(Beneficial Remedies, Treatments, and Nutrients)

SINGLE HERBS: Cayenne, Garlic, Goldenseal, Hawthorn berries, Kelp, and Oat bran.

VITAMINS: B complex, B3, B6, B9, B12, Choline, Inositol, C, and E.

ALSO: Coenzyme Q10, Guar Gum, Lecithin, and Lipotropic factors.

HELPFUL FOODS: Brewers yeast, broccoli, cabbage, spinach, fruit(citrus and other), fish liver oils, egg whites, vegetable oils, unpolished rice, and whole grains.

CHRONIC FATIGUE SYNDROME

SPECIFICS: Chronic fatigue syndrome is caused by the Epstein Barr virus (EBV). This virus is highly contagious and can be passed from one person to another by any close contact. The symptoms of chronic fatigue syndrome are anxiety, depression, extreme fatigue, irritability, headache, fever, swollen glands, sore throat, jaundice, and sleep disturbances.

(BeneficialRemedies,Treatments,andNutrients)

SINGLE HERBS: Burdock root, Dandelion, Echinacea, Goldenseal, and Pau d'Arco.

VITAMINS: Multi-vitamin complex plus A, B complex, B12, and E.

MINERALS: Calcium, Magnesium, Potassium, Selenium, and Zinc.

ALSO: Acidophilus, Coenzyme Q10, Germanium, Protein, Proteolytic enzymes, and Raw thymus.

HELPFUL FOODS: Apples, aloe vera juice, bananas, citrus fruits, beef, bran, carrots, cheese, green leafy vegetables, herring, mushrooms, nuts, soybeans, and yams.

CHRONIC OBSTRUCTIVE LUNG DISEASE
(Refer to "Emphysema")

CIRCULATION

SPECIFICS: There are many disorders associated with circulatory problems. The most common disease for sluggish circulation is Raynaud's disease, characterized by constriction and spasm of the blood vessels in the limbs.

Poor circulation can also result from varicose veins, caused by the loss of elasticity in the walls of the veins. For information on high blood pressure refer to (arteriosclerosis) or (blood pressure high).

(BeneficialRemedies,Treatments,andNutrients)

HERBAL COMBINATIONS: (H Formula) (Ginkgold).

PHYSIOLOGIC ACTION: Contains herbs which strengthen the heart and builds the vascular system. When taken with Cayenne, it improves circulation, giving a warming sensation to the entire body.

ALSO: Cayenne strengthens the pulse rate and circulation while Black Cohosh slows it down.

SINGLE HERBS: Cayenne, Black Cohosh, Bayberry, Butchers Broom, Ginkgo, and Yarrow.

VITAMINS: A, B3, C, and E.

MINERALS: Calcium, Magnesium, Potassium, and Selenium.

ALSO: Coenzyme Q10, Germanium, Lecithin, L-Carnitine, L-Cysteine, L-Methionine, and Multi-digestive enzymes.

HELPFUL JUICES: Alfalfa, beet, blackberry, grape, parsley, and pineapple juice.

CIRRHOSIS OF THE LIVER

SPECIFICS: A chronic degenerative, inflammatory, disease in which damage and hardening of the liver cells occur. Scarring of the liver cells renders the liver unable to function properly. The most common cause is excessive alcohol consumption. Other causes are malnutrition, chronic inflammation, and viral hepatitis. Damage from excessive drinking is irreversible, however further damage can be prevented by eating properly, abstaining from alcohol, and taking vitamin and mineral supplements.

(BeneficialRemedies,Treatments,andNutrients)

SINGLE HERBS: Barberry, Burdock, Celandine, Dandelion, Echinacea, Fennel, Garlic, Goldenseal, Hops, Milk Thistle, Red Clover, and Suma.

VITAMINS: A, B3, B9, B12, B complex, C, D, E, and K.

MINERALS: Magnesium, and Zinc.

ALSO: Carbohydrates, Coenzyme Q10, L-Carnitine, L-Glutathionine, L-Methionine, and Protein.

HELPFUL FOODS: Apples, beef, butter, cheese, bran, broccoli, carrots, citrus fruits, green leafy vegetables, sardines, fish liver oils, and whole grains.

CLAP
(refertoGonorrhea)

COLD FEET

(BeneficialRemedies,Treatments,andNutrients)

HERBAL COMBINATION: (Cayenne extract).

PHYSIOLOGIC ACTION: Improves pulse rate and circulation giving a warming sensation to the entire body.

SINGLE HERBS: Cayenne, Bayberry, and Kelp.

VITAMINS: Vitamin E, and Niacin.

MINERALS: A complete multi-mineral complex.

HELPFUL FOODS: Brewers yeast, kelp, soybeans, sunflower seeds, white meat of poultry, and vegetable oils.

COLDS AND COUGHS

SPECIFICS: A general inflammation of the mucous membranes of the respiratory passages caused by a virus. Symptoms include aches, pains, coughing, headache, fever, sneezing, congestion watery eyes, and difficult breathing.

(Beneficial Remedies, Treatments, and Nutrients)

HERBAL COMBINATIONS: (Fenu-Thyme) (Garlic Syrup) (Loquat Syrup) (Garlicin CF).

PHYSIOLOGIC ACTION: These herbal syrups and combinations work to soothe the throat and lungs and act as expectorants and demulcents to cut and expel mucus from the lungs. Garlicin CF is a unique formula combining the natural benefits of Garlic with other herbs such as Echinacea, Vitamin C, bioflavanoids, and Zinc.

SINGLE HERBS: Echinacea, Ginger, Pau d'Arco, and Yarrow.

HOMEOPATHIC COMBINATION: Dry Cough Formula.

VITAMINS: Multi-vitamin complex plus C.

MINERALS: Multi-mineral complex plus Zinc.

ALSO: Proteolytic enzymes, and Canaid herbal drink.

HELPFUL FOODS: Apples, citrus fruit, celery, herring, oysters, and turnip greens.

JUICES: Apple, celery, and watercress.

COLDS AND FLU
(See Colds and Cough)

SPECIFICS: The flu is a highly contagious viral infection of the respiratory tract and is spread by coughing and sneezing. Symptoms include headache, fever, aching of limbs and back, and weakness.

(Beneficial Remedies, Treatments, and Nutrients)

HERBAL COMBINATIONS: (C+F) (Herbal Influence) (ANT-PLG Syrup).

PHYSIOLOGIC ACTION: Proven herbal formulas to help relieve symptoms of colds, flu, hoarseness, colic, cramps, sluggish circulation, beginning of fevers and germinal viral infections. Herbal Influence (formerly known as Herbal Composition) this formula was created by the early American herbalist, Samuel Thomson. It contains herbs which help with fever and nauseousness.

SINGLE HERBS: Cayenne, Red Clover, Raspberry Tea, Chaparral, Rose Hips, Garlic, Honey, and Golden Seal.

HOMEOPATHIC COMBINATION: Cold and Flu Formula.

VITAMINS: A, B6, C, and P.

MINERALS: Multi-mineral complex.

ALSO: Proteolytic enzymes and Canaid herbal drink.

HELPFUL FOODS: Apples, apricots, cherries, citrus fruits, lean beef, broccoli, carrots, green leafy vegetables, melon, nuts, sweet potatoes, turnip greens, and unpolished rice.

JUICES: Apple, Carrot, Celery, Grapefruit, and Coconut juice.

COLD SORES (Herpes Simplex Virus 1)

SPECIFICS: Herpes simplex 1 results in cold sores and skin eruptions. They usually occur with a cold, fever, infection, or when the immune system is depressed. It can also cause inflammation of the eye. If the eye becomes infected see a doctor at once. By strengthening the immune system one can defend against or prevent herpes activation.

(Beneficial Remedies, Treatments, and Nutrients)

SINGLE HERBS: Echinacea, Goldenseal, Myrrh, and Red Clover.

VITAMINS: B complex, C, and E.

MINERALS: Zinc chelate.

ALSO: The amino acid L-Lysine has a direct effect on the virus.

HELPFUL FOODS: Herring, oysters, sardines, citrus fruits, red meats, and vegetable oils.

COLIC (Infants)

SPECIFICS: Colic most often occurs shortly after feeding. During an attack the baby suffers physical pain, gas, and cramps.

(BeneficialRemedies,Treatments,andNutrients)

HERBAL COMBINATION: (Catnip and Fennel Extract).

PHYSIOLOGIC ACTION: This formula works on minor spasms, acid stomach and gas. It also soothes indigestion and nerves. Excellent for children.

SINGLE HERBS: Catnip, fennel, chamomile, peppermint or any combination in a tea. Make teas very mild. No sugar. Check your own diet if nursing baby.

HOMEOPATHIC COMBINATION: Colic Formula.

COLITIS

SPECIFICS: Mucous Colitis is often associated with, and made worse by psychological stress. Emotional upset should be avoided. Various herbs with multiple properties must be used to address the complexity of this situation.

Note: Avoid citrus juices. Bananas are very soothing and healing in ulcerative colitis. Primadophilus is effective in stabilizing flora in lower bowel.

(BeneficialRemedies,Treatments,andNutrients)

SINGLE HERBS: Alfalfa, Bayberry, Chamomile, Caraway, Garlic, Reshi Mushroom, Plantain, Valerian, Wild Yam, and Yucca.

VITAMINS: A, B6, Folic acid, Pantothenic acid, B complex, C, and E.

MINERALS: Calcium, Iron, Magnesium, and Potassium.

ALSO: Multi-digestive and Proteolytic enzymes, Raw thymus glandular, and unsaturated fatty acids.

HELPFUL FOODS: Apples, bananas, lean beef, black molasses, tuna, fish liver oils, cheese, non citrus fruit, mushrooms, and sweet potatoes.

CONJUNCTIVITIS

SPECIFICS: An inflammation of the mucous membrane that lines the eyelids. The most common cause of conjunctivitis is a calcium deficiency, however a deficiency of vitamin A, B6, or riboflavin may cause conjunctivitis symptoms.

(BeneficialRemedies,Treatments,andNutrients)

VITAMINS: A, B2, B6, B complex, Niacin, C, and D.

MINERALS: Calcium, Magnesium, and Phosphorus.

HELPFUL FOODS: Apricots, citrus fruits, cherries, beef, black molasses, broccoli, carrots, butter, cheese, shell fish, tuna, and whole wheat.

CONSTIPATION (Minor)

SPECIFICS: Constipation results when the waste material moves too slowly or there is decreased frequency of bowel movements. Constipation usually arises from insufficient amounts of fiber and fluids in the diet. Other causes include lack of exercise, nervousness, stress, infections, and poor diet.

(BeneficialRemedies,Treatments,andNutrients)

HERBAL COMBINATION: (Multilax #1) or (Naturalax #1).

PHYSIOLOGIC ACTION: Helps relieve minor constipation.

Warning: Do not use when abdominal pain nausea or vomiting are present. Frequent or prolonged use of preparation may result in dependence on laxatives.

SINGLE HERBS: Cascara Sagrada, Comfrey, Flaxseed, Goldenseal, Psyllium seed, Senna, and Yucca.

HOMEOPATHIC COMBINATION: Constipation and Hemorrhoids Formula.

VITAMINS: A, B complex, C, D, and E.

MINERALS: Calcium, Magnesium, Potassium, and Zinc.

ALSO: Yu-ccan herbal drink, Vita Cleansing Tea, Swiss Kriss, Metab Herb, Psyllium Husks, Flax meal, Super D Tea. Drink lots of pure water to flush system.

HELPFUL FOODS: Bananas, prunes, citrus fruits, all dairy products except cheese, carrots, turnips, green vegetables, soybeans, vegetable oils, and kelp.

JUICES: Celery, Grapefruit, and Spinach juice.

CONSTIPATION (Chronic)

SPECIFICS: Chronic constipation is generally due to weakness of the muscles of the abdomen and the pelvic floor, which prevents adequate pressure when attempting to move the bowels. This condition is most prevalent in the elderly and persons with immobility problems.

(BeneficialRemedies,Treatments,andNutrients)

HERBAL COMBINATIONS: (Multilax #2) or (Naturalax #2) (Laxacil) (Multilax 3) (Naturalax 3) (Aloelax Formula).

PHYSIOLOGIC ACTION: There are two forms of laxatives, stimulant and bulk forming. Stimulant laxatives encourage peristalsis of the bowel. This motion empties the intestinal tract of waste. Bulk forming laxatives absorb water and toxic wastes from the intestinal walls. The natural expansion triggers peristalsis, and pushes old fecal matter through the bowel. Both forms of laxatives have benefits.

Warning: Most laxatives should not be taken during pregnancy. Psyllium husks, however, are safe.

SINGLEHERBS: Aloe Vera, Cascara Sagrada, Comfrey, Flaxseed, Goldenseal, Pepsin, Psyllium, Senna, and Yucca.

VITAMINS: A, B1, B6, Choline, Inositol, Niacin, Pantothenic acid, B complex, C, D, and E.

MINERALS: Calcium, Magnesium, Potassium, and Zinc.

Babies: Licorice tea (made weakly). Nursing mothers can pass this one to the infant.

ALSO: Fats, Fiber, and Primadophilus.

HELPFUL FOODS: Same as minor constipation.

DERMATITIS

SPECIFICS: Contact dermatitis is an allergy to something that touches the skin, that produces flaking, scaling, itching, and eventual thickening and color changes of the skin. The best way to cure this ailment is to remove the source of the allergen and cleanse the blood.

(BeneficialRemedies,Treatments,andNutrients)

HERBAL COMBINATION: (AKN).

PHYSIOLOGIC ACTION: Many skin problems are related to liver dysfunction. This formula gives support to the liver, helps to cleanse the blood, and supplies nutrients for the skin.

SINGLE HERBS: Aloe Vera (on skin), Burdock, Cleavers, Dandelion, Evening Primrose, Garlic, Golden Seal, Pau d'Arco, Yellowdock, and Yucca.

VITAMINS: A, B complex, B2, B3, B6, D, E, and Biotin B complex.

MINERALS: Sulfur ointment, Potassium, and Zinc.

ALSO: Yu-ccan herbal drink, and Protein.

HELPFUL FOODS: Raw carrots, fish liver oils, green leafy vegetables, and vegetable oils.

CONVULSION
(RefertoEpilepsy)

COPPER TOXICITY

SPECIFICS: Copper is required by the body in minute amounts. This metallic element forms the essential part of several enzymes. Poisoning is usually due to people drinking home made alcohol distilled using copper tubing, using copper cookware, copper plumbing, and insecticides. Copper toxicity can lead to depression, nephritis, eczema, damage to the central nervous system, and sickle cell anemia.

(BeneficialRemedies,Treatments,andNutrients)

SINGLE HERBS: Alfalfa and Garlic.

VITAMINS: C.

MINERALS: Calcium, Iron, Magnesium, Sulfur, and Zinc.

ALSO: L-Cysteiene, L-Lysine, and L-Methionine.

HELPFUL FOODS: Eggs, onions, pumpkin seeds, and other foods that have a high zinc content.

COUGHS

SPECIFICS: Refex action to try to clear the air-ways of mucus (phelegm) or other irritants or blockages. Most coughs are due to irritation of the airways by dust, gases, or smoke, or by mucus dripping from the back of the nose. An unproductive or dry cough does not bring up mucus or dry sputum.

(BeneficialRemedies,Treatments,andNutrients)

HERBAL COMBINATIONS: (Fenu-Thyme) (Garlic Syrup) (Loquat Syrup) (Garlicin CF)

PHYSIOLOGIC ACTION: These herbal syrups and combinations work to soothe the throat and lungs and act as expectorants and demulcents to cut and expel mucus from the lungs. Garlicin CF is a unique formula combining the natural benefits of Garlic with other herbs such as Echinacea, Vitamin C, bioflavanoids and Zinc.

HERBAL TONICS: Pie Pa Koa, Salus, Olbas, Swiss herbal candy

HOMEOPATHIC COMBINATION: Dry Cough Formula.

VITAMINS: A, B6, C, P

BENEFICIAL JUICES: Apple, and Watercress juice.

ALSO: Fenugreek Seed, Comfrey Leaves, Garlic, Honey, Rose Hips, fresh juice, short fasts, Zinc Lozenges.

HELPFUL JUICES: Apricot, apple, cherry, grape, and all citrus juices.

CRADLE CAP

SPECIFICS: A form of Siborrheic Dermatitis. A recurring condition, most prevalent in babies between the ages of three to nine months. Thick yellow scales occur in patches over the scalp and can also occur on the face, neck, and behind the ears. Cradle cap is harmless if the scalp does not become infected.

(BeneficialRemedies,Treatments,andNutrients)

TREATMENT: Apply olive oil or vitamin E on the head and brush gently.

ALSO: A mild dandruff shampoo can be used.

CRAMPS
(Refer to "Leg Cramps" or "Menstrual Cramps")

CROHN'S DISEASE

SPECIFICS: A chronic and long-lasting inflammation of a section of the digestive tract. Inflammation works through all layers of the intestinal wall and involves the adjacent lymph nodes. If left untreated, it can increase the risk of cancer. The following nutrients are beneficial to the prevention and cure of this disease.

(BeneficialRemedies,Treatments,andNutrients)

SINGLE HERBS: Echinacea, Garlic, Goldenseal, Pau d'Arco, Rose Hips, and Yerba Mate.

VITAMINS: A strong multi-vitamin plus A, B12, B complex, and E.

MINERALS: A complete mineral complex.

ALSO: Acidophlus, Aloe Vera, Essential fatty acids, and Protein.

CROUP

SPECIFICS:A respiratory infection that causes the larynx to swell, narrowing the air passage so the victim experiences difficulty breathing, tightness in the lungs, hoarseness, and a harsh high pitched cough. Treatment involves a well-balanced diet and the following supplements to promote the growth and repair of tissues.

(BeneficialRemedies,Treatments,andNutrients)

HERBAL COMBINATION: (Breath aid)(BRE).

PHYSIOLOGIC ACTION: This formula helps to restore free breathing by opening up the bronchial passages. It is especially effective for the shortness of breath, tightness of chest, and wheezing associated with croup.

SINGLE HERBS: Comfrey, Echinacea tincture, Fenugreek, and Goldenseal.

HOMEOPATHIC COMBINATION: Dry Cough Formula.

VITAMINS: A, C, and E.

MINERALS: Zinc.

ALSO: Cod liver oil, and Protein.

JUICES: Apple, celery, grapefruit, and watercress.

CYSTIC FIBROSIS

SPECIFICS: A hereditary disease that begins during infancy, though symptoms may manifest themselves later in life.
This disease affects the endocrine, and exocrine glands. The victim experiences impaired gastrointestinal absorption, and recurrent lung infections. The greatest danger is malnutrition due to underproduction of digestive juices. The following nutrients are beneficial in the treatment of this disease.

(BeneficialRemedies,Treatments,andNutrients)

SINGLE HERBS: Echinacea, Ginger, Goldenseal, and Yarrow.

VITAMINS: A, B2, B6, Pantothenic acid, C, D, E, and K.

MINERALS: Copper, Selenium, Sodium, and Zinc.

ALSO: Acidophlus, Coenzyme Q10, Germanium, Lecithin, Protein, Proteolytic enzymes, and Raw thymus.

HELPFUL FOODS: Aloe Vera, beef, bacon, bean, butter, broccoli, carrots, herring, oysters, fish liver oils, vegetable oils, and green leafy vegetables.

CYSTITIS
(refer to Kidney and Bladder)

DANDRUFF

SPECIFICS:A condition caused by dysfunctional sebaceous glands in the scalp. It can substantially be controlled by the use of B vitamin supplements and a diet of unrefined carbohydrates. A shampoo designed to control dandruff is also recommended.

(BeneficialRemedies,Treatments,andNutrients)

SINGLE HERBS: Burdock, Chaparral, Red Clover, and Yarrow. May be used as teas or rubbed on the head.

VITAMINS: A, B complex, B6, C, and E.

MINERALS: Selenium, and Zinc.

ALSO: Unsaturated fatty acids.

HELPFUL FOODS: Bran, carrots, all fruits, lean beef, herring, oysters, nuts, and whole grains.

DEAFNESS
(refer to Ear Infections)

DECUBITUS ULCERS
(refer to Bed Sores)

DEPRESSION

SPECIFICS: The body can handle minor anxiety, but long term chronic depression and fatigue causes the body to break down. Long term depression occurs when the situation that causes anxiety is not relieved. Find the cause and handle it constructively. People experiencing depression should maintain a well-balanced diet and replace the nutrients depleted during anxiety or stress.

(BeneficialRemedies,Treatments,andNutrients)

HERBAL COMBINATIONS: (Ginseng, Gotu Kola Plus) (Adren-Aid).

PHYSIOLOGIC ACTION: These excellent formulas build zest, energy, stamina, mental alertness, and reflex action. The herbs also help provide adrenal support which affect depression.

SINGLE HERBS: Bee Pollen, Cayenne, Damiana, Gotu Kola, St. John's Wort, Scullcap, Shitaki Mushroom, and Siberian Ginseng, and Yucca.

HOMEOPATHIC COMBINATION: Fatigue Formula.

VITAMINS: B3, B6, B12, B complex(stress vitamin), lots of Vit C, plus a strong multi-vitamin.

MINERALS: Mineral complex, plus Calcium, Chromium, Magnesium, and Zinc chelate.

ALSO: Bee pollen, Lithium, Primrose oil, Spirulina, L-Tryptophan and L-Tyrosine.

HELPFUL FOODS: Apples, broccoli, butter, cheese, citrus fruits, chicken, green leafy vegetables, sardines, shell fish, and whole grains.

DERMATITIS

SPECIFICS: An inflammatory, usually recurring skin reaction, that produces flaking, scaling, itching, and eventual thickening and color changes of the skin.

(BeneficialRemedies,Treatments,andNutrients)

HERBAL COMBINATION: (AKN).

PHYSIOLOGIC ACTION: Many skin problems are related to liver dysfunction. This formula gives support to the liver, helps to cleanse the blood, and supplies nutrients for the skin.

SINGLE HERBS: Aloe Vera (on skin), Burdock, Cleavers, Dandelion, Evening Primrose, Garlic, Golden Seal, Pau d'Arco, Yellowdock, and Yucca.

VITAMINS: A, B complex, B2, B3, B6, D, E, and Biotin B complex.

MINERALS: Sulfur ointment, Potassium, and Zinc.

ALSO: Yu-ccan herbal drink, and Protein.

HELPFUL FOODS: Raw carrots, fish liver oils, green leafy vegetables, and vegetable oils.

DIABETES

SPECIFICS: Diabetes is the result of insufficient production of insulin by the pancreas. Insulin is a hormone that is essential for the conversion of glucose into energy. The resulting symptoms range in severity from mental confusion to coma. Generally a well-balanced diet, rich in vitamins and minerals, is one of the most important factors in the control of diabetes.

(BeneficialRemedies,Treatments,andNutrients)

HERBAL COMBINATION: (PC).

PHYSIOLOGIC ACTION: An excellent formula to stimulate and restore natural functions of the pancreas and spleen. Contains a natural form of insulin thus relieving most symptoms associated with diabetes.

SINGLE HERBS: Buchu, Dandelion, Cayenne, Cedar Berries, Goldenseal, Licorice Root, Mullein, Suma, Juniper and Uva Ursi.

VITAMINS: A, B complex, B1, B2, B6, B12, Choline, Inositol 89 E, and P.

MINERALS: Calcium, Chromium, Iron, Potassium, Magnesium, and Zinc.

ALSO: Lecithin, Protein, and Proteolytic enzymes.

HELPFUL FOODS: Apricots, bananas, beef, chicken, blackstrap molasses, butter, cheese, herring, oysters, carrots, turnip greens, and soybeans.

DIAPER RASH

SPECIFICS: Quite similar to a heat rash. Caused by infrequent changing of diapers or undergarments. Massage the affected area daily is very helpful. Frequent sponge baths with warm water and a mild herbal soap or a soap containing vitamin E are recommended.

(Beneficial Remedies, Treatments, and Nutrients)

HERBAL OINTMENTS: (X-Itch ointment) (Derm-Aid Ointment).

SINGLE HERBS: Mullein Leaf and Slippery Elm (used internally in juice or apply as paste).

ALSO: Vitamin E, Powdered Golden Seal, or Comfrey added to baby powder.

VITAMINS: Mom can take Vitamins A, B, and C.

DIARRHEA

SPECIFICS: A condition causing frequent elimination of loose watery stools. Because of the rapid expulsion of food through the lower digestive tract, the victim does not properly absorb nutrients and can therefore develop nutrient deficiencies. Treatment for diarrhea includes a diet rich in protein, vitamins, and minerals.

(Beneficial Remedies, Treatments, and Nutrients)

HERBAL COMBINATION: (Diarid).

PHYSIOLOGICAL ACTION: This is a maximum-strength formula that relieves diarrhea and the pain and cramping that accompany it. The active ingredient is called Activated Attapulgite, a special kaolin substance with water absorbing abilities.

SINGLE HERBS: Blackberry Root, Red Raspberry, Slippery Elm, and Yucca.

HOMEOPATHIC COMBINATION: Indigestion & Gas Formula.

VITAMINS: A, B complex, B1, B2, B3, B6, C, Folic acid, and Choline.

MINERALS: Calcium, Chlorine, Iron, Magnesium, Potassium, and Sodium.

ALSO: Nutmeg and Cloves for cramps, Acidophilus, Activated Charcoal, and Digestive enzymes.

Babies and Children: Slippery Elm enema, Red Raspberry tea, fresh apple juice, banana, brown rice water, or carob.

JUICES: Carrot and Blackberry juice.

DIGESTIVE DISORDERS (Dyspepsia)

SPECIFICS: Dyspepsia is a disorder in the stomach or small or large intestine usually caused by the fermentation of food in the colon, producing carbon dioxide and hydrogen. Symptoms include abdominal pain, belching, gas, heartburn, nausea, bloating, and vomiting.

(BeneficialRemedies,Treatments,andNutrients)

HERBAL COMBINATIONS: (Multilax #2) or (Naturalax #2).

PHYSIOLOGIC ACTION: Helps intestinal gas, indigestion, heartburn, and stomach ache. Warm Peppermint tea, Cayenne, Papaya, or Aloe Vera can be taken with meals.

SINGLE HERBS: Aloe Vera, Chamomile, Cayenne, Comfrey leaves, Fennel, Ginger, Golden Seal, Licorice, Marshmallow Root, Papaya, and Yucca.

HOMEOPATHIC COMBINATION: Indigestion & Gas Formula.

VITAMINS: A, B3, B complex, and Biotin.

MINERALS: Copper, Dolomite, Iodine, Phosphorus, Potassium, and Zinc.

ALSO: Digestive Enzymes, Garlic, Bee Pollen, Calmus Root tea, Lactic Acid foods, Swedish Bitters, Primadophilus, and Yu-ccan.

HELPFUL FOODS: Avocados, bananas, red meat, bacon, chicken, cheese, oat bran, and whole grains.

DIVERTICULITIS

SPECIFICS: Diverticulitis is when the colon's mucous membranes become inflamed, resulting in the formation of small sacs (diverticula), that may be found along the small or large intestine. In very severe cases the disease can result in perforation of the colon, causing severe bleeding.

(BeneficialRemedies,Treatments,andNutrients)

HERBAL COMBINATION: (Naturalax or Multilax #2).

PHYSIOLOGIC ACTION: The most effective prevention for diverticulitis is to avoid constipation. The above combination both tones and naturally accelerates internal cleansing of the body through the bowels. This combination acts as a tonic to the entire digestive system, it strengthens the tissue of the intestinal tract, resulting in a healthier muscular reaction.

Warning: Do not take during pregnancy!

SINGLE HERBS: Alfalfa, Cayenne, Chamomile, Garlic, Papaya, Psyllium, Red Clover, and Yarrow.

VITAMINS: A, B complex, C, E, and K.

MINERALS: Multi-mineral

ALSO: Fiber (Oat bran, Glucomannan), Multi-digestive and Proteolytic enzymes, and Acidophlus.

HELPFUL FOODS: Broccoli, carrots, celery, corn, fish liver oils, all sea foods, citrus fruits, pineapples, and nuts.

JUICES: Celery and spinach juice

DROPSY

SPECIFICS: Dropsy is caused by fluid accumulation in the body. The retention of fluids appears as swelling and is often seen in the hands and feet, but may be located in any area of the body. Fluid retention is often caused by allergies.

(BeneficialRemedies,Treatments,andNutrients)

HERBAL COMBINATION: (KB).

PHYSIOLOGIC ACTION: KB acts as a mild diuretic to rid the body of excessive water. Disorders that cause edema are sodium retention, congestive heart failure, weak kidneys, varicose veins, and protein and thiamine deficiencies.

SINGLE HERBS: Alfalfa, Buchu, Dandelion tea, Juniper, lobelia, Parsley, Pau d'Arco tea, Safflower, Uva Ursi, and Yarrow.

VITAMINS: B1, B6, B complex, C, D, and E.

MINERALS: Calcium, Copper, and Potassium.

ALSO: L-Taurine, #9 and #11 tissue salts, Silicon, low Sodium, and Protein.

HELPFUL FOODS: All sea foods, red meats, chicken, cheese, fruits(citrus and other), soybeans, spinach, sprouted seeds, and whole grains.

DRUG DEPENDENCY

SPECIFICS: A chronic physiological or psychological condition marked by a dependence on drugs. Deficiencies of many nutrients occur when taking drugs. Some effects of drugs are a depressed immune system, damage to the central nervous system, brain, duodenum, pancreas, liver, and a loss of inhibition.

Note: Tobacco, alcohol, caffeine and other drug "cravings" are brought about by a physiological body dependence on the poison which develops during prolonged use. The addicts blood poison level must remain at a certain level at all times. As the poison level drops, there is a "desire" to take in more of the drug, to bring the level back again.

(BeneficialRemedies,Treatments,andNutrients)

HERBAL COMBINATIONS: (AdrenAid) (Red Clover Comb).

PHYSIOLOGIC ACTION: These herbal formulas provide support to the body while cleansing toxins. Red Clover Combination will minimize withdrawal symptoms such as headache, insomnia, sensitivity to light, irrational thinking, disorientation, and should be used with all detoxification programs.

SINGLE HERBS: Pau d'Arco, Chamomile tea, Licorice Root, and Lobelia.

VITAMINS: B complex, and C.

MINERALS: Calcium, and Potassium.

ALSO: Tyrosine, Vitamins B, C, and E, alleviates depression, fatigue, and irritability when dependent on cocaine, hashish, and marijuana.

Refer to: "Note in SMOKING" in this manual.

HELPFUL FOODS: All fruits, red meats, chicken, honey, seafood's, nuts, raw vegetables, and vegetable oils.

DYSMENORRHEA

SPECIFICS: Dysmenorrhea is associated with the hormonal changes in teenage girls and young women. Symptoms consist of pain, bloated abdomen, cramps, and discomfort during or just before a menstrual period. The best prevention for Dysmenorrhea is a nutrient rich diet, supplemented with vitamins and minerals, plus a good exercise program.

(BeneficialRemedies,Treatments,andNutrients)

HERBAL COMBINATIONS: (FC) or (FEM-MEND).

PHYSIOLOGIC ACTION: Helps regulate the menstrual cycle, relieve cramps, bloating, and strengthens and regulates the kidneys, bladder and uterus areas. Beneficial for all female and uterine complaints.

Warning: Do not use this combination while taking estrogen or oral contraceptives!

SINGLE HERBS: Dong Quai, Kelp, Red Raspberry, and Uva Ursi.

VITAMINS: B complex, B5, B6, B12, C, E, and K.

MINERALS: Calcium, Chlorine, Chromium, Iodine, Iron, Magnesium, and Manganese.

ALSO: Inositol, L-Lysine, L-Tyrosine, Methionine, Spirulina, and Primrose oil.

HELPFUL FOODS: All vegetables and vegetable oils, fish and fish liver oils, cheese, butter, apples, bananas, citrus fruits, and mushrooms.

DYSPEPSIA
(refer to Digestive Disorders)

EAR INFECTIONS

SPECIFICS: The most common type of ear infection is outer ear infection(otitis externa). Symptoms of the infection are fever, severe pain, and discharge from the ear. Middle ear infections(otitis media) are common in children and are usually caused by the spread of bacteria from the nose and throat. Symptoms include pressure in the ear and earache. Infection in the inner ear is usually caused by the spread of bacteria from a middle ear infection. Symptoms include fever, loss of hearing, dizziness, and vomiting.

(BeneficialRemedies,Treatments,andNutrients)

HERBAL COMBINATIONS: (ImmunAid) (B&B Extract) (EchinaGuard).

PHYSIOLOGIC ACTION: ImmunAid boosts immunity, thereby helping with ear infections. EchinaGuard is a liquid and Echinacea extract is excellent for small children with ear infections. B&B Extract can be placed in the ear or taken internally. It is also used to aid poor equilibrium, and nervous conditions.

SINGLE HERBS: Blue Cohosh, Echinacea, Garlic Oil, Garlic, Mullein Oil, Mullein, Skullcap, Sheep Sorrel, and St. Johns Wort.

HOMEOPATHIC COMBINATION: Earache Formula.

VITAMINS: A, B complex, and C.

MINERALS: Calcium and Zinc.

ALSO: Canaid herbal drink, Propolis, Protein, and Primadophilus. When combating ear infections, it is imperative to exclude allergen foods from the diet. This is particularly true of all dairy products.

HELPFUL FOODS: Lean red meat, carrots, green vegetables, citrus fruits, fish liver oils, herring, oysters, sardines, nuts, sprouted seeds, and sunflower seeds.

ECZEMA

SPECIFICS: A type of skin eruption characterized by tiny blisters that weep and crust. Chronic forms produce flaking, scaling, itching, and eventual thickening and color changes of the skin.

(Beneficial Remedies, Treatments, and Nutrients)

HERBAL COMBINATION: (AKN).

PHYSIOLOGIC ACTION: When toxins are not properly eliminated from the body, they may surface through the skin creating eczema. This formula has been created to support liver and gall bladder function, to ensure toxins are filtered from the blood.

SINGLE HERBS: Aloe Vera, Chickweed, Evening Primrose Oil, Pau d'Arco, Red Clover, Thisilyn (Milk Thistle), and Yellow Dock.

VITAMINS: A, B complex, C, D, Paba, Biotin, Choline, and Inositol.

MINERALS: Magnesium, Sulfur Ointment, and Zinc ointment.

HELPFUL FOODS: Apples, apricots, cherries, citrus fruits, all sea foods, lean red meat, chicken, broccoli, carrots, celery, vegetable oils, and grain sprouts.

JUICES: Carrot, Celery, and Lemon juice.

ALSO: This condition is aggravated by food allergens such as dairy and wheat. These foods should be avoided. Powders and pastes should not be applied during acute or weeping stages. After acute stage passes, ointments and salves may be applied. Herbal ointments which contain Chickweed and Calendula are particularly helpful.

EDEMA

SPECIFICS: Edema is a fluid accumulation in the body. The retention of fluids appears as swelling and is often seen in the hands and feet, but may be located in any area of the body. Fluid retention is often caused by allergies.

(BeneficialRemedies,Treatments,andNutrients)

HERBAL COMBINATION: (KB).

PHYSIOLOGIC ACTION: KB acts as a mild diuretic to rid the body of excessive water. Disorders that cause edema are sodium retention, congestive heart failure, weak kidneys, varicose veins, and protein and thiamine deficiencies.

SINGLE HERBS: Alfalfa, Buchu, Dandelion tea, Juniper, lobelia, Parsley, Pau d'Arco tea, Safflower, Uva Ursi, and Yarrow.

VITAMINS: B1, B6, B complex, C, D, and E.

MINERALS: Calcium, Copper, and Potassium.

ALSO: L-Taurine, #9 and #11 tissue salts, Silicon, low Sodium, and Protein.

HELPFUL FOODS: Fruit(citrus and other), beef, butter, cheese, egg whites, seafood, fish liver oils, broccoli, spinach, flax seed, and sunflower seeds.

EMPHYSEMA

SPECIFICS: Emphysema is caused by loss of elasticity and dilation of the lung tissue, resulting in abnormal swelling and destruction of the tiny air sacs of the lungs. Factors that contribute to the onset of emphysema are asthma, bronchitis, cigarette smoking, and exposure to air pollution.

(BeneficialRemedies,Treatments,andNutrients)

HERBAL COMBINATIONS: (Breath-Aid) (BronCare) (Garlicin CF).

PHYSIOLOGICAL ACTION: These natural formulas help to restore free breathing by dilating bronchial passages. They also offer nutritional support to the lungs.

SINGLE HERBS: Anise Seed Oil, Comfrey, Elecampane, Fenugreek, Garlic, Lobelia, Mullein, and Swedish Bitters.

VITAMINS: A, B complex, C, D, E, and Folic Acid.

ALSO: L-Cysteine, L-Methionine, Protein supplement, Multienzymes and Proteolytic enzymes.

HELPFUL FOODS: All dairy products, beef, chicken, black molasses, citrus fruits, carrots, green leafy vegetables, turnip tops, soybeans, and whole rye.

ENDOMETRIOSIS

SPECIFICS: Endometriosis is the condition of having uterine tissue in abnormal locations. The location of this uterine tissue is around the ovaries, fallopian tubes, rectum and peritoneum. Symptoms are pain in the lower back, abdomen, uterus and other pelvic organs, painful menstruation, and the passage of large clots and shreds of tissue during menses. High fat diets and genetics have been associated with the development of endometriosis.

(BeneficialRemedies,Treatments,andNutrients)

SINGLE HERBS: Black Cohosh, Blue Cohosh, Chaste Tree, Dong Quai, Peony Root, Red Raspberry.

VITAMINS: A, Beta-carotene, B complex, B6, C, and E.

MINERALS: Calcium and Magnesium.

ALSO: Omega-3 and Omega-6 oils.

HELPFUL FOODS: All fresh water fish and vegetable oils.

ENTERITIS

SPECIFICS: A chronic and long-lasting inflammation of a section of the digestive tract. Inflammation works through all layers of the intestinal wall and involves the adjacent lymph nodes. If left untreated, it can increase the risk of cancer. The following nutrients are beneficial to the prevention and cure of this disease.

(BeneficialRemedies,Treatments,andNutrients)

SINGLE HERBS: Echinacea, Garlic, Goldenseal, Pau d'Arco, Rose Hips, and Yerba Mate.

VITAMINS: A strong multi-vitamin plus A, B12, B complex, and E.

MINERALS: A complete mineral complex.

ALSO: Acidophlus, Aloe Vera, Essential fatty acids, and Protein.

ENTEROBIASIS
(refer to Parasites)

EPILEPSY

SPECIFICS: A disease characterized by seizures, caused by electrical disturbances in the nerve cells in one section of the brain.

The epileptic should maintain a well-balanced diet and avoid all refined sugars, completely eliminate all animal proteins, except milk, as they rob body of magnesium and Vitamin B6 reserves. Eat lots of raw vegetables and fruit. Epileptics require plenty of fresh air, exercise and sound sleep.

(Beneficial Remedies, Treatments, and Nutrients)

HERBAL COMBINATION: (B&B Tincture).

PHYSIOLOGICAL ACTION: The herbs in this formula have a beneficial effect on the autonomic nervous system. It helps to calm the nerves and relax the muscles.

SINGLE HERBS: Black-Cohosh, Horse Nettle, Hyssop, Irish Moss, Mistletoe, and Skullcap.

VITAMINS: A, B complex, Niacin, B6, B15, C, D, and E.

MINERALS: Calcium, Chromium, Iron, and Magnesium.

ALSO: Germanium, L-Taurine, L-Tyrosine, Proteolytic enzymes, and Digestive enzymes.

HELPFUL FOODS: Apples, apricots, bananas, cherries, grapes, melon, citrus fruits, broccoli, carrots, celery, cauliflower, green peppers, and spinach.

EPSTEIN BARR VIRUS
(refer to Fatigue, Stress-Chronic)

EXFOLIATION

SPECIFICS: An inflammatory, usually recurring skin reaction, that produces flaking, scaling, itching, and eventual thickening and color changes of the skin.

(BeneficialRemedies,Treatments,andNutrients)

HERBAL COMBINATION: (AKN).

PHYSIOLOGIC ACTION: Many skin problems are related to liver dysfunction. This formula gives support to the liver, helps to cleanse the blood, and supplies nutrients for the skin.

SINGLE HERBS: Aloe Vera (on skin), Burdock, Cleavers, Dandelion, Evening Primrose, Garlic, Golden Seal, Pau d'Arco, Yellowdock, and Yucca.

VITAMINS: A, B complex, B2, B3, B6, D, E, and Biotin B complex.

MINERALS: Sulfur ointment, Potassium, and Zinc.

ALSO: Yu-ccan herbal drink, and Protein.

HELPFUL FOODS: Raw carrots, fish liver oils, green leafy vegetables, and vegetable oils.

EYE DISORDERS

SPECIFICS: A deficiency of any one of the vitamins can lead to eye problems. Most eye problems can be prevented by supplementing the diet with vitamins and the nutrients listed.

(BeneficialRemedies,Treatments,andNutrients)

HERBAL COMBINATION: (Herbal Eye bright Formula).

PHYSIOLOGIC ACTION: Extremely valuable in strengthening and healing the eyes. Aids the body in healing lesions and eye injuries.

Warning: If symptoms persist, discontinue use.

ALSO: The herb eye bright may be used as a wash for superficial inflammations of the eye.

SINGLE HERBS: Bilberry, and Eyebright.

VITAMINS: A Multi-vitamin complex, plus A, B1, B2, B3, B5, B6, C D, and E.

MINERALS: Calcium, Copper, Manganese, Magnesium, Potassium, Selenium, and Zinc.

ALSO: Gyncydo, and Protein.

HELPFUL FOODS: Apples, citrus fruits, beets, rice bran, carrots, green leafy vegetables, herring, oysters, red meat, chicken, nuts, and soybeans.

FARMERS LUNG
(refer to Allergies)

FATIGUE, STRESS (Chronic)

SPECIFICS: The body can handle minor stress but long term stress causes the body to break down. Fatigue occurs when the situation that causes stress is not relieved. Find the cause and handle it constructively. People experiencing depression should maintain a well-balanced diet and replace the nutrients depleted during anxiety or stress.

(BeneficialRemedies,Treatments,andNutrients)

HERBAL COMBINATIONS: (AdrenAid) (Echinacea Astragalus and Reshi Combination) (ImmuneAid) (Healthy Greens).

PHYSIOLOGIC ACTION: The herbs in these combinations work to support the adrenal glands and act as a tonic boost to the immune system.

SINGLE HERBS: Astragalus, Cayenne, Echinacea, Ginkgo Bilobia, Siberian Ginseng, Ginseng, Gota Kola, Lobelia, Reshi Mushroom, Yucca, and all deep green herbs such as Barley Grass, Chlorella, Spirulina, and Garlic.

HOMEOPATHIC COMBINATION: Fatigue Formula.

VITAMINS: A, Ester C with Bioflavonoids, B complex (high potency), E, D, and folic acid.

MINERALS: Iron, Magnesium, Manganese, Potassium, Selenium, and Zinc.

ALSO: Canaid and Yu-ccan herbal drinks, Coenzyme Q 10, Fiber, and Raw Thymus.

HELPFUL FOODS: All fruits(citrus and other), black molasses, butter, cheese, beef, tuna, sardines, fish liver oils, beets, broccoli, carrots, vegetable oils, green leafy vegetables, soybeans, and sunflower seeds.

FATIGUE, (Chronic)

SPECIFICS: Recent studies have shown that a combination of Evening Primrose Oil, and Fish Oil is very beneficial in combating chronic fatigue. The original study was called, "Efamol Marine." This product is not available in the United States nor Canada. It can be replicated by combining the individual Evening Primrose Oil capsules with Fish Oil, or Fish Liver Oil.

(BeneficialRemedies,Treatments,andNutrients)

HERBAL COMBINATIONS: AdrenAid, Echinacea Astragalus and Reshi Combination, ImmuneAid, and Healthy Greens.

PHYSIOLOGICAL ACTION: The herbs in these combs. work to support the adrenal glands and acts as a tonic to the immune system

SINGLE HERBS: Astragalus, Echinacea, EchinaGuard Liquid Extract, Siberian Ginseng, Reshi Mushroom, Yucca, and all deep green herbs such as Barley Grass, Chlorella, Spirulina, & Garlic.

VITAMINS: Ester C with Bioflavonoids, B Complex, E, & D.

MINERALS: Calcium, Magnesium, Potassium, Selenium, & Zinc.

ALSO: CoQ 10, and Raw Thymus.

HELPFUL FOODS: Refer to <u>Fatigue, Stress</u> (chronic).

FATIGUE, (General)

SPECIFICS: General fatigue is characterized by the feeling of mental and physical weariness usually caused by a nutrient deficiency or physical exertion.

(Beneficial Remedies, Treatments, and Nutrients)

HERBAL COMBINATION: (Herbal UP) (Energizer) (AdrenAid).

PHYSIOLOGIC ACTION: These herbal formulas combine herbs which support the adrenals, tonify the system, and offer stamina and endurance. Many of the herbs in these formulas are used by athletes to improve performance.

SINGLE HERBS: Siberian Ginseng, Gotu Kola, and Bee Pollen.

HOMEOPATHIC COMBINATION: Fatigue Formula.

VITAMINS: Multi-vitamin and Mineral supplement, B Complex, B 12, and Vitamin C.

MINERALS: GTF Chromium, Potassium, Selenium, and Zinc.

HELPFUL FOODS: Beef, chicken, herring, oysters, shellfish, all fruits, melon, raw vegetables, sweet potatoes, turnip greens, and unpolished rice.

FEVER BLISTERS
(Refer to Cold Sores)

FEVER and FLU COMPLAINTS

SPECIFICS: Fever is any temperature above that which is normal for the individuals body. The flu is a highly contagious viral infection of the respiratory tract and is spread by coughing and sneezing. Symptoms include headache, fever, aching of limbs and back, and weakness.

(BeneficialRemedies,Treatments,andNutrients)

HERBAL COMBINATIONS: (Fenu-Thyme) (Herbal Influence) (Immune Aid).

PHYSIOLOGIC ACTION: These effective formulas help to cleanse toxins, combat infections and inflammations especially in the lymphatic system. They give support to the immune system enabling the body to combat the illness.

HOMEOPATHIC COMBINATION: Cold and Flu Formula.

VITAMINS: A, B complex, B1, B3, C, E, and P.

MINERALS: Calcium, Phosphorus, Potassium, and Sodium.

ALSO: Canaid herbal drink, Cold Care, Propolis, Red Raspberry, Elder Flowers, Garlic, Rosehip, Golden Seal, Yarrow, Red Clover, #4 tissue salts.

Catnip and Peppermint together at onset of flu.

Infants and Children: Red Raspberry or Peppermint tea.

HELPFUL FOODS: Apricots, bananas, citrus fruits, broccoli, carrots, celery, corn, green leafy vegetables, bacon, beef, chicken, and fish liver oils.

JUICES: Celery, grapefruit, lemon, and parsley juice.

FIBROCYSTIC DISEASE OF THE BREAST

SPECIFICS: In fibrocystic disease, round cysts either firm or soft that move freely are produced. The cysts become filled with fluid, fibrous tissue encircles the cysts and thickens, forming a firm lump. The most common cause of this disease is iron deficiency. Other factors include hormone imbalance and abnormal breast milk production.

(BeneficialRemedies,Treatments,andNutrients)

SINGLE HERBS: Echinacea, Goldenseal, Squaw vine, Mullein, Pau d'Arco, and Red Clover.

VITAMINS: A, B1, B6, B complex, and C.

MINERALS: A comprehensive multi-mineral formula.

ALSO: Coenzyme Q10, Germanium, and Proteolytic enzymes.

HELPFUL FOODS: Black molasses, fish liver oils, red meat, all fruits, nuts, and vegetables.

FLATULENCE

(refertoDigestiveDisorders)

FLATWORM

SPECIFICS: Flatworms live in the gastrointestinal tract. Early signs include diarrhea, loss of appetite, and rectal itching. If not eliminated they will result in the loss of weight, colon disorders, and anemia. Causes include ingestion of eggs or larvae from partially cooked meat and improper disposal of human waste.

(BeneficialRemedies,Treatments,andNutrients)

HERBAL COMBINATIONS: (Para-X) (Para-VF).

PHYSIOLOGIC ACTION: Useful in destroying and eliminating parasites, such as worms. Also helps relieve many kinds of skin problems. The Para-VF is a liquid and is useful for children and the elderly who cannot swallow capsules.

Warning: Do not use during pregnancy!

SINGLE HERBS: Black Walnut, Garlic, Pumpkin Seeds, Sage, Swedish Bitters, and Wormwood.

VITAMINS: Folic Acid.

MINERALS: Iron and Zinc.

Children: Chamomile tea or raisins soaked in Senna tea for older children may be helpful.

HELPFUL FOODS: Asparagus, brewers yeast, broccoli, lettuce, lima beans, liver, mushrooms, nuts, and spinach.

FOOD ALLERGIES
(refer to Allergies)

FOOD POISONING

SPECIFICS: When a person consumes food containing harmful bacteria or viruses. Symptoms for common food poisoning include cramps, diarrhea, nausea, and vomiting.

(BeneficialRemedies,Treatments,andNutrients)

SINGLE HERBS: Pau d'Arco.

VITAMINS: C and E.

MINERALS: Multi-mineral complex.

ALSO: Acidophlus, L-Cysteine, L-Methionine and Fiber.

HELPFUL FOODS: Bran, broccoli, soybeans, spinach, sweet potatoes, turnip greens, citrus fruits, vegetable oils, and whole wheat.

FRACTURE (Broken Bone)

SPECIFICS: A fracture is called "simple" when the skin remains intact and "open" when the broken bone protrudes through the skin.

(BeneficialRemedies,Treatments,andNutrients)

HERBAL COMBINATION: (BF + C).

PHYSIOLOGIC ACTION: A special formula to aid the body's healing processes involved with broken bones, athletic injuries, sprained limbs, and related inflammation and swelling. A tonic used after acute and chronic diseases to help rebuild the body.

SINGLE HERBS: Comfrey Root, Black Walnut, Horsetail, Kelp, Lobelia, Skullcap, and White Oak Bark.

HOMEOPATHIC COMBINATION: Injury and Backache Formula.

VITAMINS: A, Pantothenic acid, C, and D.

MINERALS: Calcium, Magnesium, and Potassium.

ALSO: Silicon and Protein.

HELPFUL FOODS: Apples, bananas, citrus fruits, butter, cheese, and other dairy products, raw vegetables, vegetable oils, fish liver oils, flax seed, nuts, and sprouts.

NOTE: Avoid the consumption of red meat and products containing caffeine. Phosphorus can lead to bone loss, so preserved foods should be limited due to their high phosphorus content.

FRIGIDITY

SPECIFICS: The lack of desire for or inability to become aroused during sexual intercourse. Frigidity may be psychological or organic in nature. A balanced diet is important. Do not consume animal fats, fried foods, junk foods, or sugar!

(BeneficialRemedies,Treatments,andNutrients)

HERBAL COMBINATION: (APH).

PHYSIOLOGIC ACTION: Stimulates male and female sexual impulses as well as strengthens and increases sexual power and helps fight fatigue.

SINGLE HERBS: Damiana, Ginkgo, Ginseng and Gotu Kola.

VITAMINS: E, Paba, Folic acid, and Lecithin.

MINERALS: Zinc, Iodine, and Calcium.

ALSO: L-Arginine, L-Tyrosine, Proteolytic enzymes, Melbrosia (for men), Tropical Impulse tea, Loving Mood, Bee pollen, Sesame seeds, and Ginseng.

HELPFUL FOODS: High quality vegetable oil, fertile eggs, raw milk.

JUICES: Celery and parsley juice.

FUNGUS INFESTATIONS
(Athletesfoot, ringworm, thrush)

SPECIFICS: Fungus infestations are highly contagious and live off dead skin cells. Victims of fungus infestations should eat a well-balanced diet, supplemented by megadoses of vitamins A, B, and C.

(BeneficialRemedies, Treatments, andNutrients)

VITAMINS: A, B, C, and E.

ALSO: Primadophilus, Black Walnut, Garlic, Caprinex, and Pau d'Arco.

HELPFUL FOODS: Beef, chicken, tuna, carrots, black walnut, raw fruits, spinach, turnip greens, and sweet potatoes.

NOTE: Avoid dairy products and processed foods.

GALLBLADDER DISORDERS

SPECIFICS: The gallbladder is a small pear shaped organ located directly under the liver that contains bile. When this organ becomes inflamed, the person suffers severe pain in the right abdomen, accompanied by nausea and vomiting. Too much refined carbohydrate or too little protein in the diet prevents adequate bile production.

(BeneficialRemedies, Treatments, andNutrients)

HERBAL COMBINATION: (KB).

PHYSIOLOGIC ACTION: Extremely valuable in healing and strengthening the kidneys, bladder and genito-urinary area. Useful to stop bed-wetting, but is a diuretic when congestion of the kidneys is indicated. Helps remove bladder, uterine and urethral toxins.

Warning: Intended for occasional use only. May cause green-yellow discoloration of urine.

SINGLE HERBS: Alfalfa, Barberry root, Catnip, Dandelion, Fennel, Ginger root, Horsetail, and Wild Yam.

VITAMINS: A, B complex, Choline, Inosetol, C, D, and E.

MINERALS: Multi-mineral complex.

ALSO: Acidophilus, Cranberry juice, Lecithin, Protein, Propolis, Multi-enzymes, Uratonic, Unsaturated fatty acids, Watermelon, 3-way herb teas, and other Diuretic tablets.

HELPFUL FOODS: Red meats, chicken, tuna, fish liver oil, fruit(citrus and other), green leafy vegetables, soybeans, sunflower seeds, sweet potatoes, and wheat bran.

JUICES: Blackcherry, carrot, celery, cucumber, pomegranate, and radish juice.

GANGRENE

SPECIFICS: Gangrene is the reduced or stopped blood flow which results in oxygen deprived tissue. It may be caused by frostbite, poor circulation, hardening of the arteries, diabetes, or could be the result of a wound or injury.

(BeneficialRemedies,Treatments,andNutrients)

SINGLE HERBS: Barberry, Black Cohosh, Cayenne, Echinacea, Ginkgo Biloba, Golden Seal, Kelp, and Licorice.

VITAMINS: Multi-vitamin plus A, C, and E.

MINERALS: Calcium, Magnesium, Potassium, and Zinc.

ALSO: DMG, Coenzyme Q10, Germanium, and Proteolytic enzymes.

HELPFUL FOODS: Apples, bananas, citrus fruits, broccoli, carrots, green and green leafy vegetables, cheese, herring, oysters, fish liver oils, and aloe vera.

GARDNERELLA VAGINALIS
(refer to Vaginitis)

GAS (Intestinal)

SPECIFICS: A disorder in the small or large intestine usually caused by the fermentation of food in the colon, producing carbon dioxide and hydrogen. Symptoms include abdominal pain, belching, gas, heartburn, nausea, bloating, and vomiting.

(BeneficialRemedies,Treatments,andNutrients)

HERBAL COMBINATION: (LG).

PHYSIOLOGIC ACTION: Excellent formula for relieving intestinal gas; also cleanses liver and gall bladder.

SINGLE HERBS: Catnip, Ginger, Peppermint, and Horseradish are helpful for colon gas.

HOMEOPATHIC COMBINATION: Indigestion & Gas Formula.

VITAMINS: B complex, B1, and B5.

ALSO: Eucarbon, Primadophilus, #8 tissue salts, and activated charcoal.

HELPFUL FOODS: Brewers yeast, beets, all seeds and nuts, milk and dairy products, beef, whole grain breads and cereals, and sprouted seeds.

GASTRITIS

SPECIFICS: Gastritis is a disease in which the mucous lining of the stomach becomes inflamed and irritated. Diet and lifestyle influence this condition. It is important to avoid all food irritants such as spices, fried foods, and fiber. Alcohol, aspirin, and coffee irritate the stomach lining. Avoid acidic foods such as tomatoes and citrus fruits. Stress reduction is important in the treatment of gastritis.

(BeneficialRemedies,Treatments,andNutrients)

SINGLE HERBS: Calamus, Chamomile, Dandelion, Marshmallow, Meadowsweet, and Swedish Bitters.

VITAMINS: A, B complex, B6, B12, C, D, and E.

MINERALS: Calcium, and Iron.

ALSO: Lecithin, and Linoleic acid.

HELPFUL FOODS: Raw vegetables, vegetable oils, fish and fish liver oils, black molasses, yogurt, cheese and other dairy products.

GERMAN MEASLES
(refer to Measles)

GINGIVITIS

SPECIFICS: Gingivitis is an inflammation of the bones and gums that surround and support the teeth. This disease accounts for the loss of more teeth than cavities, caused by improper cleaning of teeth and gums, poorly fitting dentures, loose fillings, or an inadequate diet.

(BeneficialRemedies,Treatments,andNutrients)

SINGLE HERBS: Chamomile, Echinacea, Lobelia, Myrrh Gum, and White Oak Bark.

VITAMINS: A, B complex, C, D, P, Niacin, and Folic Acid.

MINERALS: Calcium, Copper, Magnesium, Manganese, Phosphorus, Potassium, Silicon, Sodium, and Zinc.

ALSO: Coenzyme Q10, Protein, and Unsaturated fatty acids.

HELPFUL FOODS: Green leafy vegetables, nuts, oat bran, apples, apricots, bananas, citrus fruits, and seafood.

JUICES: Beet greens, celery, green kale, and parsley juice.

GLAND INFECTIONS

SPECIFICS: The lymph glands act as a filter, removing poisons from the blood stream. If the lymph glands are overworked, you will feel run down due to an overload of toxins. A person should cleanse his or her blood at least once every six months.

(BeneficialRemedies,Treatments,andNutrients)

HERBAL COMBINATION: (IGL).

PHYSIOLOGIC ACTION: Combats infection and reduces inflammation from the body, especially the lymphatic system, ears, throat, lungs, breasts, and organs of the body.

VITAMINS: C.

ALSO: Propolis, Golden Seal, Pau d'Arco, Saw Palmetto, and Echinacea.

HELPFUL FOODS: Apples, black currants, cherries, strawberries, citrus fruits, cabbage, green bell peppers, guavas, persimmons, turnip greens, and tomatoes.

JUICES: Carrot and Blackberry juice.

GLAND PROBLEMS

SPECIFICS: When the body is under stress, the nutrients in the glands are depleted and the glands, like all body parts, need nutritional replenishment. If one gland malfunctions and is not treated, it puts more stress on all of the other glands. Maintain a well-balanced diet, high in vitamins, minerals and multi glandulars.

(BeneficialRemedies,Treatments,andNutrients)

HERBAL COMBINATIONS: (GL) (IF).

PHYSIOLOGIC ACTION: Effective for swollen lymph nodes and in helping the body fight glandular weakness and infections.

SINGLE HERBS: Alfalfa, Calendula, Echinacea, Golden Seal, Lobelia, Mullein, Saw Palmetto, and Skullcap.

VITAMINS: A, B5, B complex, C, and E.

MINERALS: Calcium, Magnesium, and Potassium.

ALSO: Multi Glandulars and Primrose oil.

HELPFUL FOODS: Apples, bananas, grapes, citrus fruits, broccoli, carrots, cheese, red meat, fish, chicken, soybeans, sweet potatoes, and turnip greens.

JUICES: Carrot, tomato, and pineapple.

GLANDULAR FEVER

SPECIFICS: An infectious disease believed to be caused by a virus. It affects the respiratory system, liver, the lymph tissues, and glands. The disease can be transmitted through communal drinking utensils, kissing, and blood transfusions. A well-balanced diet, adequate in protein, is essential for the prevention of glandular fever.

(Beneficial Remedies, Treatments, and Nutrients)

SINGLE HERBS: Dandelion, Echinacea, Goldenseal, Pau d'Arco, and Sheep Sorrel.

VITAMINS: A, B complex, B1, B2, B5, B6, C, Biotin, and Choline.

MINERALS: Potassium.

ALSO: Canaid herbal drink, a nondairy form of Acidophilus, Germanium, Raw thymus, Raw glandular complex, and Protein.

HELPFUL FOODS: Aloe Vera, bananas, melons, citrus fruits, nuts, oat bran, green leafy vegetables, sweet potatoes, turnip greens, carrots, and fish liver oils.

GLAUCOMA (Hypertension of the eye)

SPECIFICS: Glaucoma is characterized by an increase in pressure of the fluid within the eyeball and a hardening of the surface of the eyeball. The main causes of this disease are related to stress and nutritional problems. It is believed that restoration of vision lost due to nerve degeneration cannot occur. However the vitamins and herbs listed can be effective in controlling and preserving the remaining sight.

(Beneficial Remedies, Treatments, and Nutrients)

HERBAL SUPPLEMENTATION: Eyebright Formula, KB, Bilberry, and Extress.

PHYSIOLOGIC ACTION: These herbs work to restore balance to the system. They supply nutrition to the eye, while helping to remove excessive fluids and toxins. They also help to reduce problems associated with stress.

Note: It is important to keep in contact with your doctor while working with this serious eye problem.

HERB COMBINATION: (Eyebright Comb).

VITAMINS: A, B2, B5, B complex, C, D, and E.

MINERALS: A comprehensive multi-mineral formula.

ALSO: Germanium.

WARNING: Avoid the use of antihistamines, tranquilizers, the herb licorice, and high amounts of niacin.

HELPFUL FOODS: Aloe Vera, carrot juice, all fruits, raw vegetables, melon, nuts, seeds, soybeans, sprouted seeds, and sweet potatoes.

GLUTEN ENTEROPATHY

SPECIFICS: Gluten enteropathy is an intestinal disorder caused by the intolerance to a protein in wheat, barley, and rye called gluten. Treatment includes eating a well-balanced gluten-free diet, high in proteins, calories, and normal in fats. Exclude all cereal grains except corn and rice.

(Beneficial Remedies, Treatments, and Nutrients)

VITAMINS: A, B6, B12, B complex, C, D, E, and K.

MINERALS: Calcium, Iron, Magnesium, and Potassium.

HELPFUL FOODS: Apples, bananas, beets, black molasses, carrots, cheese, butter, goats milk, all fruit, kelp, and green leafy vegetables.

GOITER

SPECIFICS: Goiter is the enlargement of the thyroid gland located at the base of the neck. Thyroid disorders are caused by a lack of iodine in the diet, resulting in insufficient thyroxin production or a disorder in the body that requires more thyroxin than the thyroid can produce.

(Beneficial Remedies, Treatments, and Nutrients)

SINGLE HERBS: Kelp is an excellent source of iodine.

VITAMINS: A, B6, B complex, Choline, C, and E.

MINERALS: Calcium and Iodine.

ALSO: Protein.

HELPFUL FOODS: Beef, fish liver oils, dulse and other seaweed, broccoli, carrots, pineapple, citrus fruits, cheese, milk, soybeans, and spinach.

GONORRHEA

SPECIFICS: Gonorrhea is transmitted through sexual intimacy or from the mother to the newborn infant as it passes through the infected birth canal. Complications of gonorrhea may result in sterility in both sexes. Penicillin or another antibiotic is the usual treatment. In addition to medical treatment, an afflicted person should maintain a high nutrient diet to help repair the tissue damage that has occurred.

(Beneficial Remedies, Treatments, and Nutrients)

SINGLE HERBS: Echinacea, Goldenseal, Pau d'Arco and Suma.

VITAMINS: B complex and K.

MINERALS: Zinc.

ALSO: Acidophilus, Coenzyme Q10, Germanium, and Protein.

HELPFUL FOODS: All red meats, fruits, aloe vera, kelp, herring, oysters, liver, nuts, and yogurt.

GOUT

SPECIFICS: This disease occurs when there is an excess of uric acid in the blood and deposits of uric acid salts in the tissue around the joints. Obesity and an improper diet increase an individual's susceptibility to gout. All purine-rich foods need to be avoided, such as anchovies, herring, sardines, mushrooms, mussels, and liver. Treatment requires a low purine diet, generous in vitamins and minerals.

(Beneficial Remedies, Treatments, and Nutrients)

HERBAL COMBINATION: (Yucca AR) (Rheum Aid).

PHYSIOLOGIC ACTION: This formula is effective in helping to reduce swelling and inflammation in body joints and connective tissues. Also helps relieve stiffness and pain.

SINGLE HERBS: Burdock, Dandelion Root, Lobelia, Stinging nettle, Safflower, Pau d'Arco, and Yucca.

VITAMINS: A, B complex, B5, C, and E.

MINERALS: Calcium, Magnesium, and Potassium.

ALSO: Yu-ccan herbal drink, Primadophilus, Protein, and diet play a vital function in the treatment of this malady. Foods containing Uric Acids, such as meat, and rich pastries need to be avoided.

HELPFUL FOODS: Raw vegetables, fish liver oils, dairy products, green leafy vegetables, and whole wheat.

JUICES: Celery and parsley juice.

GRIPPE
(refer to Colds and Flu)

GROWTH PROBLEMS

SPECIFICS: Growth problems occur when there is a malfunction in the thyroid gland or the pituitary gland. The pituitary gland is responsible for the distribution of the growth hormone (somatotropin). An overproduction as well as an underproduction of somatotropin will cause growth abnormalities. Growth problems are also caused by a malfunction of the thyroid gland. Malnutrition plays a significant role in growth and development.

(Beneficial Remedies, Treatments, and Nutrients)

SINGLE HERBS: Kelp.

VITAMINS: A multi-vitamin plus B complex, and B6.

MINERALS: Calcium and Magnesium.

ALSO: Cod liver oil, L-Lysine, L-Ornithine, Protein, Raw pituitary glandular, and Unsaturated fatty acids.

HELPFUL FOODS: Apples, bananas, citrus fruits, cantaloupe, beef, eggs, cheese and other dairy products, kelp, nuts, wheat germ, and wheat bran.

GYNECOLOGICAL PROBLEMS

SPECIFICS: Menstruation is the cyclical process that continuously prepares the uterus for pregnancy, starting at puberty and continuing through menopause. If this cycle is interrupted or irregular many gynecological problems can occur. Most problems are due to a deficiency of nutrients, this allows infections and viruses to invade the system. (Refer to Premenstrual Syndrome -PMS).

(BeneficialRemedies,Treatments,andNutrients)

HERBAL COMBINATION: (Fem-Mend).

PHYSIOLOGIC ACTION: Menstrual regulator, tonic for genito-urinary system. Helpful for severe menstrual discomforts. Acts as an aid in rebuilding a malfunctioning reproductive system (Uterus, ovaries, fallopian tubes, etc.).

SINGLE HERBS: Aloe Vera, Blessed Thistle, Comfrey Root, Garlic, Ginger, Golden Seal Root, Red Raspberry, Slippery Elm Bark, Uva Ursi, and Yellow Dock Root.

VITAMINS: A, B complex, C, and E.

MINERALS: A complete multi-mineral.

HELPFUL FOODS: Beef, fish and fish liver oils, broccoli, carrots, fruit(citrus and other), green leafy vegetables, liver, nuts, soybeans, and sweet potatoes.

HAIR PROBLEMS

SPECIFICS: Good hygiene and a well-balanced diet is most important for healthy hair. Most hair problems such as balding, graying, dry and brittle hair, etc. can be prevented by nutritional means. There is no known cure to hair loss in males due to heredity. If one is a victim of hair problems due to acute illness, pregnancy, surgery, poor circulation, or stress, the following nutrients can be helpful.

(BeneficialRemedies,Treatments,andNutrients)

SINGLE HERBS: Aloe Vera, Horsetail, Kelp, Rosemary, Sage, Nettle, Yarrow and Yucca.

VITAMINS: A, B complex, B3, B5, B6. C, Biotin, Folic Acid, and Inositol.

MINERALS: Copper, Iodine, and Magnesium.

ALSO: Coenzyme Q10, L-Cysteine, L-Methionine, Primadophilus, Protein, Raw thymus glandular, Unsaturated fatty acids, Yu-ccan herbal drink.

HELPFUL FOODS: Apples, pineapple, raisins, citrus fruits, dulse and other seaweed, nuts, beef, seafood, turnip greens, broccoli, and carrots.

JUICES: Blackcherry juice.

HALITOSIS (Bad breath)

SPECIFICS: Halitosis is generally attributed to putrefactive bacteria living on undigested food. Nutrients necessary for efficient digestion are essential. Other causes are poor dental hygiene (gum or tooth decay), nose or throat infection, excessive smoking, liver malfunction, and constipation.

(BeneficialRemedies,Treatments,andNutrients)

SINGLE HERBS: Chlorophyll, Myrrh, Parsley, Peppermint, Rosemary, Sage, and Yucca.

VITAMINS: A, B complex, B3, B6, C, and Paba.

MINERALS: Magnesium, and Zinc.

ALSO: Yu-ccan herbal drink, Primadophilus and Digestive enzymes.

HELPFUL FOODS: Apples, citrus fruits, green leafy vegetables, turnip greens, yellow corn, nuts, and unpolished rice.

HANGNAILS
(refer to Nail Problems)

HANGOVER

SPECIFICS: A chronic physiological or psychological condition marked by overindulgence of alcohol. Deficiencies of many nutrients occur when alcohol itself satisfies the body's caloric needs. If the person knows that he or she will be drinking to excess in advance, it is advisable to take vitamin C and a B complex before the party begins. The following vitamins and minerals will also be useful if taken before retiring for the night and the morning after.

(BeneficialRemedies,Treatments,andNutrients)

VITAMINS: A, B complex, B1, B2, B6, B12, Choline, Folic acid, Niacin, Pangamic acid, Pantothenic acid, C, D, E, and K.

MINERALS: Calcium, Chromium, Iron, Magnesium, Manganese, Selenium, and Zinc.

HARDENING OF ARTERIES

SPECIFICS: The thickening and hardening of the walls of the arteries is due to the gradual build-up of calcium and fatty deposits on the inside of the artery walls. This buildup will slow or restrict the circulation of the blood causing high blood pressure. Symptoms of hardening of arteries are cramping of muscles, chest pains and pressure, and hypertension. The main causes are poor diet, drug abuse, alcoholism, smoking, heredity, obesity, and stress.

(BeneficialRemedies,Treatments,andNutrients)

HERBAL COMBINATION: (Garlicin HC).

PHYSIOLOGIC ACTION: A combination of herbs which supports the cardiovascular system. Helps to strengthen the heart, while building and cleansing the arteries and veins.

SPECIFICS: Recent animal studies suggest that vitamin C deficiency could be involved in the causation of arteriosclerosis. E.F.A.s (essential fatty acids) play a fundamental role in keeping cell membranes fluid and flexible.

SINGLEHERBS: Cayenne, Comfrey, Evening Primrose Oil, Fish Oil, Garlic, Golden Seal, and Rose Hips.

VITAMINS: B complex, C, E, Niacin, Inositol, and Choline.

MINERALS: Calcium and Magnesium

ALSO: (E.F.A.s) — Fish oils and cold pressed vegetable oils.

HELPFULFOODS: Fish and fish liver oils, vegetable oils, oat bran, high fiber fruits, kelp, green tea, yogurt, and legumes.

JUICES: Alfalfa, beet, blackberry, grape, parsley, and pineapple juice.

HASHIMOTO'S THYROIDITIS
(refertoHypothyroidism)

HAY FEVER (Allergic rhinitis)

SPECIFICS: A reaction of the mucous membranes of the nose, eyes, and air passages to animal hair and skin, dust, feathers, pollen, and other irritants. Symptoms include sneezing, itchy eyes, nervous irritability, and a watery discharge from the nose and eyes.

(BeneficialRemedies,Treatments,andNutrients)

HERBAL COMBINATIONS: (HAS Original and Fast Acting Formulas) (Allergy Care).

PHYSIOLOGIC ACTION: These herbal formulas contain a natural extract of Pseudoepheda, in a base of herbs, which help to restore free breathing without causing drowsiness. HAS original is for those sensitive to Ephedra.

SINGLE HERBS: EchinaGuard, Nettle tea, Elder Flowers, Eye Bright, Golden Seal, Golden Rod, Swedish Bitters, and Yarrow

HOMEOPATHIC COMBINATION: Allergy Formula.

VITAMINS: A, B complex, B6, Ester C with Bioflavanoids, and E.

ALSO: Coenzyme Q10, Bee pollen granules or tablets, and Pollen-rich unprocessed raw honey.

HELPFUL FOODS: Apple, papaya, broccoli, carrots, green leafy vegetables, soybeans, sweet potatoes, turnip greens, fish and fish liver oils, red meat, and vegetable oils.

JUICES: Carrot, celery, and papaya juice.

Note: It is recommended that one reduces consumption of dairy products, white flour products, sugar, and canned foods.

HEADACHE

SPECIFICS: Most common headaches are caused by stress and tension, fevers brought on by allergies or infection, or disturbances of the digestive tract and circulatory system. The following nutrients are beneficial in the treatment the common headache.

(Beneficial Remedies, Treatments, and Nutrients)

SINGLE HERBS: Chamomile and Feverfew.

PHYSIOLOGIC ACTION: Chamomile will prevent migraine headaches. Feverfew reduces fever. Feverfew has been historically used for chills and pain that accompany fever. Because of its anecdotal claims for migraine sufferers, it is presently being researched at the London Migraine Clinic.

HOMEOPATHIC COMBINATION: Tension Headache Formula.

VITAMINS: A, B1, B2, B3, B6, B12, B complex, C, D, E, and F.

MINERALS: Calcium, Iron, Magnesium, Potassium, and Zinc.

ALSO: Acidophilus and Coenzyme Q10.

HELPFUL FOODS: Almonds, apples, avocados, bananas, black molasses, carrots, broccoli, spinach, cheese and other dairy products, herring, and oysters.

HEART ATTACK
(refer to Myocardial infraction)

HEART DISEASE

SPECIFICS: The heart is the most important organ of the circulatory system. If the coronary arteries supplying the heart with blood become plugged or hardened, the flow of oxygen to the heart will be reduced causing severe pain (angina).

Most heart problems are caused by cardiovascular disease. Refer to arteriosclerosis in this manual.

(Beneficial Remedies, Treatments, and Nutrients)

HERBAL COMBINATIONS: (H) (Garlicin HC).

PHYSIOLOGIC ACTION: Promotes elasticity of arteries. Helps eliminate cholesterol; also aids in rebuilding the heart, strengthening and regulating the beat of the heart, and improving circulation in general.

SINGLE HERBS: Barberry, Cayenne, Garlic, Hawthorn Berries, Lobelia, and Shepherds Purse.

VITAMINS: A, B1, B5, B15, C, D, E, Lecithin, Biotin, Inositol, Choline, and Folic acid.

MINERALS: Calcium, Copper, Iodine, Iron, Magnesium, and Potassium.

HELPFUL FOODS: Fish and fish liver oils, vegetable oils, oat bran, high fiber fruits, kelp, legumes, green tea, yogurt, and legumes.

JUICES: Alfalfa, beet, blackberry, grape, parsley, and pineapple juice.

HEART BURN

SPECIFICS: A burning sensation in the stomach that occurs when hydrochloric acid backs up into the esophagus. Heartburn is caused by allergies, enzyme deficiency, gallbladder problems, hiatal hernia, ulcers, or excessive consumption of spicy and fatty foods.

(Beneficial Remedies, Treatments, and Nutrients)

HERBAL COMBINATION: (Motion Mate).

SINGLE HERBS: Chamomile, Chewable Papaya, Meadowsweet, and Marshmallow Root.

ALSO: Digestive enzymes (especially Pancreatic enzymes), bone meal, and primadophilus.

HELPFUL FOODS: Raw fruits and vegetables.
JUICES: Carrot, fig, and parsley juice.

HEEL SPUR

SPECIFICS: A painful pointed growth on the bone, most commonly located on the heel. Bone spurs are usually caused by calcium deposits and are common in people who have alkaloses, arthritis, neuritis, and tendonitis.

(Beneficial Remedies, Treatments, and Nutrients)

VITAMINS: B6, B complex, and C.
MINERALS: Calcium and Magnesium.
ALSO: Bioflavonoids and Proteolytic enzymes.
HELPFUL FOODS: Apples, citrus fruits, sardines, fish liver oils, broccoli, sweet potatoes, turnip greens, unpolished rice, and yellow corn.

HEMOPHILIA

SPECIFICS: A hereditary blood disease that is found only in men. The blood of hemophiliacs fails to clot or coagulation as time is prolonged. Transfusion of fresh whole blood or plasma is required to provide necessary coagulation in emergencies.

(Beneficial Remedies, Treatments, and Nutrients)

SINGLE HERBS: Barley Grass, Beet Powder, Black Current, Chlorophyll, Chlorella, Comfrey, Dandelion, Fenugreek, Kelp, and Yellowdock.
VITAMINS: A multi-vitamin and additional C and E.
MINERALS: Complete multi-mineral.
ALSO: Desiccated liver.
HELPFUL FOODS: Red meats, liver, citrus fruits, vegetable oils, and whole wheat.

HEMORRHOIDS

SPECIFICS: Hemorrhoids are swollen or ruptured veins located around the anus that may protrude out of the rectum. The most common cause is strain on the abdominal muscles due to constipation, improper lifting, and pregnancy. Prevention and treatment include an improved diet containing fluids and fiber and exercise.

(BeneficialRemedies,Treatments,andNutrients)

HERBAL COMBINATION: (Yellow Dock Formula).

PHYSIOLOGIC ACTION: Effective formula for hemorrhoids, colitis, and blood purifier. Also revitalizes prolapsed uterus, kidneys, and bowl.

SINGLE HERBS: Butchers Broom, Collinsonia Root, Horse chestnut, Lobelia, Stone Root, and Yellow Dock.

HOMEOPATHIC COMBINATION: Constipation and Hemorrhoids Formula.

VITAMINS: A, B complex, Choline, Inositol, B6, C, E, and P.

MINERALS: Multi-mineral complex plus Calcium.

ALSO: Coenzyme Q10, Bulk forming laxatives such as Laxacil, or Psyllium seed husks are recommended to take pressure from the colon. Combination "Hem Relief" ointment, Pile ointment and suppositories, or Circu Caps Witch Hazel Compresses.

HELPFUL FOODS: Apricots, cherries, grapes, citrus fruits, broccoli, carrots, green leafy vegetables, oats, soybeans, beef, fish, and whole wheat bread.

JUICES: Celery, grapefruit, and spinach juice.

HEPATITIS

SPECIFICS: An inflammation of the liver caused by infection or toxic agents. The liver is unable to eliminate poisons and it cannot store and process certain nutrients that are vital for the body. Recovery from hepatitis requires a diet adequate in all nutrients, abstention from alcohol, and rest.
Sensitivity to toxic materials may persist so B complex, C, and E should be continued long after recovery.

(BeneficialRemedies,Treatments,andNutrients)

SINGLE HERBS: Dandelion, Goldenseal, Milk Thistle, and Red Clover.

VITAMINS: A, B complex, B6, Pangamic acid, Pantothenic acid, C, and E.

MINERALS: Zinc.

ALSO: Coenzyme Q10, Fluids, Germanium, Lecithin, Multienzymes, Protein, Raw liver extract, and Unsaturated fatty acids.

HELPFUL FOODS: Aloe Vera, broccoli, carrots, spinach, turnip greens, soybeans, sweet potatoes, garlic, herring, oysters, fish liver oils, and vegetable oils.

JUICES: Grapefruit, sauerkraut, and tomato juice.

HERPES SIMPLEX (I and II)

SPECIFICS: Herpes simplex 1 results in cold sores and skin eruptions. It can also cause inflammation of the eye. If the eye becomes infected see a doctor at once. Herpes simplex 2 is sexually transmitted and results in lesions on the penis in men and infection inside the vagina in women. After entering the body the herpes virus never leaves. By strengthening the immune system one can defend against or prevent herpes activation.

(BeneficialRemedies,Treatments,andNutrients)

SINGLE HERBS: Echinacea, Goldenseal, Myrrh, Red Clover, and Turkish Rhubarb.

VITAMINS: B complex, C, and E.

MINERALS: Zinc chelate.

ALSO: Canaid herbal drink strengthens the immune system and the amino acid L-Lysine has a direct effect on the virus.

HELPFUL FOODS: Raw vegetables, all fruits and melons, vegetable oils, soybeans, and whole grains.

HIATAL HERNIA

SPECIFICS: Over fifty percent of the population, over the age of forty, experience hiatal hernia. This condition is caused by a hole in the diaphragm muscles. Heartburn and ulcers can occur due to the leakage of stomach acid back into the lower esophagus.

The victim suffers from discomfort behind the breastbone, heartburn, and a burning sensation in the throat caused by the acid coming up into the throat.

(BeneficialRemedies,Treatments,andNutrients)

SINGLE HERBS: Aloe Vera juice, Comfrey, Goldenseal, and Red Clover.

VITAMINS: Multi-vitamin plus A, B complex, B12, and C.

MINERALS: Multi-mineral plus Zinc.

ALSO: Pancreatin, Papaya, and Proteolytic enzymes.

HELPFUL FOODS: Beef, broccoli, carrots, green leafy vegetables, all fruit, melon, nuts, herring, oysters, fish liver oils, and unpolished rice.

HOOKWORMS

SPECIFICS: Hookworms live in the gastrointestinal tract. Early signs include diarrhea, loss of appetite, and rectal itching. If not eliminated they will result in the loss of weight, colon disorders, and anemia. Causes include ingestion of eggs or larvae from partially cooked meat, improper disposal of human waste, and walking barefoot on contaminated soil.

(Beneficial Remedies, Treatments, and Nutrients)

HERBAL COMBINATIONS: (Para-X) (Para-VF).

PHYSIOLOGIC ACTION: Useful in destroying and eliminating parasites, such as worms. Also helps relieve many kinds of skin problems. The Para-VF is liquid and is useful for children and the elderly, who cannot swallow capsules.

Warning: Do not use during pregnancy!

SINGLE HERBS: Black Walnut, Garlic, Pumpkin Seeds, Sage, Sheep Sorrel, Swedish Bitters, and Wormwood.

VITAMINS: Folic Acid.

Children: Chamomile tea or raisins soaked in Senna tea, for older children, may be helpful.

HELPFUL FOODS: Asparagus, brewers yeast, lettuce, liver, mushrooms, nuts, lima beans, and wheat germ.

HORMONE REGULATION

SPECIFICS: A hormonal imbalance is always experienced at the point at which women stop ovulating, the end of their reproductive years, or during puberty. Symptoms include difficult breathing, dizziness, headache, heart palpitations, hot flashes, and depression. The following nutrients will help regulate the hormones and alleviate the symptoms in both cases.

(Beneficial Remedies, Treatments, and Nutrients)

FEMALE HERBAL COMBINATIONS: (MP) or (Change-O-Life).

PHYSIOLOGIC ACTION: This herbal formula is effective in regulating hormonal imbalance. Its greatest benefit is for the relief of the symptoms of menopause. Also good for youth during puberty.

SINGLE HERBS: Blessed Thistle, Damiana, Dong Quai, Mistletoe, and Vitex Agnus Castus.

HOMEOPATHIC COMBINATION: Menopause Formula.

MALE HERB COMBINATION: (APH).

PHYSIOLOGIC ACTION: Stimulates sexual impulses and strengthens and increases sexual power. Helps eliminate fatigue and increases longevity.

SINGLE HERBS: Damiana, Fo-Ti, Gota Kola, Sarsaparilla Root, Saw Palmetto, and Siberian Ginseng.

MINERALS: Potassium.

HELPFUL FOODS: All vegetables, bananas, cantaloupe, citrus fruits, milk, mint leaves, potatoes, sunflower seeds, tomatoes, watercress, and whole wheat.

HORMONE IMBALANCE
(Refer to Menopause)

HOT FLASHES
(refer to Menopause)

HOUSEMAID'S KNEE

SPECIFICS: Housemaid's knee is an inflammation of the bursae, liquid filled sacs found in the joints, tendons, muscles, and bones. This disorder is caused by prolonged kneeling on a hard surface, causing swelling, tenderness, and extreme pain. During infection, elevated doses of A, C, and E are beneficial in the treatment of bursitis.

(Beneficial Remedies, Treatments, and Nutrients)

HERBAL COMBINATIONS: (Rheum-Aid) (Cal-Silica) (Kalmin).

PHYSIOLOGIC ACTIONS: These herbal combinations contain herbs which exhibit anti-inflammatory and relaxing effects. Help to build nerve tissue and relieve stiffness and pain.

SINGLE HERBS: Alfalfa, Chaparral, and Comfrey. Mullein is often used as a poultice to give relief externally.

VITAMINS: A, B12, B complex, C, E, and P.

MINERALS: Calcium and Magnesium.

ALSO: Alkaline diet, Coenzyme Q10, Germanium, Proteolytic enzymes, and a protein supplement.

HELPFUL FOODS: Apples, apricots, cherries, citrus fruits, sardines, tuna, fish liver oils, spinach, and sweet potatoes.

HYPERACTIVITY

SPECIFICS: A disorder of certain mechanisms in the central nervous system. This disorder is usually caused by a diet high in refined carbohydrates, a result of boredom, or feelings of insecurity.

(BeneficialRemedies,Treatments,andNutrients)

HERBAL COMBINATION: (Wild Lettuce and Valerian Extract).

PHYSIOLOGIC ACTION: This excellent formula is a natural sedative. Promotes overall calming of the nerves and restores a sense of control and balance without causing drowsiness.

ALSO: Ginkgo or Ginkgold. Although this herb is often used to promote circulation, it also has a positive effect on the nervous system. Used in conjunction with the following single herbs and with a balanced, chemical free diet, good results can be expected.

SINGLE HERBS: Evening Primrose Oil, Lobelia, Oat Extract, Skullcap, St. John's Wort, Valerian, Wild Lettuce, and Yucca.

VITAMINS: High potency B vitamins, B3, B5, B6, and C.

NOTE: Yeast free B vitamins may be required if yeast intolerance is present.

MINERALS: High doses of all minerals.

HELPFUL FOODS: Red meats, chicken, green leafy vegetables, nuts, turnip greens, and unpolished rice.

NOTE: Avoid all foods with artificial flavoring and coloring. Processed foods should be eliminated from the diet. Foods which contain natural salicylates such as apples, tomatoes, and oranges need to be avoided. Carbonated drinks will worsen the condition.

HYPERTENTION

SPECIFICS: The main cause of hypertention is arteriosclerosis. This condition is due to the gradual build-up of calcium and fatty deposits on the inside of the artery walls. This buildup will slow or restrict the circulation of the blood causing high blood pressure. Symptoms of high blood pressure are cramping of muscles, chest pains and pressure, and hypertension. Causes for high blood pressure are poor diet, drug abuse, alcoholism, smoking, heredity, obesity, and stress.

(BeneficialRemedies,Treatments,andNutrients)

HERBAL COMBINATIONS: (Cayenne-Garlic) (Garlicin HC) (BP)

PHYSIOLOGIC ACTION: In addition to lowering the blood pressure, the above will help to relieve colds, influenza, and general infections, strengthen the heart and improves blood circulation.

SINGLE HERBS: Cayenne, Garlic, Kelp, Hawthorn, Mistletoe, Valerian Root, Yarrow, and Yucca.

VITAMINS: A, B complex (stress) B3, B5, B15, C, D, E, P, Inositol, Choline, and Lecithin

MINERALS: Calcium, Magnesium, and Potassium.

HELPFUL FOODS: Apples, apricots, bananas, cherries, broccoli, carrots, green leafy vegetables, soybeans, sunflower seeds, vegetable oils, and fish liver oils.

JUICES: Carrot, celery, grape, and lime juice.

HYPERTHYROIDISM

SPECIFICS: When the body is under stress, the nutrients in the glands are depleted and the glands, like all body parts, need nutritional replenishment. If one gland malfunctions and is not treated, it puts more stress on all of the other glands. Maintain a well-balanced diet, high in vitamins, minerals and multi glandulars.

(BeneficialRemedies,Treatments,andNutrients)

HERBAL COMBINATIONS: (GL) (IF).

PHYSIOLOGIC ACTION: Effective for swollen lymph nodes and in helping the body fight glandular weakness and infections.

SINGLE HERBS: Alfalfa, Calendula, Echinacea, Golden Seal, Lobelia, Mullein, Saw Palmetto, and Skullcap.

VITAMINS: A, B5, B complex, C, and E.

MINERALS: Calcium, Magnesium, and Potassium.

ALSO: Multi Glandulars and Primrose oil.

HELPFUL FOODS: Apples, bananas, grapes, citrus fruits, broccoli, carrots, cheese, red meat, fish, chicken, soybeans, sweet potatoes, and turnip greens.

JUICES: Carrot, tomato, and pineapple.

HYPOCALCEMIA
(refer to Calcium Deficiency)

HYPOGLYCEMIA

SPECIFICS: Hypoglycemia is caused by the over secretion of insulin by the pancreas, resulting in an abnormally low level of glucose or sugar in the blood. Hypoglycemia can contribute to allergies, arthritis, asthma, epilepsy, impotence, and mental disorders. A proper diet is the main factor in maintaining proper blood sugar levels.

(Beneficial Remedies, Treatments, and Nutrients)

HERBAL COMBINATIONS: (HIGL) (AdrenAid).

PHYSIOLOGIC ACTION: Stimulates the adrenals and the pancreas to help restore sugar levels, helps correct glandular imbalances, eliminates toxins, assists the body in handling stressful conditions, and promotes a feeling of well-being.

Note: Some people who have hypoglycemia cannot handle Golden Seal, as it tends to lower the blood sugar level. Safflower is good to take before exercise.

VITAMINS: A, B1, B2, B3, B6, B9, B12, B complex, C, and E.

MINERALS: Magnesium and Potassium.

ALSO: Bee Pollen, Juniper, Glyco-lite, Acidophilus. Low animal protein, small meals high in natural complex carbohydrates.

HELPFUL FOODS: All vegetables, apples, apricots, bananas, citrus fruits, oat bran, vegetable oils, and whole wheat bread.

HYPOTENTION
(refer to Blood Pressure Low)

HYPOTHYROIDISM

SPECIFICS: A disorder that occurs when there is an underproduction of hormones by the thyroid gland, resulting in lowered cellular metabolism. In this disorder, the brain cells are effected and intellectual capacity is impaired. Problems with the thyroid gland can be the cause of many recurring illnesses, infections, and chronic fatigue.

(BeneficialRemedies,Treatments,andNutrients)

HERBAL COMBINATION: (T).

PHYSIOLOGIC ACTION: Rich in natural vitamins and minerals, this excellent formula helps revitalize and promote healing of the thyroid glands, thus restoring metabolism balance. Helps the body store up needed vitality and energy.

SINGLE HERBS: Black Walnut, Irish Moss, Kelp, Mullein, and Parsley.

VITAMINS: B1, B5, C, D, E, and F.

MINERALS: Chlorine, Iodine, Potassium, and Zinc.

ALSO: Brewer's yeast, Essential fatty acids, Lecithin, Protein, and Thyroid glandular.

HELPFUL FOODS: Broccoli, carrots, green leafy vegetables, soybeans, turnip greens, sweet potatoes, vegetable oils, fish liver oils, citrus fruits, and melons.

JUICES: Celery and clam juice.

ICTERUS
(refer to Jaundice)

ILEITIS
(refer to Crohn's disease)

IMPETIGO

SPECIFICS: This condition is best looked after with a good blood cleanser and a vitamin and mineral rich diet.

(BeneficialRemedies,Treatments,andNutrients)

HERBAL COMBINATIONS: (Red Clover Combination) (Yellow Dock Formula) (AKN).

PHYSIOLOGIC ACTION: These herbal formulas effectively aid the body's cleansing systems, thus helps eliminate ulcers of the skin, impetigo, etc.

SINGLEHERBS: Echinacea, Licorice Root, and Red Clover.

VITAMINS: A, C, D, E. Vitamin A and E applied topically. Vitamin A is necessary for the health of the skin tissue and vitamins C, D, and E, may be helpful in aiding the skin in its recovery from impetigo.

HELPFULFOODS: Citrus fruits, fish liver oils, and vegetable oils.

IMMUNE DEFICIENCY

SPECIFICS: When the immune system weakens, you become more susceptible to infections and viruses. The key factors in the treatment and prevention of immune deficiency are proper nutrition and good supplementation.

(BeneficialRemedies,Treatments,andNutrients)

HERBAL COMBINATION: (EchinaGuard).

PHYSIOLOGIC ACTION: Stimulates the immune response systems. Especially helpful in rebuilding the body during convalescence and as a preventative.

SINGLE HERBS: Echinacea root, Chaparral, Korean White Ginseng, Goldenseal root, Pau d'Arco, and Rosemary.

VITAMINS: A multi-vitamin plus B6, B12, C, and E.

MINERALS: A strong mineral complex.

ALSO: Canaid herbal drink strengthens the immune system. L-Cysteine, L-Methionine, L-Lysine, L-Ornithine, Propolis, Proteolytic enzymes, and Primadophilus.

HELPFUL FOODS: Beef, broccoli, fruit(citrus and other), nuts, soybeans, spinach, sweet potatoes, turnip greens, unpolished rice, and whole grains.

IMPOTENCE

SPECIFICS: The inability to achieve or maintain an erection. Impotence may be psychological or organic in nature. A balanced diet is important. Do not consume animal fats, fried foods, junk foods, or sugar!

(BeneficialRemedies,Treatments,andNutrients)

HERBAL COMBINATION: (APH).

PHYSIOLOGICACTION: Stimulates male and female sexual impulses as well as strengthens and increases sexual power and helps fight fatigue.

SINGLE HERBS: Damiana, Ginkgo, Ginseng and Gotu Kola.

VITAMINS: E, Paba, Folic acid, and Lecithin.

MINERALS: Zinc, Iodine, and Calcium.

ALSO: L-Arginine, L-Tyrosine, Proteolytic enzymes, Melbrosia (for men), Tropical Impulse tea, Loving Mood, Bee pollen, Sesame seeds, and Ginseng.

HELPFUL FOODS: High quality vegetable oil, fertile eggs, raw milk.

JUICES: Celery and parsley juice.

INDIGESTION
(refer to Digestive Disorders)

INFERTILITY

SPECIFICS: The inability to become pregnant or the inability to carry a pregnancy full-term. The following supplements are essential to correcting hormonal imbalance. Because there are so many causes of infertility, it is recommended that you get a qualified doctors opinion.

(Beneficial Remedies, Treatments, and Nutrients)

SINGLE HERBS: Dong Quai, and Gotu Kola.

VITAMINS: A, B6, B complex, and E.

MINERALS: A complete mineral complex.

ALSO: Astrelin, Gerovital H-3, L-Tyrosine, Proteolytic enzymes, and Raw ovarian concentrate.

HELPFUL FOODS: Beef, chicken, fish and fish liver oils, fruit, melons, nuts, soybeans, vegetable oils, green leafy vegetables, and whole grain vegetables.

INFLUENZA
(refer to Colds and Flu)

INSOMNIA

SPECIFICS: Insomnia is classified as habitual sleeplessness, repeated night after night. Some of the causes of insomnia are asthma, depression, compulsive personality or schizophrenic tendencies, and deficiencies of vitamins, minerals, and enzymes.

(BeneficialRemedies,Treatments,andNutrients)

HERBAL COMBINATIONS: (E-Z Sleep) (Silent Night).

PHYSIOLOGIC ACTION: Soothing mild relaxant. Promotes natural restful and refreshing sleep.

SINGLE HERBS: Catnip, Hops, Lady Slipper, Skullcap, Passionflower, Pau d'Arco, and Valerian root.

HOMEOPATHIC COMBINATION: Insomnia Formula.

VITAMINS: B1, B3, B5, B6, D, and E.

MINERALS: Calcium, Iron, Magnesium, and Potassium.

ALSO: Protein and Tryptophan.

HELPFUL FOODS: Apples, apricots, bananas, citrus fruits, sprouted seeds, sunflower seeds, whole rye and wheat, and yellow corn.

JUICES: Celery and lettuce juice.

INTESTINAL PARASITES

SPECIFICS: There are several types of parasites that can live in human intestines. The most common parasites are hookworms, pinworms, roundworms, and tapeworms. Worms irritate the intestinal lining causing poor absorption of vital nutrients.

(BeneficialRemedies,Treatments,andNutrients)

HERBAL COMBINATIONS: (Para-X) (Para-VF).

PHYSIOLOGIC ACTION: Useful in destroying and eliminating parasites, such as worms. The Para-VF is liquid and is useful for children and the elderly who cannot swallow capsules.

Warning: Do not use during pregnancy!

SINGLE HERBS: Black Walnut, Garlic, Pumpkin Seeds, Sage, Sheep Sorrel, Swedish Bitters, and Wormwood.

VITAMINS: A, B1, B2, B6, B12, B complex, D, and K.

MINERALS: Calcium and Iron.

Children: Chamomile tea or raisins soaked in Senna tea, for older children, may be helpful.

HELPFUL FOODS: Raw vegetables and fruits, vegetable oils, and fish liver oils.

IRRITABLE BLADDER
(refer to Kidney and Bladder)

IRRITABLE BOWEL SYNDROME

SPECIFICS: A common gastrointestinal disorder caused by irregular and uncoordinated muscular contractions of the intestine. This interferes with the movement of waste through the bowels causing the formation of excess toxins and mucus in the bloodstream and bowels.

(Beneficial Remedies, Treatments, and Nutrients)

HERBAL COMBINATION: (Multilax #1) or (Naturalax #1).

PHYSIOLOGIC ACTION: Helps relieve minor constipation.

Warning: Do not use when abdominal pain nausea or vomiting are present! Frequent or prolonged use of preparation may result in dependence on laxatives.

ALSO: Yu-ccan herbal drink, Vita Cleansing Tea, Swiss Kriss, Metab Herb, Psyllium Husks, Flax meal, Super D Tea. Drink lots of pure water to flush system.

HELPFUL FOODS: Citrus fruits and bananas.

JAUNDICE (NON INFECTIOUS)

SPECIFICS: Jaundice is not in itself a disease, but a sign of a liver, kidney, or blood disorder, which causes a build-up of bilirubin in the blood. Bilirubin is the presence of pigments from worn out blood cells that are deposited in the tissues, causing the skin and whites of the eyes to become abnormally yellow, rather than being excreted in bile as waste products.

(Beneficial Remedies, Treatments, and Nutrients)

HERBAL COMBINATION: (LG).

PHYSIOLOGIC ACTION: This herbal combination helps to correct malfunctioning of the liver and gall bladder. It is a liver detoxifier, and a bile stimulant.

SINGLE HERBS: Birch Leaves, Dandelion, Fennel, Horse Tail, Irish Moss, Parsley, and Rose Hips.

VITAMINS: A, B6, C, D, and E.

MINERALS: Calcium, Magnesium, and Phosphorus.

ALSO: Lecithin, Protein, and Unsaturated fatty acids.

HELPFUL FOODS: Apples, bananas, broccoli, carrots, cheese and other dairy products, tuna, fish liver oils, red meat, vegetable oils, and sprouted seeds.

JUICES: Sauerkraut and tomato juice.

JET LAG

SPECIFICS: Siberian ginseng, taken on a regular basis for about a week before the trip, seems to have a balancing effect on the system, lessening the effects of Jet Lag. A good vitamin supplement is also helpful.

(Beneficial Remedies, Treatments, and Nutrients)

SINGLE HERBS: Gota Kola and Korean Ginseng.

VITAMINS: Stress B Complex, Multi-Vitamin, C, and E.

MINERALS: Multi-mineral complex.

HELPFUL FOODS: All fruits, spinach, sweet potatoes, turnip greens, and unpolished rice.

KIDNEY AND BLADDER DISORDERS

SPECIFICS: There are many problems that may occur in the kidneys and bladder, however most of the problems are caused by infection. The symptoms of urinary tract infections are loss of appetite, chills, fever, frequency of urination, back pain, nausea, and vomiting.

(Beneficial Remedies, Treatments, and Nutrients)

HERBAL COMBINATION: (KB).

PHYSIOLOGIC ACTION: Extremely valuable in healing and strengthening the kidneys, bladder, and genito-urinary area. Useful to stop bed-wetting, but is a diuretic when congestion of the kidneys is indicated. Helps remove bladder, uterine, and urethral toxins.

Warning: Intended for occasional use only. May cause green-yellow discoloration of urine.

SINGLE HERBS: Alfalfa, Barberry root, Catnip, Dandelion, Fennel, Ginger root, Goldenrod, Horsetail, Uva Ursi, and Wild Yam.

VITAMINS: A, B complex, C, D, E, and Choline.

MINERALS: Calcium, Magnesium, and Potassium.

ALSO: Digestive enzymes, Lecithin, L-Arginine, L-Methionine, Propolis, Uratonic, Watermelon, 3-way herb teas, and other Diuretic tablets.

HELPFUL FOODS: All vegetables, apples, bananas, broccoli, carrots, cheese and other dairy products, tuna, and fish liver oils, red meat, and sprouted seeds.

JUICES: Asparagus, black currant, cranberry, celery, juniper berry, parsley, and pomegranate juice.

KIDNEY FUNCTIONS

SPECIFICS: The kidney is essential to the regulation of the body's acid base balance and fluid balance. Kidney failure is the inability of the kidneys to filter waste products from the blood and excrete them in the urine, to regulate the blood pressure, and to control the body's water and salt balance.

(BeneficialRemedies,Treatments,andNutrients)

HERBAL COMBINATION: Garlic and Parsley.

PHYSIOLOGIC ACTION: Promotes urine flow and strengthens kidneys. Also revitalizes and strengthens liver and spleen.

ALSO: Propolis, cranberry juice, 3-way herb teas, and uratonic.

HELPFUL FOODS: Refer to Kidney and Bladder in this manual.

KIDNEY AND BLADDER STONES

SPECIFICS: Kidney and bladder stones are abnormal accumulations of mineral salts, combined mostly with calcium, which form in the kidney, but can lodge anywhere along the course of the urinary tract. Symptoms include increased urination that may contain blood or pus, chills, fever, and pain radiating from the upper back to the lower abdomen.

(BeneficialRemedies,Treatments,andNutrients)

HERBAL COMBINATION: (PR).

PHYSIOLOGIC ACTION: PR combination helps dissolve kidney stones. PR helps keep kidneys flushed out (toxins and buildup of waste and sediments). Juniper keeps kidneys flushed out. Parsley acts as a diuretic. Magnesium helps prevent stones from forming. Thyme helps prevent buildup and dissolves stones if already present.

SINGLE HERBS: Corn silk, Dandelion, Ginkgo Biloba extract, Goldenrod, Juniper, Parsley, Sheep Sorrel, Thyme, and Uva Ursi.

VITAMINS: A, B2, B5, B6, C, E, F, and Choline.

MINERALS: Magnesium and Potassium.

ALSO: Canaid herbal drink and Proteolytic enzymes.

HELPFUL FOODS: All vegetable oils, apples, bananas, broccoli, carrots, cheese and other dairy products, tuna, fish liver oils, red meat, sprouted seeds, unpolished rice, and whole wheat.

JUICES: Apple, beet root, lemon, and radish juice.

LABOR AND DELIVERY

SPECIFICS: The process by which an infant moves from the uterus to the outside world. The first stage of labor covers the period from the onset until the woman's cervix is fully dilated. The second stage lasts from full dilatation of the cervix until the birth of the baby. The third stage lasts from the delivery until the afterbirth is expelled.

(BeneficialRemedies,Treatments,andNutrients)

SINGLE HERBS: Red Raspberry.

SPECIFICS: Red Raspberry is essential during labor. It coordinates the uterine contractions often making labor shorter.

LACTOSE INTOLERANCE

SPECIFICS: The inability to properly digest milk and milk products due to a shortage of the enzyme called lactase in the system. Symptoms range from mild abdominal discomfort to bloating, diarrhea, flatulence, and stomachache.

(BeneficialRemedies,Treatments,andNutrients)

VITAMINS: A complete multi-vitamin.

MINERALS: Calcium.

HELPFUL FOODS: Broccoli, tofo, kale, salmon, and sardines.

LEAD POISONING

SPECIFICS: Lead is one of the most widely used and one of the most toxic metal contaminants in the world today. A cumulative poison that is retained in bones, brain, central nervous system, and glands. Victims of lead poisoning experience hyperactivity, severe gastrointestinal colic, their gums turn blue, and muscle weakness. Lead poisoning can eventually lead to blindness, loss of memory, mental retardation, and paralysis of the limbs. If you suspect lead poisoning you should drink distilled water and make sure that your diet is high in fiber, supplemented with pectin.

(BeneficialRemedies,Treatments,andNutrients)

SINGLEHERBS: Alfalfa and Kelp.

VITAMINS: A, B1, B6, B complex, C, and E.

MINERALS: Chromium, Iron, Selenium, and Zinc.

ALSO: Lecithin, L-Cysteine, L-Cystine, L-Glutathionine, L-Lysine, and L-Methionine.

HELPFUL FOODS: Beef, black molasses, oat bran, chicken, herring and oysters, shellfish, mushrooms, fruit(citrus and other), whole rye, and whole wheat.

LEG CRAMPS

SPECIFICS: An involuntary spasm or contraction of the muscle in the leg. Most cramps occur at night after a day of unusual exertion, when the limbs are cool. Leg cramps are caused by impaired blood circulation or a nutritional deficiency.

(BeneficialRemedies,Treatments,andNutrients)

HERBAL COMBINATION: (Ca-T).

PHYSIOLOGIC ACTION: Effectively calms nerves and aids sleep, in addition to rebuilding the nerve sheath, veins, and artery walls.

SINGLEHERBS: Comfrey Herb, Horsetail Grass, Oat Straw, and Skullcap.

VITAMINS: B complex, B1, B2, B5, C, D, and E.

MINERALS: Calcium, Magnesium, and Phosphorus.

ALSO: #12 tissue salts, Protein, and Unsaturated fatty acids.

HELPFUL FOODS: Red meat, butter, cheese, citrus fruits, soybeans, rice, sunflower seeds, nuts, whole grains, and sweet potatoes.

LEG ULCERS

SPECIFICS: Leg ulcers are caused by poor circulation of blood to the legs. Restricted blood flow causes open sores to develop on deteriorated patches of skin.

(BeneficialRemedies,Treatments,andNutrients)

HERBAL COMBINATIONS: (H Formula) (Ginkgold).

PHYSIOLOGIC ACTION: Contains herbs which strengthen the heart and builds the vascular system. When taken with Cayenne, it improves circulation, giving a warming sensation to the entire body.

SINGLE HERBS: Cayenne, Bayberry, Butchers Broom, Ginkgo, and Yarrow.

VITAMINS: A, B3, B12, C, and E.

MINERALS: Calcium, Iron, Magnesium, and Potassium.

ALSO: Coenzyme Q10, Germanium, Lecithin, and Protein.

HELPFUL FOODS: Aloe Vera juice, apples, apricots, bananas, all vegetables, citrus fruit, cheese, fish, and beef.

LEGIONNAIRES' DISEASE

SPECIFICS: A lung and bronchial tube infection caused by the bacterial infection called (legionella pneumophilia). At this time modern science knows very little about this disease. It is believed that the bacteria are transmitted through the air, the bacteria which is found at excavation sites, or in newly plowed soil could be transmitted through the skin.

(BeneficialRemedies,Treatments,andNutrients)

SINGLE HERBS: Pau d'Arco, plus Catnip, Echinacea, Eucalyptus, Garlic, and Goldenseal.

VITAMINS: A strong multi-vitamin plus A, B complex, and C.

MINERALS: Multi-mineral complex plus Zinc.

ALSO: L-Carnitine, L-Cystine, and Raw thumus.

HELPFUL FOODS: Apples, apricots, cherries, citrus fruits, melons, lean beef, broccoli, carrots, green leafy vegetables, nuts, sweet potatoes, turnip greens, and unpolished rice.

LEUKEMIA

SPECIFICS: Leukemia is a fatal blood disease caused by an overproduction of white blood cells. Acute leukemia is marked by a sudden onset of symptoms and usually occurs in children and young adults. Chronic leukemia is found only in adults and the symptoms develop slower. A well-balanced diet containing all vitamins and minerals will help maintain strength and may possibly extend their lifetime.

(BeneficialRemedies,Treatments,andNutrients)

SINGLE HERBS: Pau d'Arco, Swedish Bitters, and Nettle.

VITAMINS: B complex, B12, C, and E.

MINERALS: Copper, Iron, and Zinc.

ALSO: Canaid herbal drink.

HELPFUL FOODS: Aloe Vera, apples, bananas, broccoli, oat bran, carrots, citrus fruits, green leafy vegetables, soybeans, sweet potatoes, turnip greens, vegetable oils, lean red meat, and fish liver oils.

Refer to "Cancer" in the manual.

LEUKORRHEA

SPECIFICS: Leukorrhea is a white vaginal discharge often caused by a one celled microorganism called Trichomonas vaginalis, or by a yeast fungus called monilia.

(BeneficialRemedies,Treatments,andNutrients)

HERBAL COMBINATION: (Cantrol).

PHYSIOLOGIC ACTION: An excellent well-balanced formula of herbs and supplements which balance the system while killing yeast. It includes caprylic acid and anti-oxidants for the control and eventual elimination of yeast fungus.

SINGLE HERBS: Black Walnut, Caprinex, Garlicin, Pau d'Arco, and Yucca.

Note: Drink three cups of Pau d'Arco tea daily. This herb is a natural antibiotic agent.

VITAMINS: A, B complex, Biotin, D, and E.

MINERALS: Calcium and Magnesium.

ALSO: Yu-ccan herbal drink, Linseed Oil, Candida Cleanse, Caprilic Acid, and Primadophilus.

HELPFUL FOODS: Egg yolk, apricot, citrus fruits, beef kidney, beef liver, vegetable and fish oils.

LIVER and GALLBLADDER DISORDERS

SPECIFICS: The liver is the largest organ of the body and is located under the diaphragm just above the stomach. It is responsible for detoxifying harmful substances such as alcohol, food additives, pesticides, and environmental pollutants. The liver also produces cholesterol, enzymes, lecithin, and bile. The following nutrients are beneficial in the treatment of liver and gallbladder disorders.

(BeneficialRemedies,Treatments,andNutrients)

HERBAL COMBINATION: (LG).

PHYSIOLOGIC ACTION: Helps the cleansing of the liver and gall bladder; restores new energy to these organs. Also can be taken to relieve intestinal gas.

SINGLE HERBS: Bayberry Root, Catnip, Fennel Seed, Ginger Root, and Peppermint.

VITAMINS: A, B1, B2, B6, Choline, Niacin, Pantothenic acid, C, and E.

MINERALS: Copper and Sulfur for the Liver. Magnesium and Sulfur for the Gallbladder.

ALSO: Acidophilus, Calamus Root tea, Chlorophyll, Digestive enzymes, and Hydrochloric acid.

HELPFUL FOODS: All vegetables, apples, bananas, broccoli, carrots, cheese and other dairy products, tuna and fish liver oils, red meat, and sprouted seeds.

JUICES: Beet root, blackcherry, carrot, cucumber, pineapple, and radish juice.

LIVER DISORDERS

SPECIFICS: Refer to liver and gallbladder disorders.

(BeneficialRemedies,Treatments,andNutrients)

HERBAL COMBINATIONS: (Thisilyn) (Milk Thistle Extract).

PHYSIOLOGIC ACTION: Protects liver. Anti-oxidant quality prevents free radical damage in the liver.

SINGLE HERBS: Dandelion and Horsetail.

VITAMINS: A, B Complex, B1, B2, B3, B6, Choline, C, and E.

ALSO: Digestive Enzymes, Lecithin, and Primadophilus.

HELPFUL FOODS: Apples, bananas, broccoli, carrots, cheese and other dairy products, tuna and fish liver oils, red meat, vegetable oils, and sprouted seeds.

JUICES: Sauerkraut and tomato juice.

LOWER BOWEL PROBLEMS

SPECIFICS: Constipation results when the waste material moves too slowly or there is decreased frequency of bowel movements. Constipation usually arises from insufficient amounts of fiber and fluids in the diet. Other causes include lack of exercise, nervousness, stress, infections, and poor diet.

(BeneficialRemedies,Treatments,andNutrients)

HERBAL COMBINATIONS: (Multilax #2) or (Naturalax #2)

PHYSIOLOGIC ACTION: Accelerates natural cleansing of the body and improves intestinal absorption by gentle evacuation of bowels. Cleans out old toxic fecal matter, mucus and encrustation's from the colon wall, and helps normalize the peristaltic action and rebuild the bowel structure. Use until the bowel is cleansed, healed, and functioning normally.

SINGLE HERBS: Cascara Sagrada, Golden Seal Root, Lobelia, Red Raspberry, Senna, and Yucca.

VITAMINS: A multi-vitamin plus the B complex.

MINERALS: A strong multi-mineral complex.

ALSO: Yu-ccan herbal drink, Flax seeds, Psyllium seeds, Whey powder, Yogurt, soaked Prunes and Figs, and Licorice tea.

HELPFUL FOODS: Brewers yeast, cabbage, cantaloupe, egg yolk, beef heart, brains, kidney, liver, rice bran, milk, nuts, peas, and soybeans.

JUICES: Celery, grapefruit, and spinach juice.

LUMBAGO
(refer to Back Pain)

LUPUS

SPECIFICS: An inflammatory auto immune mechanism disease that affects many organs. Discoid lupus is a skin disease and systemic lupus affects the joints and organs of the body. Both types have remissions and flare up cycles.

(BeneficialRemedies,Treatments,andNutrients)

SINGLE HERBS: Echinacea, Goldenseal, Pau d'Arco, Red Clover, Turkish Rhubarb, and Yucca.

VITAMINS: C.

MINERALS: Calcium, Magnesium, and Zinc.

ALSO: Canaid strengthens the immune system. Acidophilus, L-Cysteine, L-Cystine, L-Methionine, Proteolytic enzymes, and Unsaturated fatty acids.

HELPFUL FOODS: Broccoli, yellow corn, sweet potatoes, turnip greens, citrus fruits, cheese, butter, milk, shell fish, herring, and oysters.

LYME DISEASE

SPECIFICS: Lyme disease is caused by a tick that is carried by mice, lizards, and the white tailed deer. Tick bites often go undetected and the first sign of lyme disease is a rash a few days after the tick bite. Symptoms include backache, headache, stiff neck, nausea, and vomiting. If left untreated, lyme disease can lead to damage to the central nervous system and cardiovascular system.

(BeneficialRemedies,Treatments,andNutrients)

SINGLEHERBS: Echinacea, Goldenseal, Milk thistle, Pau d'Arco, Red Clover, and Suma.

VITAMINS: Multi-vitamin plus A, C, and E.

MINERALS: Zinc.

ALSO: Chlorophyll and Germanium.

HELPFUL FOODS: Aloe Vera, broccoli, carrots, citrus fruits, garlic, vegetable oils, and fish liver oils.

MACULAR DEGENERATION

SPECIFICS: Macular degeneration is one of the leading causes of decreased visual acuity. This condition is characterized by the degeneration of the macula or the central area of the retina. Factors that contribute to the development of this disease include cigarette smoking, poor nutrition, hypertension, and atherosclerosis. Consumption of saturated fats, white sugar, and refined carbohydrates should be avoided.

(BeneficialRemedies,Treatments,andNutrients)

SINGLEHERBS: Gingko Biloba, Bilberry, and Hawthorn.

VITAMINS: A, Beta-carotene, C, and E.

MINERALS: Selenium and Zinc.

ALSO: Bioflavonoids, Omega-3, and Omega-6.

HELPFUL FOODS: Broccoli, carrots, citrus fruits, garlic, strawberries, vegetable oils, and fish liver oils.

MALABSORPTION SYNDROME

SPECIFICS: This disorder is due to an incorrect diet over a long period of time. This condition will cause anemia and osteoporosis if not addressed in time. The problem is always due to malnutrition. Treatment is a diet high in all nutrients, vitamins, and minerals.

(BeneficialRemedies,Treatments,andNutrients)

SINGLE HERBS: Kelp and Horsetail.

VITAMINS: B12, B complex, and C.

MINERALS: Multi-mineral complex plus Zinc.

ALSO: Acidophilus, Essential fatty acids, Liver, and Protein.

HELPFUL FOODS: All fruits(citrus and other), green leafy vegetables, turnip greens, nuts, unpolished rice, herring, oysters, and red meats.

JUICES: Blackberry, grape, and parsley juice.

MANIC DEPRESSION

SPECIFICS: A mental disorder in which a disturbance of mood is the major symptom. Mood swings may be accompanied by extreme negative delusions or by grandiose ideas. The main causes of this ailment are drugs, inherited tendency, and malnutrition.

(BeneficialRemedies,Treatments,andNutrients)

VITAMINS: B complex, B12, and Folic Acid.

MINERALS: Lithium.

ALSO: Omega-6 oils, L-phenylalanine, and L-tryptophan.

HELPFUL FOODS: Liver, red meat, eggs, asparagus, citrus fruits, turnip greens, sprouted seeds, cheese and other dairy products, sunflower seeds, wheat germ, and whole grains.

MARBLE BONE DISEASE

SPECIFICS: Marble bone disease is a gradual loss in the total mass of bone, leaving the remaining bone fragile or brittle. The major cause of this disease is a calcium-phosphorus imbalance or an inability to absorb sufficient amounts of calcium through the intestine. The best prevention and treatment is a diet that is adequate in vitamin C and D, protein, calcium, magnesium, and phosphorus.

(BeneficialRemedies,Treatments,andNutrients)

SINGLE HERBS: Feverfew, Horsetail, and Oatstraw,

VITAMINS: B12, C, D, and E.

MINERALS: Calcium, Copper, Fluoride, Magnesium, and Phosphorus.

ALSO: L-Lysine, L-Arginine, Protein, Multidigestive enzymes with Betaine hydrochloride, and Proteolytic enzymes.

HELPFUL FOODS: All dairy products, red meats, chicken, sardines, tuna, herring, oysters, all fruit, soybeans, nuts, broccoli, corn, rice, and whole wheat.

MASTITIS   (Breast infection)

SPECIFICS: Mastitis is the result of a plugged duct. If the mother should stop nursing the baby, the duct will remain full and could worsen the problem by allowing the duct to overfill. A few of the milder antibiotics can be taken while nursing. The following nutrients should be taken by the nursing mother.

(BeneficialRemedies,Treatments,andNutrients)

VITAMINS: A good multi-vitamin, plus B complex, C, and D.
MINERALS: Calcium, Manganese, and Iron.

ALSO: Acidophlus and Protein.

HELPFUL FOODS: Tuna, red meat, beets, broccoli, peas, turnip greens, sprouted seeds, cheese and other dairy products, sunflower seeds, and whole rye.

MEASLES

SPECIFICS: The two main varieties of measles are German measles and common measles.

German measles is a contagious, but mild virus, however if contracted during the first four months of pregnancy it can cause serious birth defects.

Common measles may have many serious complications, such as bronchitis, croup, middle ear infection, or pneumonia.

(BeneficialRemedies,Treatments,andNutrients)

HERBAL COMBINATION: (Fenu-Thyme) (ANT-PLG Syrup).

PHYSIOLOGIC ACTION: Helps the body to resist infectious diseases and reduce fever. Acts as a support to the immune system during such illnesses as chicken pox, mumps, and measles.

SINGLE HERBS: Garlic, Catnip tea, Turkey Rhubarb, and Pau d'Arco.

VITAMINS: A, C, and E.

MINERALS: Calcium, Magnesium, and Zinc.

ALSO: Canaid herbal drink helps to strengthen the immune system. Raw thymus and Proteolytic enzymes.

HELPFUL FOODS: Bananas, citrus fruits, melons, herring, fish liver oils, carrots, broccoli, green leafy vegetables, sweet potatoes, and turnip greens.

MELANOMA

SPECIFICS: The most dangerous form of skin cancer. Melanoma is life threatening, but can be cured if discovered and treated early. In this type of skin cancer, a tumor is produced from the pigment producing cells of the deeper layers of the skin. Most often it begins as a lesion that looks like a mole. The most common cause of melanoma is overexposure to the suns ultraviolet rays.

(Beneficial Remedies, Treatments, and Nutrients)

SINGLE HERBS: Kelp and Pau d'Arco.

VITAMINS: A, B complex, B12, Niacin, Folic Acid, C, and E.

MINERALS: A strong Multi-mineral plus Potassium, Calcium, and Magnesium.

ALSO: Coenzyme Q10, L-Cysteine, L-Methionine, L-Taurine, Essential fatty acids, Germanium, Primadophilus, Proteolytic enzymes, and Raw glandular complex with extra Raw thymus.

HELPFUL FOODS: Aloe Vera, apples, bananas, broccoli, bran, carrots, citrus fruits, green leafy vegetables, soybeans, sweet potatoes, turnip greens, vegetable oils, lean red meat, and fish liver oils.

MEMORY AID

SPECIFICS: Most memory lapses are caused by a deficiency of vitamins and minerals. Other causes may be due to cerebral dysfunction, nervous disturbances, and strokes.

(Beneficial Remedies, Treatments, and Nutrients)

HERBAL COMBINATIONS: (SEN) or (Remem).

PHYSIOLOGIC ACTION: This formula contains remarkable rejuvenating properties that nourish the brain cells and tissues and improves their ability to perform mental functions.

SINGLE HERBS: Cayenne, Ginkgo, Gotu Kola, Korean Ginseng, and Lobelia.

VITAMINS: Multi-vitamin complex plus Choline.

MINERALS: A good multi-mineral complex.

ALSO: Lecithin.

HELPFUL FOODS: Brewers yeast, egg yolk, green leafy vegetables, liver, and wheat germ.

MENIERE'S SYNDROME

SPECIFICS: A disease of the inner ear characterized by loss of hearing, ringing in the ears, nausea, vomiting, and dizziness. Meniere's syndrome is often caused by impaired blood flow to the brain from clogged arteries and poor circulation.

(BeneficialRemedies,Treatments,andNutrients)

HERBAL COMBINATIONS: (H Formula) (Ginkgold).

PHYSIOLOGIC ACTION: Contains herbs which strengthen the heart and builds the vascular system. When taken with Cayenne, it improves circulation and pulse rate, giving a warming sensation to the entire body.

SINGLE HERBS: Cayenne, Black Cohosh, Bayberry, Butchers Broom, Ginkgo, and Yarrow

VITAMINS: A, B complex, B3, B6, C, and E.

MINERALS: Calcium, Magnesium, Manganese, and Potassium.

ALSO: Bio-Strath, Coenzyme Q10, and Lecithin.

HELPFUL FOODS: All vegetables and vegetable oils, apples, bananas, citrus fruits, beets, broccoli, carrots, oat bran, soya beans, and whole wheat.

MENINGITIS

SPECIFICS: This disease occurs when the three layers of membranes lying between the skull and the brain, called the "meninges", become infected. Medical attention should be sought promptly, if untreated complications such as brain damage and paralysis can occur.

Symptoms include drowsiness, chills, high fever, headache, nausea, and a stiff neck. A well-balanced diet high in vitamins, minerals, and protein will help the body ward off infection and repair damaged tissue.

(BeneficialRemedies,Treatments,andNutrients)

SINGLE HERBS: Catnip and Garlic.

VITAMINS: Multi-vitamin plus A, C, and D.

MINERALS: A high potency mineral complex, Calcium, and Zinc.

ALSO: Germanium, Protein, and Raw thymus.

HELPFUL FOODS: Aloe Vera juice, butter, cheese and other dairy products, citrus fruit, tuna, beef, sardines, herring, oysters, and sweet potatoes.

MENOPAUSE

SPECIFICS: Menopause is the point at which women stop ovulating, the end of their reproductive years. It usually lasts from three to five years and is experienced by most women around the age of fifty. Symptoms include difficult breathing, dizziness, headache, heart palpitations, hot flashes, and depression.

(BeneficialRemedies,Treatments,andNutrients)

HERBAL COMBINATIONS: (Change-O-Life) or (MP).

PHYSIOLOGIC ACTION: For both male and female health to the pancreas, pituitary, and other glandular areas. Maintains a healthy hormone balance in the body, especially during puberty and menopause.

SINGLE HERBS: Black Cohosh, Blessed Thistle, Damiana, Licorice Root, Quan Yin, Sarsaparilla, and Siberian Ginseng,

HOMEOPATHIC COMBINATION: Menopause Formula.

VITAMINS: A, B complex, B3, C, D, and E.

MINERALS: Calcium, Magnesium, Potassium, and Selenium.

ALSO: Enzymes with hydrochloric acid, Germanium, L-Arginine, L-Lysine, and Melbrosia.

HELPFUL FOODS: All vegetables and vegetable oils, fish and fish liver oils, cheese, butter, apples, bananas, citrus fruits, and mushrooms.

MENSTRUATION

SPECIFICS: Menstruation is the cyclical process that continuously prepares the uterus for pregnancy, starting at puberty and continuing through menopause.

(BeneficialRemedies,Treatments,andNutrients)

HERBAL COMBINATIONS: (FC) or (FEM-MEND).

PHYSIOLOGIC ACTION: Helps regulate the menstrual cycle, relieve cramps, bloating and vaginitis, ease inflammation of the vagina and uterus, and strengthen and regulate the kidneys, bladder and uterus areas. Beneficial for all female and uterine complaints.

Warning: Do not use this combination while taking estrogen or oral contraceptives!

SINGLE HERBS: Red Raspberry and Uva Ursi.

HOMEOPATHIC COMBINATION: PMS Formula.

VITAMINS: B complex, B6, C, E.

MINERALS: A complete multi-mineral.

HELPFUL FOODS: Dulse, pineapples, citrus fruits, broccoli, soybeans, spinach, sweet potatoes, turnip greens, vegetable oils, nuts, unpolished rice, and whole wheat.

MENSTRUAL CRAMPS
(refer to Premenstrual Syndrome - PMS)

MERCURY POISONING

SPECIFICS: Mercury is found in the soil, water, our food supply and is even more toxic than lead. It is accumulated and retained in the brain and central nervous system. Large amounts of mercury can cause depression, dizziness, fatigue, memory loss and weakness.

(BeneficialRemedies,Treatments,andNutrients)

SINGLE HERBS: Alfalfa, Kelp, and Garlic.

PHYSIOLOGIC ACTION: Garlic acts as a detoxifier and alfalfa and kelp help the body to remove the toxins.

VITAMINS: A, B complex, C, and E.

MINERALS: Selenium.

ALSO: L-Cysteine, L- Cystine, L- Glutathione, L- Methionine, and Hydrochloric acid.

HELPFUL FOODS: Apples, garlic, onions, fruit and vegetable juices, oat bran, and whole grains.

MIGRAINE HEADACHES

SPECIFICS: A migraine headache begins with a throbbing pain that usually begins at the back of the head and spreads to the entire side of the head or is centered above or behind one eye. Most migraines are caused by allergies, constipation, stress, or liver malfunction. Note - Avoid the following: salt, dairy products, red meat, and fried foods.

(BeneficialRemedies,Treatments,andNutrients)

SINGLE HERBS: Chamomile, Feverfew, Ginkgo Biloba, and Yucca.

PHYSIOLOGIC ACTION: Chamomile will prevent migraine headaches. Ginkgo Biloba enhances cerebral circulation. Feverfew reduces fever. Feverfew has been historically used for chills and pain that accompany fever. Because of its anecdotal claims for migraine sufferers, it is presently being researched at the London Migraine Clinic.

HOMEOPATHIC COMBINATION: Migraine Headache Formula.

VITAMINS: B complex, B3, B5, B12, Paba, and Niacin, C, and F.

MINERALS: Calcium, Magnesium, and Potassium.

ALSO: Unsaturated fatty acids.

HELPFUL FOODS: Almonds, apples, avocados, bananas, all vegetables and vegetable oils, citrus fruits, whole grains, and unpolished rice.

MITRAL VALVE PROLAPSE

SPECIFICS: A mitral valve prolapse is a common condition that is usually detected if a heart murmer and/or click is heard, and is generally considered a benign heart valve abnormality.

(BeneficialRemedies,Treatments,andNutrients)

VITAMINS: Multi-vitamin.

MINERALS: Multi-mineral plus extra Magnesium.

ALSO: Coenzyme Q10.

MONONUCLEOSIS

SPECIFICS:An infectious disease believed to be caused by a virus. It affects the respiratory system, liver, the lymph tissues, and glands. The disease can be transmitted through communal drinking utensils, kissing , and blood transfusions. A well-balanced diet, adequate in protein, is essential for the prevention of mononucleosis.

(BeneficialRemedies,Treatments,andNutrients)

SINGLE HERBS: Dandelion, Echinacea, Goldenseal, Pau d'Arco, and Sheep Sorrel.

VITAMINS: A, B complex, B1, B2, B5, B6, C, Biotin, and Choline.

MINERALS: Potassium.

ALSO: Canaid herbal drink, a nondairy form of Acidophilus, Germanium, Raw thymus, Raw glandular complex, and Protein.

HELPFUL FOODS: Aloe Vera, bananas, melons, citrus fruits, nuts, oat bran, green leafy vegetables, sweet potatoes, turnip greens, carrots, and fish liver oils.

MORNING SICKNESS

SPECIFICS: About half of all pregnant women experience nausea and vomiting from the 5th week to the 12th week of pregnancy. Morning sickness may be due to either a dairy product intolerance or a nutrient deficiency.

(BeneficialRemedies,Treatments,andNutrients)

SINGLE HERBS: Red Raspberry and Peppermint.

PHYSIOLOGIC ACTION: Red Raspberry or Peppermint Tea often overcomes nausea. Alfalfa, Chamomile, Catnip, and Ginger tea may also be helpful. Sometimes small, frequent meals instead of a larger one is beneficial.

VITAMINS: A multi-vitamin plus B6, C, and K.

ALSO: Eliminate alcohol from your diet. Avoid cigarette smoke, yours and other people's. Do not use white sugar, refined carbohydrates, coffee and other stimulants.

HELPFUL FOODS: Broccoli, kale, lettuce, spinach, turnip greens, and strawberries.

MOTION SICKNESS

SPECIFICS:Motion induced nausea can indicate the presence of

many diseases including inner ear infection, low blood sugar, food poisoning, and nutrient deficiency. The most common cause is a deficiency of the vitamin "B6" and the mineral "magnesium". Ginkgo is excellent for chronic dizziness and light headedness.
Natural remedies have been used with great success in cases of motion sickness. Do not eat junk foods, heavily processed meals, or alcohol before or during the trip.

(BeneficialRemedies,Treatments,andNutrients)

HERBAL COMBINATION: (Motion Mate).

PHYSIOLOGIC ACTION: In a recent university study, ginger root caps proved more effective than either a drug or placebo at controlling motion induced nausea. Also queasy travelers have found taking B complex at night and just before the trip is most effective.

SINGLE HERBS: Ginger Root Caps and Ginkgo.

VITAMINS: B complex, plus B6.

MINERALS: Magnesium.

ALSO: Charcoal tablets.

HELPFUL FOODS: Fruits, lean beef, nuts, unpolished rice, whole grains, and yellow corn.

MOUTH AND TONGUE DISORDERS
(Canker, Thrush, Pyorrhea)

SPECIFICS: Nearly all mouth and tongue disorders such as sore mouth, tongue, and gums are attributed to a deficiency of the B vitamins. The gums become puffy, tender, and the oral membranes become susceptible to canker sores with the deficiency of vitamin C and niacin.

(BeneficialRemedies,Treatments,andNutrients)

SINGLE HERBS: Aloe Vera, Golden Seal, Myrrh, Red Raspberry, and White Oak Bark.

VITAMINS: A, B complex, B2, B3, B12, C, and E.

MINERALS: Iron, Magnesium, Phosphorus, and Zinc.

ALSO: Chlorophyll, Lysine, and Primadophilus.

HELPFUL FOODS: All fruits, carrots, corn, broccoli, herring, oysters, red meat, soybeans, and spinach.

MULTIPLE SCLEROSIS

SPECIFICS: MS is a degenerative and progressive disorder of the central nervous system that destroys the myelin sheaths which cover the nerves, causing an inflammatory response. A strong immune system helps avoid infection and a diet rich in vitamin and mineral supplements is beneficial for the MS patient.

Note: Limit the consumption of saturated fats, sugar, and processed foods.

(BeneficialRemedies,Treatments,andNutrients)

SINGLE HERBS: Evening Primrose Oil, Kelp, Oat Extract, Skullcap, and St. John's Wort.

VITAMINS: B complex, B1, B2, B3, B5, B6, B12, C, E, F, and Inositol.

MINERALS: Calcium, Copper, Iron, Magnesium, Manganese, Selenium, and Zinc.

ALSO: Acidophilus, Bonemeal, Coenzyme Q10, Germanium, Digestive enzymes, Proteolytic enzymes, Lecithin, L-Leucine, L-Isoleucine, L-Valine, and Protein.

HELPFUL FOODS: Apples, apricots, cherries, grapes, citrus fruits, cheese, beets, broccoli, green leafy vegetables, soy beans, spinach, red meat, mushrooms, and garlic.

MUMPS

SPECIFICS: A contagious viral infection that causes swelling of one or both parotid glands at the jaw angles below the ears. Mumps usually infect children between the ages of three and twelve, however they can occur after puberty and cause serious complications such as sterility in the ovaries and testes.

(BeneficialRemedies,Treatments,andNutrients)

HERBAL COMBINATION: (ANT-PLG).

PHYSIOLOGIC ACTION: An effective formula that helps cleanse toxins and reduce infection. This combination is a natural aid in fighting contagious diseases.

SINGLE HERBS: Bayberry Root Bark, Echinacea, Ginger Root, Lobelia, and Mullein.

VITAMINS: A, B complex, C, and E.

MINERALS: A complete multi complex.

ALSO: Germanium and Acidophilus.

HELPFUL FOODS: Bananas, citrus fruits, melons, herring, fish liver oils, carrots, broccoli, green leafy vegetables, sweet potatoes, and turnip greens.

MUSCLE CRAMPS

SPECIFICS: An involuntary spasm or contraction of the muscle. Most cramps occur at night after a day of unusual exertion, when the limbs are cool. Muscle cramps are caused by impaired blood circulation or a calcium and magnesium imbalance.

(Beneficial Remedies, Treatments, and Nutrients)

HERBAL COMBINATION: (Ca-T).

PHYSIOLOGIC ACTION: Effectively calms nerves and aids sleep in addition to rebuilding the nerve sheath, vein, and artery walls.

SINGLE HERBS: Comfrey Herb, Dong Quai, Elderberry, Ginkgo Biloba, Horsetail Grass, Oat Straw, Saffron, and Skullcap.

VITAMINS: A, B complex, B1, B3, B5, C, D, and E.

MINERALS: Calcium, Magnesium, and Zinc.

ALSO: #12 tissue salts, Coenzyme Q10, and Lecithin.

HELPFUL FOODS: Red meat, butter, cheese, citrus fruits, soybeans, rice, sunflower seeds, nuts, whole grains, and sweet potatoes.

MUSCLE INJURIES
(refer to Athletic Injuries)

MUSCLE WEAKNESS

SPECIFICS: Almost every nutrient is involved in muscle contraction, relaxation, and repair. A deficiency interferes with the metabolism of amino acids and increases the need for oxygen in the blood. This in turn, causes a gradual, progressive weakness throughout the muscles of the body.

(Beneficial Remedies, Treatments, and Nutrients)

SINGLE HERBS: Gota Kola and Ginseng.

VITAMINS: A complete multi-vitamin plus additional E.

MINERALS: Manganese, Potassium, and Zinc.

ALSO: Protein and Unsaturated fatty acids.

HELPFUL FOODS: All vegetables and vegetable oils, bananas, herring, oysters, and whole wheat.

MUSCULAR DYSTROPHY

SPECIFICS: In muscular dystrophy the essential fatty acids that form the structural part of the muscle are destroyed and the nutrients necessary for muscle function are reduced. The disease is considered to be largely hereditary, except for one type that occurs in adults between the ages of forty to fifty. The victims diet should be adequate in all essential nutrients including proteins and vegetable oils.

(BeneficialRemedies,Treatments,andNutrients)

SINGLE HERBS: Saw Palmetto.

VITAMINS: A, B complex, B3, B5, B6, B12, C, E, and Choline.

MINERALS: Potassium.

ALSO: Protein and Unsaturated fatty acids.

HELPFUL FOODS: All fruits, all vegetables and vegetable oils, whole grains and seeds, red meat, sardines, herring, oysters, and fish liver oils.

MYALGIA
(refer to Muscle Cramps)

MYASTHENIA GRAVIS

SPECIFICS: Myasthenia usually effects muscles in the face and neck. This disease is caused by underproduction of acetylcholine, a substance that transmits nerve impulses to the muscles. Many nutrients are required for the production of acetylcholine, and in many cases recovery from the ailment has occurred with the use of a proper diet.

(BeneficialRemedies,Treatments,andNutrients)

SINGLE HERBS: Dong Quai and Korean Ginseng.

VITAMINS: B complex, B1, B2, B6, B12, Choline, Folic acid, Inositol, Pantothenic acid, C, and E.

MINERALS: Magnesium, Manganese, and Potassium.

ALSO: Lecithin and Protein.

HELPFUL FOODS: Apples, bananas, grapes, citrus fruits, beets, broccoli, yellow corn, soybeans, and nuts.

MYCOSES

SPECIFICS: Diseases of the skin or other organs caused by the multiplication and spread of fungi. Victims of mycoses should eat a well-balanced diet, supplemented by megadoses of vitamins A, B, and C.

(BeneficialRemedies,Treatments,andNutrients)

VITAMINS: A, B, C, and E.

ALSO: Primadophilus, Black Walnut, Garlic, Caprinex, and Pau d'Arco.

HELPFUL FOODS: Beef, chicken, tuna, carrots, black walnut, raw fruits, spinach, turnip greens, and sweet potatoes.

NOTE: Avoid dairy products and processed foods.

MYOCARDIAL INFARCTION

SPECIFICS: When the heart is temporarily deprived of oxygen due to the thickening, hardening, and narrowing of the coronary arteries. A coronary may be triggered by complete or partial blockage of the coronary arteries. Recent animal studies suggest that vitamin C deficiency could, be involved in the causation of myocardial infarction. E.F.A.s (essential fatty acids) play a fundamental role in keeping cell membranes, fluid and flexible.

(BeneficialRemedies,Treatments,andNutrients)

HERBAL COMBINATION: (Garlicin HC).

PHYSIOLOGIC ACTION: A combination of herbs which supports the cardiovascular system. Helps to strengthen the heart, while building and cleansing the arteries and veins.

SINGLE HERBS: Cayenne, Comfrey, Evening Primrose Oil, Fish Oil, Garlic, Golden Seal, and Rose Hips.

VITAMINS: B complex, C, E, Niacin, Inositol, and Choline.

MINERALS: Calcium and Magnesium

ALSO: Coenzyme Q10, L-Carnitine, L-Cysteine, L-Methionine, Multidigestive enzymes, DMG, Fish oils, and cold pressed vegetable oils.

HELPFUL FOODS: Apples, lean beef, broccoli, fruits(citrus and other),sprouted seeds, sunflower seeds, sweet potatoes, sardines, tuna, turnip greens, and yellow corn.

NAIL PROBLEMS

SPECIFICS: Nail changes or abnormalities are often the result of nutritional deficiencies. A well-balanced diet supplying all essential nutrients is recommended.

Vitamin A deficiency causes dryness and brittleness.

Vitamin B deficiency causes fragility.

Vitamin C deficiency causes hangnails.

Iron deficiency causes thinning and flattening.

Zinc deficiency causes white spots.

(Beneficial Remedies, Treatments, and Nutrients)

SINGLE HERBS: Horsetail.

VITAMINS: A, B complex, and C.

MINERALS: Calcium, Magnesium, Iron, and Zinc.

ALSO: L-Cysteine, L-Methionine, Protein, and Silicon.

HELPFUL FOODS: All dairy products, red meat, chicken, tuna, salmon, sardines, all vegetables, and vegetable oils.

JUICES: Beet greens, celery, kale, and parsley juice.

NAUSEA AND VOMITING

SPECIFICS: Both illnesses can indicate the presence of one of many diseases, and both are produced by a deficiency of magnesium and/or vitamin B6.

(Beneficial Remedies, Treatments, and Nutrients)

HERBAL COMBINATION: (Herbal Influence).

PHYSIOLOGIC ACTION: Herbal Influence (formerly known as Herbal Composition) was created by the early American herbalist, Samuel Thomson. It contains herbs which help with fever and nauseousness.

SINGLE HERBS: Cayenne, Red Clover, Raspberry Tea, Chaparral, Rose Hips, Garlic, Honey, and Golden Seal.

VITAMINS: A, B6, C, and P.

MINERALS: Magnesium.

HELPFUL FOODS: Apples, apricots, avocados, citrus fruits, broccoli, carrots, peas, sweet potatoes, turnip greens, yellow corn, red meats, rice, and buck wheat.

JUICES: Carrot and blackberry juice.

NEPHRITIS
(refer to Kidney and Bladder)

NERVOUS DISORDERS

SPECIFICS: Nervous disorders are generally a direct result of stress. The body can handle some stress but long term stress causes the body to break down. Long term stress occurs when the situation that causes anxiety is not relieved. Find the cause and handle it constructively. People experiencing stress should maintain a well-balanced diet and replace the nutrients depleted during stress.

(BeneficialRemedies,Treatments,andNutrients)

HERBAL COMBINATIONS: (Calm-aid) or (Ex stress comb).

PHYSIOLOGIC ACTION: A proven formula that is soothing, strengthening, and healing to the whole nervous system to relieve nervous tension and rebuild the nerve sheaths. Excellent aid for insomnia, chronic nervousness, and stress-related conditions.

SINGLE HERBS: Evening Primrose Oil, Hops, Mistletoe, Skullcap, Valerian, and Yucca.

VITAMINS: B complex, B1, B2, B3, B5, B6, and C.

MINERALS: Calcium, Iodine, Iron, Magnesium, Phosphorus, Potassium, Silicon, and Sodium.

HELPFUL FOODS: Dulse, flax seed, sea salt, fruit(citrus and other), bacon, beef, chicken, all dairy products, all vegetables, and whole rye.

JUICES: Radish and prune juice.

NETTLE RASH

SPECIFICS: If the sap of nettles touches the skin, it can cause persistent itching, rash, swelling, and blistering in sensitive people. The following nutrients will help alleviate the symptoms.

(BeneficialRemedies,Treatments,andNutrients)

SINGLE HERBS: Echinacea, Goldenseal, and Lobelia.

VITAMINS: A, C, and E.

MINERALS: Zinc.

HELPFUL FOODS: Broccoli, carrots, citrus fruits, melon, fish liver oils, and vegetable oils.

NEURITIS

SPECIFICS: Neuritis is the inflammation or deterioration of a nerve or a group of nerves. It is caused by an injury to a nerve, diabetes, infection, or the deficiency of the vitamin B complex. The best treatment for neuritis is to make sure the patient gets optimum nutrition.

(BeneficialRemedies,Treatments,andNutrients)

SINGLE HERBS: Black Cohosh, Lobelia, Lady Slipper, Skullcap, and Valerian Root.

VITAMINS: B1, B2, B6, B12, Niacin, and Pantothenic acid.

MINERALS: Mineral complex, plus Calcium and Magnesium.

ALSO: Lecithin, Protein, and Proteolytic enzymes.

HELPFUL FOODS: Brewers yeast, cheese, all fruit, nuts, oat bran, and unpolished rice.

JUICES: Cucumber, Endive, and Pineapple juice.

NIGHT BLINDNESS

SPECIFICS: The inability to see well in dim light. The condition may be an inherited functional defect of the retina but the most common cause is a deficiency of vitamin A. Night blindness can usually be prevented by supplementing the diet with vitamins and the nutrients listed.

(BeneficialRemedies,Treatments,andNutrients)

HERBAL COMBINATION: (Herbal Eye bright Formula).

PHYSIOLOGIC ACTION: Extremely valuable in strengthening and healing the eyes. Aids the body in healing lesions and eye injuries.

Warning: If symptoms persist, discontinue use.

ALSO: The herb eye bright may be used as a wash for superficial inflammations of the eye.

SINGLE HERBS: Bilberry, and Eyebright.

VITAMINS: A Multi-vitamin complex, plus A, B1, B2, B3, B5, B6, C D, and E.

MINERALS: Calcium, Copper, Manganese, Magnesium, Potassium, Selenium, and Zinc.

ALSO: Gyncydo, and Protein.

HELPFUL FOODS: Apples, citrus fruits, beets, rice bran, carrots, green leafy vegetables, herring, oysters, red meat, chicken, nuts, and soybeans.

NOCTURIA

SPECIFICS: The disturbance of a person's sleep by the need to pass urine. Common causes are infection, cystitis (inflammation of the bladder), and enlargement of the prostate gland (obstructs the normal outflow of urine and causes the bladder to empty incompletely). Rarer causes of nocturia include diabetes insipidus, diabetes mellitus, and chronic kidney failure.

(BeneficialRemedies,Treatments,andNutrients)

HERBAL COMBINATION: (KB).

PHYSIOLOGIC ACTION: Extremely valuable in healing and strengthening the kidneys, bladder, and genito-urinary area. Useful to stop bed-wetting, but is a diuretic when congestion of the kidneys is indicated. Helps remove bladder, uterine, and urethral toxins.

Warning: Intended for occasional use only. May cause green-yellow discoloration of urine.

SINGLE HERBS: Alfalfa, Barberry root, Catnip, Dandelion, Fennel, Ginger root, Goldenrod, Horsetail, Uva Ursi, and Wild Yam.

VITAMINS: A, B complex, C, D, E, and Choline.

MINERALS: Calcium, Magnesium, and Potassium.

ALSO: Digestive enzymes, Lecithin, L-Arginine, L-Methionine, Propolis, Uratonic, Watermelon, 3-way herb teas, and other Diuretic tablets.

HELPFUL FOODS: All vegetables, apples, bananas, broccoli, carrots, cheese and other dairy products, tuna, and fish liver oils, red meat, and sprouted seeds.

JUICES: Asparagus, black currant, cranberry, celery, juniper berry, parsley, and pomegranate juice.

NUTRITIONAL DISORDERS

SPECIFICS: Nutritional disorders are usually caused by a deficiency or excess of one or more of the elements of nutrition. Inadequate intake of protein and calories may occur in individuals that have an intense fear of becoming obese. Recent studies show that some nutritional disorders may be caused by a severe zinc deficiency. When trying to stimulate the appetite, consider the aroma and appearance of foods, as well as the nutritional value.

(BeneficialRemedies,Treatments,andNutrients)

SINGLE HERBS: Catnip, Fennel, Ginger, Ginseng, Gotu Kola, Kelp, Papaya, Peppermint, and Saw Palmetto.

VITAMINS: Multi-vitamins plus A, B12, B complex, D, and E.

MINERALS: Multi-minerals plus Potassium, Selenium, and Zinc.

ALSO: Acidophilus, Bio-Strath, Brewer's yeast, Liver, Protein, and Proteolytic enzymes.

HELPFUL FOODS: Butter, bran, beef, bananas, herring, sunflower seeds, soybeans, spinach, tuna, and nuts.

OBESITY

SPECIFICS: A person who has twenty percent excess body fat over the norm for their age, build, and height is considered obese. Losing weight is a matter of consciously regulating the types and amount of food eaten and increasing daily activity. Some hormonal disorders are accompanied by obesity, but the overwhelming majority of obese people do not suffer from such disorders.

(BeneficialRemedies,Treatments,andNutrients)

HERBAL COMBINATIONS: (SKC) or (Herbal Slim).

PHYSIOLOGIC ACTION: This effective formula cleanses the bowels and eliminates excess water. Helps control appetite, dissolves excess fat, reduces tension, stress, and anxiety associated with dieting.

SINGLE HERBS: Chickweed, Hawthorn Berries, Kelp, Licorice Root, Papaya Leaves, Saffron, and Yucca.

VITAMINS: B2, B5, B6, B12, B complex, C, E, Choline, Folic Acid, Inositol, and Pantothenic acid.

MINERALS: Calcium, Magnesium, and Phosphorus.

ALSO: Yu-ccan herbal drink, Lecithin, Protein, and Unsaturated fatty acids.

HELPFUL FOODS: Shell fish, white meat of chicken, tuna, citrus fruits, green leafy vegetables, and sprouted seeds.

JUICES: Beet greens, Celery, and Parsley juice.

OPTIC NEURITIS

SPECIFICS: Optic neuritis is the inflammation or deterioration of the optic nerve in the eye, causing gradual or sudden blurred vision. The eye may be painful and temporary blindness may occur in severe cases. The best treatment for optic neuritis is to make sure the patient gets rest and optimum nutrition.

(BeneficialRemedies,Treatments,andNutrients)

SINGLE HERBS: Black Cohosh, Lobelia, Lady Slipper, Skullcap, and Valerian Root.

VITAMINS: B1, B2, B6, B12, Niacin, and Pantothenic acid.

MINERALS: Mineral complex plus Calcium and Magnesium.

ALSO: Lecithin, Protein, and Proteolytic enzymes.

HELPFUL FOODS: All dairy products, beef, yellow corn, fruit, nuts, oat bran, and unpolished rice.

OSTEOARTHRITIS

SPECIFICS: Osteoarthritis is a degenerative joint disease involving the deterioration of the cartilage at the ends of the bones, causing the cartilage to become rough resulting in friction. This form of arthritis usually affects the weight bearing joints, such as the hips and knees.

(BeneficialRemedies,Treatments,andNutrients)

HERBAL COMBINATION: (Rheum-Aid) or (Yucca -AR).

PHYSIOLOGIC ACTION: Relieves symptoms associated with bursitis, calcification, gout, rheumatoid arthritis, rheumatism, and osteoarthritis. Helps the body reduce or eliminate swelling and inflammation in the joints and connective tissue. Also helps to relieve stiffness and pain.

SINGLE HERBS: Alfalfa, Black Cohosh, Burdock, Cayenne, Celery seed, Chaparral, Devil's Claw, Valerian root, and Yucca.

VITAMINS: Niacin, B5, B6, B12, B complex, C, D, E, F, and P.

MINERALS: A strong Multi-mineral complex plus Calcium and Magnesium.

ALSO: Cod liver oil, Green Magma, Aqua life, Seatone, Bromelain, Goats milk, and Mung beans.

HELPFUL FOODS: Almonds, apples, apricots, avocados, cherries, broccoli, soybeans, spinach, sprouted seeds, sweet potatoes, buckwheat, whole wheat, red meat, citrus fruit, and all dairy products.

JUICES: Cherry, papaya, and pineapple juice.

OSTEOMALACIA

SPECIFICS: A disease of malnutrition caused by a deficiency of calcium, phosphorus, and vitamin D. This causes the bones to become soft, resulting in deformities. It is most likely to occur at times of body stress, when pregnant, or breast feeding.

(BeneficialRemedies,Treatments,andNutrients)

SINGLE HERBS: Horsetail.

VITAMINS: A, B12, C, and D.

MINERALS: Calcium, Magnesium, and Phosphorus.

ALSO: Cod liver oil, Lecithin, Hydrochloric acid, Silica, and Digestive enzymes.

HELPFUL FOODS: Beef, butter, cheese, tuna, fish liver oils, green leafy vegetables, turnip greens, fruit(citrus and other), nuts, and sunflower seeds.

OSTEOPOROSIS (Brittle bones)

SPECIFICS: Osteoporosis is a gradual loss in the total mass of bone, leaving the remaining bone fragile or brittle. The major cause of osteoporosis is a calcium-phosphorus imbalance or an inability to absorb sufficient amounts of calcium through the intestine. The best prevention and treatment is a diet that is adequate in vitamin C and D, protein, calcium, magnesium, and phosphorus.

(BeneficialRemedies,Treatments,andNutrients)

SINGLE HERBS: Feverfew, Horsetail, and Oatstraw,

VITAMINS: B12, C, D, and E.

MINERALS: Calcium, Copper, Fluoride, Magnesium, and Phosphorus.

ALSO: L-Lysine, L-Arginine, Protein, Multidigestive enzymes with Betaine hydrochloride, and Proteolytic enzymes.

HELPFUL FOODS: All dairy products, red meats, chicken, sardines, tuna, herring, oysters, all fruit, soybeans, nuts, broccoli, corn, rice, and whole wheat.

OTITIS EXTERNA

SPECIFICS: The most common type of ear infection, also known as swimmers ear. This ailment is caused by generalized infection causing inflammation of the outer ear canal. Symptoms of the infection are fever, severe pain, and discharge from the ear.

(BeneficialRemedies,Treatments,andNutrients)

HERBAL COMBINATIONS: (ImmunAid) (B&B Extract) (EchinaGuard).

PHYSIOLOGIC ACTION: ImmunAid boosts immunity, thereby helping with ear infections. EchinaGuard is a liquid and Echinacea extract is excellent for small children with ear infections. B&B Extract can be placed in the ear or taken internally. It is also used to aid poor equilibrium, and nervous conditions.

SINGLE HERBS: Blue Cohosh, Echinacea, Garlic Oil, Garlic, Mullein Oil, Mullein, Skullcap, Sheep Sorrel, and St. John's Wort.

HOMEOPATHIC COMBINATION: Earache Formula.

VITAMINS: A, B complex, and C.

MINERALS: Calcium and Zinc.

ALSO: Canaid herbal drink, Propolis, Protein, and Primadophilus. When combating ear infections, it is imperative to exclude allergen foods from the diet. This is particularly true of all dairy products.

HELPFUL FOODS: Lean red meat, carrots, green vegetables, citrus fruits, fish liver oils, herring, oysters, sardines, nuts, sprouted seeds, and sunflower seeds.

PAIN (Headaches, Tension)

SPECIFICS: Pain is a localized sensation that can range from mild discomfort to an excruciating and unbearable experience. It is the result of stimulation of special sensory nerve endings usually following injury or caused by disease.

(Beneficial Remedies, Treatments, and Nutrients)

HERBAL COMBINATION: (A-P).

PHYSIOLOGIC ACTION: Helps relieve pain in any part of the body. A natural way to ease chronic pain, headaches, childbirth after-pains, aching teeth, nervous tension, spasms, and intestinal gas.

SINGLE HERBS: Pau d'Arco.

HOMEOPATHIC COMBINATION: Tension Headache Formula.

MINERALS: Calcium.

ALSO: DLPA (amino acid), and Lobelia.

HELPFUL FOODS: All dairy products, beef, cod liver oil, tuna, beets, broccoli, carrot, celery, peanuts, sunflower seeds, soybeans, and sprouted seeds.

JUICES: Carrot, celery, lettuce, and tomato juice.

PANCREATITIS

SPECIFICS: An inflammation of the pancreas, caused by an obstruction of the pancreatic duct from cancer scarring or stones. The pancreas secretes insulin and digestive enzymes, and for this reason pancreatitis often causes diabetes and digestive disorders.

(BeneficialRemedies,Treatments,andNutrients)

HERBAL COMBINATION: (PC).

PHYSIOLOGIC ACTION: Helps eliminate mucus and sedimentation, arrest infection, and stimulate and restore the natural functions of the pancreas. Also used for blood-sugar problems and healing the spleen.

SINGLE HERBS: Dandelion, Golden Seal, Juniper Berries, and Uva Ursi.

VITAMINS: A, B complex, C, E, Choline, and Inositol.

MINERALS: Chromium, Potassium, and Zinc.

ALSO: Coenzyme Q10, Germanium, Lecithin, Proteolytic enzymes, and Raw pancreas concentrate.

HELPFUL FOODS: All vegetables, vegetable oils, bananas, citrus fruits, herring, oysters, shellfish, fish liver oils, soybeans, and spinach.

JUICES: Beet root and radish juice.

PARASITES

SPECIFICS: Parasites live in the gastrointestinal tract. Early signs include diarrhea, loss of appetite, and rectal itching. If not eliminated they will result in the loss of weight, colon disorders, and anemia. Causes include ingestion of eggs or larvae from partially cooked meat, improper disposal of human waste, and walking barefoot on contaminated soil.

(BeneficialRemedies,Treatments,andNutrients)

HERBAL COMBINATIONS: (Para-X) (Para-VF).

PHYSIOLOGIC ACTION: Useful in destroying and eliminating parasites, such as worms. Also helps relieve many kinds of skin problems. The Para-VF is liquid and is useful for children and the elderly who cannot swallow capsules.

Warning: Do not use during pregnancy!

SINGLE HERBS: Black Walnut, Garlic, Pumpkin Seeds, Sage, Sheep Sorrel, Swedish Bitters, and Wormwood.

VITAMINS: Folic Acid.

MINERALS: A multi-mineral complex.

Children: Chamomile tea or raisins soaked in Senna tea for older children may be helpful.

HELPFUL FOODS: Asparagus, brewers yeast, broccoli, lettuce, lima beans, liver, mushrooms, nuts, and spinach.

PARKINSONS DISEASE

SPECIFICS: A degenerative disease affecting the nervous system that causes muscle tremor, stiffness, and weakness. The cause of the disease is unknown, but malnutrition is believed to be a major underlying factor. A low protein diet of raw, organic foods is best for patients with Parkinson's Disease.

(BeneficialRemedies,Treatments,andNutrients)

SINGLEHERBS: Ginseng, Damiana, and Cayenne

VITAMINS: B complex, plus B2, B6, C, and E.

MINERALS: Calcium Lactate, and Magnesium.

ALSO: Brewer's yeast, Lecithin, Multidigestive enzymes, L-Glutamic acid, and L-Tyrosine.

HELPFUL FOODS: Apples, apricots, cherries, grapes, citrus fruits, oat bran, broccoli, carrots, yellow corn, vegetable oils, and unpolished rice

PELLAGRA

SPECIFICS: A vitamin deficiency disease, caused by the long term shortage of B vitamins. A diet with niacin, thiamine, riboflavin, folic acid, and vitamin B12 will cure the disease.

(BeneficialRemedies,Treatments,andNutrients)

VITAMINS: B complex, plus extra B1, B2, B3, B12, and Folic acid.

MINERALS: Calcium and Zinc.

ALSO: Protein and Tryptophan.

HELPFUL FOODS: Avocados, bananas, broccoli, figs, legumes, nuts, potatoes, tomatoes, and prunes.

JUICES: Blackberry, grape, and parsley juice.

PEPTIC ULCERS

SPECIFICS:Peptic ulcers occur along the gastrointestinal tract and result when, during stress, the stomach is unable to secrete sufficient mucus, to protect against the strong acid essential for digestion. Symptoms of an ulcer are choking sensations, nausea, lower back pain, and stomach pain. Most ulcers are aggravated by the level of anxiety of the individual before eating.

(BeneficialRemedies,Treatments,andNutrients)

HERBAL COMBINATION: (Myrrh – Gold Seal Plus).

SINGLE HERBS: Cayenne (stomach ulcers only), Golden Seal, Myrrh, Pau d'Arco, Red Raspberry, Slippery Elm Bark, Valerian, and White Oak Bark.

VITAMINS: A, B complex, B2, B5, B6, B12, C, D, E, P, Choline, and Folic acid.

MINERALS: Calcium, Manganese, and Zinc,

ALSO: Acidophilus, Adrenal glandular extract, Bioflavonoids, Bromelain, Chlorophyll, Raw Cabbage, Glutamine, Goat's milk, Brewer's yeast, and Halibut oil.

Refer to "Digestive Disorders" in this manual.

HELPFUL FOODS: Avocados, bananas, green leafy vegetables, red meat, bacon, chicken, cheese, fish liver oils, vegetable oils, oat bran, and whole grains.

JUICES: Aloe Vera, celery, grapefruit, potato, and spinach juice.

PERIODONTITIS

SPECIFICS:Periodontitis(a gum disease) accounts for the loss of more teeth than cavities. Periodontitis is an inflammation of the bones and gums that surround and support the teeth. This disease is caused by improper cleaning of teeth and gums, poorly fitting dentures, loose fillings, or an inadequate diet.

(BeneficialRemedies,Treatments,andNutrients)

SINGLE HERBS: Chamomile, Echinacea, Lobelia, Myrrh Gum, and White Oak Bark.

VITAMINS: A, B complex, C, D, P, Niacin, and Folic Acid.

MINERALS: Calcium, Copper, Magnesium, Manganese, Phosphorus, Potassium, Silicon, Sodium, and Zinc.

ALSO: Coenzyme Q10, Protein, and Unsaturated fatty acids.

HELPFUL FOODS: Green leafy vegetables, nuts, oat bran, apples, apricots, bananas, citrus fruits, and seafood.

JUICES: Beet greens, celery, green kale, and parsley juice.

PERNICIOUS ANEMIA

SPECIFICS: Pernicious anemia is caused from a deficiency of the vitamin B12, which in turn causes the gradual reduction in the number of blood cells, because the bone marrow is unable to produce mature red blood cells. This disease may be fatal without treatment. A highly nutritious diet, supplemented with large amounts of desiccated liver, and B12 injections are the recommended treatment.

(BeneficialRemedies,Treatments,andNutrients)

VITAMINS: B complex, B1, B2, B12, Folic acid, Niacin, C, and E.

MINERALS: Cobalt, Copper, Iron, and Magnesium.

ALSO: Protein and L-Tryptophan.

HELPFUL FOODS: Apples, peaches, brewers yeast, citrus fruits, clams, eggs, kidney, soybeans, spinach, sweet potatoes, turnip greens, red meat, whole rye, and wheat.

JUICES: Grape juice.

PERTUSSIS
(refertoWhoopingCough)

PHLEBITIS

SPECIFICS: An Inflammation of the vein wall (usually found in the legs) and can be a complication of varicose veins. Prevention and treatment require a diet rich in vitamins B, C, and E, plus regular exercise.

(BeneficialRemedies,Treatments,andNutrients)

HERBAL COMBINATIONS: (H Formula) (Garlicin HC).

PHYSIOLOGIC ACTION: The herbs in these combinations are known to strengthen and support the cardiovascular system. Supplementing the body with niacin (B3) may be useful to help prevent clot formation. Vitamin C can help strengthen the blood vessel walls. Some research indicates that vitamin E may dilate the blood vessels, thus discouraging the formation of varicose veins and phlebitis.

SINGLE HERBS: Ginkgo, Horse Chestnut, and Yarrow.

VITAMINS: B complex, Niacin, Pantothenic acid, C, and E.

MINERALS: A multi-mineral complex.

HELPFUL FOODS: Beef, broccoli, fruit(citrus and other), nuts, green leafy vegetables, turnip greens, vegetable oils, and unpolished rice.

PILES
(refer to Hemorrhoids)

PINK EYE

SPECIFICS: A highly contagious inflammation of the mucous membrane that lines the eyelids. The most common cause of pink eye is a calcium deficiency, however allergies, bacteria, and a deficiency of vitamin A, B6, or riboflavin may cause pink eye symptoms.

(Beneficial Remedies, Treatments, and Nutrients)

HERBS: Hot compresses made from Chamomile or Fennel tea may be helpful for irritation.

VITAMINS: A, B2, B6, B complex, Niacin, C, and D.

MINERALS: Calcium, Magnesium, Phosphorus, and Zinc.

HELPFUL FOODS: Apricots, citrus fruits, cherries, beef, black molasses, broccoli, carrots, butter, cheese, shell fish, tuna, and whole wheat.

PINWORMS
(refer to Parasites)

PLEURITIS

SPECIFICS: A type of skin eruption characterized by tiny blisters that weep and crust. Chronic forms produce flaking, scaling, itching, and eventual thickening and color changes of the skin.

(Beneficial Remedies, Treatments, and Nutrients)

HERBAL COMBINATION: (AKN).

PHYSIOLOGIC ACTION: When toxins are not properly eliminated from the body, they may surface through the skin creating pleuritis.

This formula has been created to support liver and gall bladder function, to ensure toxins are filtered from the blood.

SINGLE HERBS: Aloe Vera, Chickweed, Evening Primrose Oil, Pau d'Arco, Red Clover, Thisilyn (Milk Thistle), and Yellow Dock.

VITAMINS: A, B2, B3, B5, B6, C, F, P, Biotin, and Paba.

MINERALS: Iron, Silicon, and Sulfur.

ALSO: Yu-ccan herbal drink, Whey powder, and Brewers yeast.

HELPFUL FOODS: Almonds, avocados, apricots, citrus fruits, red meat, seafood's, broccoli, carrots, radish, sweet potatoes, turnip greens, and fish liver oils.

PNEUMONIA

SPECIFICS: An inflammation in the lungs, characterized by the tiny air sacs in the lung area becoming inflamed and filled with mucus and pus. The primary causes of pneumonia are allergies, bacteria, chemical irritants, and viruses.

(Beneficial Remedies, Treatments, and Nutrients)

HERBAL COMBINATIONS: (Garlicin) (C+F) (Herbal Influence).

PHYSIOLOGIC ACTION: Proven herbal formulas to help relieve symptoms of colds, flu, hoarseness, colic, cramps, sluggish circulation, beginning of fevers, and germinal viral infections.

Herbal Influence (formerly known as Herbal Composition) was created by the early American herbalist, Samuel Thomson. It contains herbs which help with fever and nauseousness.

SINGLE HERBS: Boneset, Comfrey, EchinaGuard, Eucalyptus, Fenugreek, Licorice, & Mullein.

VITAMINS: A, B complex, Ester C with Bioflavonoids, E, K, and P.

MINERALS: Zinc.

ALSO: Coenzyme Q10, Germanium, L-Carnitine, L-Cysteine, Proteolytic enzymes, and Raw thymus extract.

HELPFUL FOODS: Apricots, citrus fruits, buckwheat, soybeans, nuts, broccoli, carrots, green leafy vegetables, garlic, kelp, herring, and oysters.

JUICES: Aloe Vera juice.

POISON IVY

SPECIFICS: If the sap of the poison ivy touches the skin, it can cause persistent itching, rash, swelling, and blistering in sensitive people. The following nutrients will help alleviate the symptoms.

(BeneficialRemedies,Treatments,andNutrients)

SINGLE HERBS: Echinacea, Goldenseal, and Lobelia.

VITAMINS: A, C, and E.

MINERALS: Zinc.

HELPFUL FOODS: Broccoli, carrots, citrus fruits, melon, fish liver oils, and vegetable oils.

POLIO

SPECIFICS: Polio is a virus infection of the spinal cord, which destroys the nerves controlling muscular movement. During the infectious stage, the rapid tissue destruction causes a depletion of protein and potassium.

(BeneficialRemedies,Treatments,andNutrients)

VITAMINS: A, B complex, and C.

MINERALS: Calcium, Magnesium, Potassium, and Sodium.

ALSO: Protein.

HELPFUL FOODS: Bacon, beef, chicken, cheese and other dairy products, eggs, seafood's, apples, bananas, citrus fruits, peanuts, and unpolished rice.

POLYMYALGIA RHEUMATICA

SPECIFICS: This disorder causes pain in the joints, stiffness of muscles, and minor aches and twinges

(BeneficialRemedies,Treatments,andNutrients)

HERBAL COMBINATIONS: (Yucca-AR) or (Rheum-Aid).

PHYSIOLOGIC ACTION: Excellent formulas for relieving symptoms associated with polymyalgia rheumatica. It helps to reduce or eliminate swelling, inflammation in joints, connective tissues, and relieves stiffness and pain.

SINGLE HERBS: Alfalfa, Chaparral, Cayenne, Fennel, Garlic, Pau d'Arco, Red Clover, Red Raspberry, and Yucca.

HOMEOPATHIC COMBINATION: Arthritis Pain Formula.

VITAMINS: B complex, B5, B15, C, and E.

MINERALS: Calcium, Magnesium, Phosphorus, Potassium, and Zinc.

ALSO: Digestive enzymes, Yu-ccan herbal drink, Hydrochloric acid, and Protein.

HELPFUL FOODS: Almonds, apricots, beef, butter, broccoli, buckwheat, all fruits, cheese, sardines, soybeans, spinach, safflower, goats milk, and mung beans.

POLYPS

SPECIFICS: Benign growths found on the epithelial lining of the cervix, bladder, or large intestine.

(BeneficialRemedies,Treatments,andNutrients)

SINGLE HERBS: Pau d'Arco.

VITAMINS: Multi-vitamin complex plus A, C, and E.

MINERALS: Calcium.

ALSO: Aerobic bulk cleanse, Coenzyme Q10, and Germanium.

HELPFUL FOODS: Carrots, citrus fruits, melon, oat bran, soybeans, green leafy vegetables, vegetable oils, dairy products, and garlic.

POOR CIRCULATION

SPECIFICS: There are many disorders associated with circulatory problems. The most common disease for sluggish circulation is Raynaud's Disease, characterized by constriction and spasm of the blood vessels in the limbs. Poor circulation can also result from varicose veins, caused by the loss of elasticity in the walls of the veins.

(BeneficialRemedies,Treatments,andNutrients)

HERBAL COMBINATIONS: (H Formula) (Ginkgold).

PHYSIOLOGIC ACTION: Contains herbs which strengthen the heart and build the vascular system. When taken with Cayenne, it improves circulation, giving a warming sensation to the entire body.

Note: Cayenne strengthens the pulse rate and circulation, while Black Cohosh slows it down.

SINGLE HERBS: Cayenne, Black Cohosh, Bayberry, Butchers Broom, Ginkgo, Hawthorn berries, Horsetail, Rose Hips, and Yarrow.

VITAMINS: A, B complex, B1, B3, B6, B12, C, and E.

MINERALS: Calcium, Magnesium, Potassium, and Zinc.

ALSO: Chlorophyll, Coenzyme Q10, Germanium, Lecithin, L-Carnitine, and Multidigestive enzymes.

HELPFUL FOODS: Apples, lean beef, broccoli, fruits(citrus and other),sprouted seeds, sunflower seeds, sweet potatoes, sardines, tuna, turnip greens, and yellow corn.

JUICES: Alfalfa, blackberry, beetroot, parsley, and pineapple juice.

POSTURAL HYPOTENSION
(refertoBloodPressureLow)

PREMENSTRUAL SYNDROME (PMS)

SPECIFICS: A disorder that effects menstruating women before the menstrual cycle begins. The most common causes are candidiasis, food allergies, hormone imbalance, fluid retention, and low blood sugar. Symptoms can include one or all of the following; depression, cramps, headache, changes in personality, nervousness, fatigue, insomnia, breast swelling, and bloated abdomen. The best prevention for PMS is a nutrient rich diet, supplemented with vitamins and minerals, plus a good exercise program.

(BeneficialRemedies,Treatments,andNutrients)

HERBAL COMBINATIONS: (FC) or (FEM-MEND).

PHYSIOLOGIC ACTION: Helps regulate the menstrual cycle, relieve cramps, bloating and vaginitis, ease inflammation of the vagina and uterus, and strengthen and regulate the kidneys, bladder and uterus areas. Beneficial for all female and uterine complaints.

Warning: Do not use this combination while taking estrogen or oral contraceptives!

SINGLE HERBS: Dong Quai, Kelp, Red Raspberry, and Uva Ursi.

HOMEOPATHIC COMBINATION: PMS Formula.

VITAMINS: B complex, B5, B6, B12, C, D, and E.

MINERALS: Calcium, Chlorine, Chromium, Iodine, Iron, Magnesium, and Manganese.

ALSO: Inositol, L-Lysine, L-Tyrosine, Methionine, Spirulina, and Primrose oil.

HELPFUL FOODS: All vegetables and vegetable oils, fish and fish liver oils, cheese, butter, apples, bananas, citrus fruits, and mushrooms.

PRE-NATAL PREPARATION

SPECIFICS: Pre-natal preparation includes involves regular tests on the woman and the fetus to detect defects, disease, or potential hazards, and advising the woman on the general aspects of pregnancy , such as a well balanced diet and exercise, with the aim of making sure that the baby and mother are healthy at delivery.

(BeneficialRemedies,Treatments,andNutrients)

HERBAL COMBINATION: (Healthy Greens).

PHYSIOLOGIC ACTION: A complete combination of vitamins and minerals containing digestive aids to ensure proper assimilation.

SINGLE HERBS: Blessed Thistle, Chamomile, Chlorella, Lobelia, and Red Raspberry.

VITAMINS: A, B complex, B12, C, D, and E.

MINERALS: A multi-mineral complex, plus Calcium, Magnesium, and Phosphorus.

ALSO: Bone meal, brewer's yeast, and kelp.

HELPFUL FOODS: All fruits (citrus and other), all dairy products, carrots, corn, soybeans, spinach, sprouted seeds, sweet potatoes, nuts, tuna, and red meat.

PRESBYOPIA

SPECIFICS: Presbyopia is one of the leading causes of decreased visual acuity in the elderly. This condition is characterized by the eye lens becoming less flexible. Poor nutrition will accelerate the deterioration of your eyes. Improved nutrition will not reverse the condition but it will slow the progress of this ailment. Consumption of saturated fats, white sugar, and refined carbohydrates should be avoided.

(BeneficialRemedies,Treatments,andNutrients)

SINGLE HERBS: Gingko Biloba, Bilberry, and Hawthorn.

VITAMINS: A, Beta-carotene, C, and E.

MINERALS: Selenium and Zinc.

ALSO: Bioflavonoids, Omega-3, and Omega-6.

HELPFUL FOODS: Broccoli, carrots, citrus fruits, garlic, strawberries, vegetable oils, and fish liver oils.

PROLAPSUS

SPECIFICS:The displacement of all or part of an organ or tissue from its normal position. This condition is caused by weakening and slackness of the various muscles, ligaments, and connective tissues.

(BeneficialRemedies,Treatments,andNutrients)

HERBAL COMBINATION: (Yellow dock Combination).

PHYSIOLOGIC ACTION: Helps revitalize a prolapsed uterus, kidneys, and bowel. It also has been proven effective for hemorrhoids, colitis, and as a good purifier.

SINGLE HERBS: Black Walnut hull, Calendula flower, Marshmallow root, Mullein, White Oak bark, and Yellow Dock root.

HELPFUL JUICES: Beet root, black cherry, carrot, celery, cucumber, and radish juice.

PROSTATE and KIDNEY DISORDERS

SPECIFICS:Prostatitis is the inflammation of the prostrate gland, that is usually caused in older males by a gradual enlargement over a period of years, and in younger men by a bacterial infection from another area of the body, which has invaded the prostate. Prostatitis can partially or totally block the flow of urine, resulting in urine retention. Symptoms of prostatitis are fever, frequent urination accompanied by a burning sensation, pain between the scrotum and rectum, and blood or pus in the urine. Treatment consists of regularity in sexual habits, the following nutrients, and lots of walking and other exercise.

(BeneficialRemedies,Treatments,andNutrients)

HERBAL COMBINATION: (PR).

PHYSIOLOGIC ACTION: This formula helps cleanse sedimentation and arrest infection in the prostate and dissolve kidney stones to restore these glands to the natural functions.

SINGLE HERBS: Cayenne, Bee Pollen, Garlic, Golden Seal, Juniper Berries, Siberian Ginseng, and Uva Ursi.

Note: ProActive is an herbal extract of Saw Palmetto.

VITAMINS: A, B complex, B6, C, E, and F.

MINERALS: Calcium, Magnesium, and Zinc.

ALSO: Bee pollen, Brewer's yeast, Essential fatty acids, Lecithin, and Pumpkin seeds.

HELPFUL FOODS: All vegetables, apples, bananas, broccoli, carrots, cheese and other dairy products, tuna, and fish liver oils, red meat, and sprouted seeds.

JUICES: Black currant, celery, and pomegranate juice.

PRURITUS ANI

SPECIFICS: A form of contact dermatitis, characterized by a burning sensation and itching of the rectum. Pruritus is associated with a deficiency of vitamins A, B complex, and Iron.

(BeneficialRemedies,Treatments,andNutrients)

VITAMINS: A and B complex.

MINERALS: Iron.

ALSO: Acidophilus.

HELPFUL FOODS: Black molasses, brewers yeast, fish liver oils, vegetable oils, and red meat.

PSORIASIS

SPECIFICS: A hereditary disease that appears as patches of silvery scales or red areas on limbs, ears, and back. Attacks are triggered by inadequate diet, illness, viral and bacterial infection, sunburn, nervous tension, and stress. Since diet and stress are key factors in this skin disorder, certain allergen foods need to be completely avoided. Dairy products and wheat are especially harmful in many instances. Fat should be kept to a minimum.

(BeneficialRemedies,Treatments,andNutrients)

HERBAL COMBINATIONS: (AKN) (Evening Primrose) (Thisilyn).

PHYSIOLOGIC ACTION: The above herbs taken in combination has a dramatic effect on this disorder.

SINGLE HERBS: Chickweed, Dandelion, Goldenseal, Kelp, Lobelia, Skullcap, St. Johns Wort, and Yellow dock.

VITAMINS: A, B5, B6, B12, B complex, C, D, E, and Folic Acid.

MINERALS: Calcium, Magnesium, Sulfur ointment, and Zinc.

ALSO: Lecithin, Lipotropic factors, Proteolytic enzymes, and Unsaturated fatty acids.

HELPFUL FOODS: Apples, apricots, cherries, grapes, citrus fruits, all vegetables, beef, chicken, herring, oysters, tuna, salmon, and sardines.

EDEMA

SPECIFICS: Pulmonary edema is a fluid accumulation in the lungs. This ailment is usually caused left-sided heart failure, which results a in back-pressure of fluid in the lungs. Pulmonary edema may also be caused by allergies, chest infection, inhalation of irritant gases, or to any of the causes of generalized edema.

(BeneficialRemedies,Treatments,andNutrients)

HERBAL COMBINATION: (KB).

PHYSIOLOGIC ACTION: KB acts as a mild diuretic to rid the lungs of excessive water.

SINGLE HERBS: Alfalfa, Buchu, Dandelion tea, Juniper, lobelia, Parsley, Pau d'Arco tea, Safflower, Uva Ursi, and Yarrow.

VITAMINS: B1, B6, B complex, C, D, and E.

MINERALS: Calcium, Copper, and Potassium.

ALSO: L-Taurine, #9 and #11 tissue salts, Silicon, low Sodium, and Protein.

HELPFUL FOODS: Fruit(citrus and other), beef, butter, cheese, egg whites, seafood, fish liver oils, broccoli, spinach, flax seed, and sunflower seeds.

PYORRHEA

SPECIFICS: An infectious disease of the gums and tooth sockets. This disease is characterized by the loosening of the teeth, the formation of pus, and tender or sore gums.

(BeneficialRemedies,Treatments,andNutrients)

SINGLE HERBS: Golden Seal and Myrrh.

PHYSIOLOGIC ACTION: Use these powders on tooth brush, or make a tea, which is one teaspoon of each the Golden Seal and Myrrh, in one pint of boiling water. Steep. Rinse mouth and gargle with it freely, also, brush gums with the tea.

VITAMINS: A, B complex, B1, B2, B6, B12, C, D, and E.

MINERALS: Calcium, Magnesium, and Zinc.

ALSO: Protein. Also rub the gums, morning and evening, with vitamin E.

HELPFUL FOODS: Apples, citrus fruits, broccoli, carrots, green leafy vegetables, soybeans, sprouted seeds, seafood, red meat, and fish liver oils.

QUINSY

SPECIFICS: An abscess around the tonsil occurring as a complication of tonsillitis. The most effective prevention and treatment for tonsillitis and quinsy is a proper diet, high in vitamins, minerals, and protein.

(BeneficialRemedies,Treatments,andNutrients)

HERBAL COMBINATION: (IF) (IGL).

PHYSIOLOGIC ACTION: Effective formulas that help cleanse toxins, combat infections, and reduce infection. Especially effective for healing the lymphatic system.

SINGLE HERBS: Bayberry Root, Echina Guard, Echinacea, Ginger Root and Pau d'Arco.

VITAMINS AND MINERALS: A complete, one a day multi complex.

ALSO: Canaid herbal drink.

HELPFUL FOODS: Beef, broccoli, fruit(citrus and other), nuts, soybeans, spinach, sweet potatoes, turnip greens, unpolished rice, and whole grains.

RAYNAUD'S DISEASE

SPECIFICS: The most common disease for sluggish circulation is Raynaud's disease, characterized by constriction and spasm of the blood vessels in the limbs, resulting in hands and feet that are hypersensitive to the cold.

(BeneficialRemedies,Treatments,andNutrients)

HERBAL COMBINATIONS: (H Formula) (Ginkgold).

PHYSIOLOGIC ACTION: Contains herbs which strengthen the heart and build the vascular system. When taken with Cayenne, it improves circulation, giving a warming sensation to the entire body.

SINGLE HERBS: Cayenne, Bayberry, Butchers Broom, Garlic, Ginkgo Biloba, Pau d'Arco, and Yarrow.

VITAMINS: A, B3, B6, C, and E.

MINERALS: Calcium, Magnesium, and Potassium.

ALSO: Chlorophyll, Coenzyme Q10, Germanium, and Lecithin.

HELPFUL FOODS: Brewers yeast, broccoli, carrots, kelp, soybeans, sunflower seeds, white meat of poultry, and vegetable oils.

RENAL CALCULI
(refer to Kidney and Bladder Stones)

RESTLESS LEG SYNDROME

SPECIFICS: Characterized by unpleasant burning, prickling, tickling, or aching sensations in the muscles of the legs. Symptoms are most common during prolonged sitting or at night in bed. This ailment is most likely to occur in individuals that who consume large amounts of coffee, heavy smokers, and people with rheumatoid arthritis.

(Beneficial Remedies, Treatments, and Nutrients)

SINGLE HERBS: Alfalfa, Black Cohosh, Burdock, Cayenne, Celery seed, Chaparral, Devil's Claw, Valerian root, and Yucca.

HOMEOPATHIC COMBINATION: Arthritis Pain Formula.

VITAMINS: Niacin, B5, B6, B12, B complex, C, E, and Folic acid.

MINERALS: A strong Multi-mineral complex, plus Calcium, Magnesium, and Potassium.

ALSO: Cod liver oil, Green Magma, Aqua life, Seatone, and Omega-3 oils..

HELPFUL FOODS: Almonds, apricots, beef, butter, broccoli, buckwheat, all fruits, cheese, sardines, soybeans, spinach, sprouts, safflower, goats milk, and peanuts.

JUICES: Parsley and celery juice; cherry and pineapple juice.

RHEUMATIC FEVER

SPECIFICS: Rheumatic fever is an infection, caused by streptococcal bacteria. It most often effects children aged three to eighteen. A salt restricted diet, containing bioflavonoids and all essential nutrients has been found valuable for treating and preventing rheumatic fever.

(Beneficial Remedies, Treatments, and Nutrients)

SINGLE HERBS: Birch leaves, Catnip, Dandelion, Fenugreek, Garlic, Lobelia, and Thyme.

VITAMINS: A, B2, B6, B complex C, D, and E.

MINERALS: Zinc.

ALSO: Bioflavonoids, Coenzyme Q10, Germanium, Primadophilus, Protein, and Proteolytic enzymes.

HELPFUL FOODS: Beef, chicken, oysters, herring, tuna, carrots, green leafy vegetables, fruit(citrus and other), soybeans, sprouted seeds, and whole wheat.

JUICES: Aloe Vera and citrus juices.

RHEUMATISM

SPECIFICS: Rheumatism is a general term referring to pain in the joints and stiffness of muscles.

(BeneficialRemedies,Treatments,andNutrients)

HERBAL COMBINATIONS: (Yucca-AR) or (Rheum-Aid).

PHYSIOLOGIC ACTION: Excellent formulas for relieving symptoms associated with bursitis, calcification, gout, rheumatoid arthritis, rheumatism, and osteoarthritis. It helps to reduce or eliminate swelling, inflammation in joints, connective tissues, and relieves stiffness and pain.

SINGLE HERBS: Alfalfa, Chaparral, Cayenne, Fennel, Garlic, Pau d'Arco, Red Clover, Red Raspberry, and Yucca.

HOMEOPATHIC COMBINATION: Arthritis Pain Formula.

VITAMINS: B complex, B5, B15, C, and E.

MINERALS: Calcium, Magnesium, Phosphorus, Potassium, and Zinc.

ALSO: Digestive enzymes, Yu-ccan herbal drink, Hydrochloric acid, and Protein.

HELPFUL FOODS: Almonds, apricots, beef, butter, broccoli, buckwheat, all fruits, cheese, sardines, soybeans, spinach, safflower, goats milk, and mung beans.

JUICES: Cucumber, parsley and celery juice; cherry and pineapple juice.

RICKETS

SPECIFICS: A disease of malnutrition caused by a deficiency of calcium, phosphorus, and vitamin D. This causes the bones to become soft, resulting in deformities.

(BeneficialRemedies,Treatments,andNutrients)

SINGLE HERBS: Horsetail.

VITAMINS: A, B12, C, and D.

MINERALS: Calcium, Magnesium, and Phosphorus.

ALSO: Cod liver oil, Lecithin, Hydrochloric acid, Silica, and Digestive enzymes.

HELPFUL FOODS: Apples, citrus fruits, melon, cheese and other dairy products, beef, chicken, seafood's, all vegetables, nuts, and sunflower seeds.

JUICES: Dandelion and orange juice.

RINGING IN EARS
(refer to Tinnitus)

RINGWORM

SPECIFICS: A highly contagious, yeast-like, fungal infection, that lives off dead skin cells. Ring worm victims should eat a well-balanced diet, supplemented by megadoses of vitamins A, B, and C.

(Beneficial Remedies, Treatments, and Nutrients)

HERBAL COMBINATION: (Black Walnut extract).

PHYSIOLOGIC ACTION: High in organic iodine, this herb has proven effective against fungal infections such as ringworm and athletes foot.

SINGLE HERBS: Black Walnut, Golden Seal, and Pau d'Arco.

VITAMINS: A, B complex, and C.

MINERALS: Zinc.

ALSO: Acidophilus, Caprinex (caprylic acid), Germanium, and Unsaturated fatty acids. Rub skin with Black Walnut extract, Apple Cider Vinegar or Castor Oil, several times a day.

HELPFUL FOODS: Egg yolk, apricot, citrus fruits, beef kidney, beef liver, vegetable and fish oils.

ROUNDWORMS

SPECIFICS: Roundworms live in the gastrointestinal tract. Early signs include diarrhea, loss of appetite, and rectal itching. If not eliminated they will result in the loss of weight, colon disorders, and anemia. Causes include ingestion of eggs or larvae from partially cooked meat, improper disposal of human waste, and walking barefoot on contaminated soil.

(Beneficial Remedies, Treatments, and Nutrients)

HERBAL COMBINATIONS: (Para-X) (Para-VF).

PHYSIOLOGIC ACTION: Useful in destroying and eliminating parasites, such as worms. Also helps relieve many kinds of skin problems. The Para-VF is a liquid and is useful for children and the elderly who cannot swallow capsules.

Warning: Do not use during pregnancy!

SINGLE HERBS: Black Walnut, Garlic, Pumpkin Seeds, Sage, Sheep Sorrel, Swedish Bitters and Wormwood.

VITAMINS: Folic Acid.

MINERALS: Multi-mineral complex.

Children: Chamomile tea or raisins soaked in Senna tea, for older children, may be helpful.

HELPFUL FOODS: Asparagus, brewers yeast, broccoli, lettuce, lima beans, liver, mushrooms, nuts, and spinach.

RUBELLA
(refer to Measles)

SCARS
(refer to Skin Problems)

SCIATICA

SPECIFICS: Sciatica refers to painful spasms along the sciatic nerve which runs from the back of the thigh, down the inside of the leg to the ankle. Causes of sciatica are ruptured discs or sprained joints in the lower back, inflammation of sciatic nerve, or neuritis.

(Beneficial Remedies, Treatments, and Nutrients)

SINGLE HERBS: Pau d'Arco.

VITAMINS: B1, B12, B complex, D, and E.

MINERALS: Multi-mineral.

HELPFUL FOODS: Beef, tuna, butter, cheese, vegetable oils, sprouted seeds, soybeans, and sunflower seeds.

SCURVY

SPECIFICS: A malnutrition disease caused by vitamin D deficiency. A well-balanced diet, high in calcium, iron, protein, and vitamin D is recommended.

(BeneficialRemedies,Treatments,andNutrients)

VITAMINS: A, B complex, C, and D.

MINERALS: Calcium, Iron, and Magnesium.

ALSO: Protein.

HELPFUL FOODS: Broccoli, carrots, green leafy vegetables, citrus fruits, apples, apricots, cherries, grapes, pineapple, and turnip greens.

SEBORRHEA

SPECIFICS: Seborrhea is a disorder of the glands that secrete oil (sebaceous glands). This disease is, nearly always, caused by a nutrient deficiency.

(BeneficialRemedies,Treatments,andNutrients)

SINGLE HERBS: Chaparral, Dandelion, Goldenseal, and Red Clover.

VITAMINS: A, B complex, B6, and E.

MINERALS: Multi-mineral complex.

ALSO: Acidophilus, Coenzyme Q10, Lecithin, Protein supplement, and Unsaturated fatty acids.

HELPFUL FOODS: Carrots, green leafy vegetables, turnip greens, vegetable oils, fish liver oils, beef, all fruits, soybeans, nuts, and unpolished rice.

JUICES: Carrot, tomato, and pineapple juice.

SEBORRHEIC DERMATITIS

SPECIFICS: A red, scaly, itchy rash that develops on the back, chest, face, and chest.

(BeneficialRemedies,Treatments,andNutrients)

HERBAL COMBINATION: (AKN).

PHYSIOLOGIC ACTION: Many skin problems are related to liver dysfunction. This formula gives support to the liver, helps to cleanse the blood, and supplies nutrients for the skin.

SINGLE HERBS: Aloe Vera (on skin), Burdock, Cleavers, Dandelion, Evening Primrose, Garlic, Golden Seal, Pau d'Arco, Yellowdock, and Yucca.

VITAMINS: A, B complex, B2, B3, B6, D, E, and Biotin B complex.

MINERALS: Sulfur ointment, Potassium, and Zinc.

ALSO: Yu-ccan herbal drink, and Protein.

SEIZURES
(refer to Epilepsy)

SENILITY

SPECIFICS: Senility occurs in old age and is usually caused by cerebral dysfunction, nervous disturbances, and strokes.

(Beneficial Remedies, Treatments, and Nutrients)

HERBAL COMBINATIONS: (SEN) or (Remem).

PHYSIOLOGIC ACTION: An excellent combination to nourish the brain cells and tissues. Improves their ability to perform mental functions.

Note: Often a nutritional deficiency is the cause.

SINGLE HERBS: Dandelion, Ginkgo, Ginseng, Gotu Kola, Licorice, and Yellow Dock.

VITAMINS: A, B3, B complex, C, and E.

MINERALS: Choline and Zinc.

ALSO: Coenzyme Q10, Germanium, Lecithin, and Protein.

HELPFUL FOODS: Aloe Vera, avocados, citrus fruits, broccoli, carrots, garlic, olives, soybeans, spinach, sweet potatoes, whole wheat, oat bran, herring, and oysters.

JUICES: Carrot, celery, and prune juice.

SHINGLES (Herpes Zoster)

SPECIFICS: Shingles is an infection caused by a virus of the nerve endings in the skin. It usually occurs on the skin of the abdomen under the ribs. If shingles develop near the eyes, the cornea may become affected, causing blindness. B vitamins are necessary for the proper functioning of the nerves. Vitamins A and C promote healing of skin lesions and heavy doses of vitamin C can limit infection of lesions.

(Beneficial Remedies, Treatments, and Nutrients)

SINGLE HERBS: Yucca.

VITAMINS: A, B1, B6, B12, B complex, C, and D.

MINERALS: Calcium and Magnesium.

ALSO: L-Lysine and Protein.

HELPFUL FOODS: Red meat, butter, cheese, fruit(citrus and other), vegetable oils, nuts, sprouted seeds, and tuna.

SICKLE - CELL ANEMIA

SPECIFICS: Sickle-cell anemia is caused from a deficiency of folic acid, which in turn causes the red blood cells to become bent (sickled) and hard, clogging the circulatory system, depriving the body tissues of oxygen.
The recommended treatment is a highly nutritious diet, supplemented with large amounts of desiccated liver, vitamin C, and folic acid.

(BeneficialRemedies,Treatments,andNutrients)

VITAMINS: B complex, B1, B2, B12, Folic acid, Niacin, C, and E.

MINERALS: Cobalt, Copper, Iron, and Magnesium.

ALSO: Protein and L-Tryptophan.

HELPFUL FOODS: Citrus fruits, apples, red meat, clams, kidney, soybeans, spinach, sweet potatoes, whole wheat, and whole rye.

JUICES: Asparagus, lettuce, lima beans, spinach, and deep green vegetable juices.

SINUSITIS

SPECIFICS: Sinusitis is an inflammation of one or more of the nasal sinus cavities, that accompanies upper respiratory infection. Sinusitis may be the result of colds or viral and bacterial infections of the nose, throat, and upper respiratory tract.

(BeneficialRemedies,Treatments,andNutrients)

HERBAL COMBINATIONS: (HAS) (Zand Decongest Herbal Formula) (Garlicin CF) (Fenu-Thyme) (Sinustop).

PHYSIOLOGIC ACTION: Promote sinus drainage and shrink swollen membranes. The above are all recommended natural sinus decongestants that help relieve nasal congestion and pressure associated with sinusitis.

SINGLE HERBS: Anis, Comfrey, Elderberry, Eyebright, Fenugreek, Golden Seal, Horehound, Lobelia, Marshmallow, Mullein, Red Clover, and Rose Hips.

HOMEOPATHIC COMBINATION: Sinusitis Formula.

VITAMINS: A, B complex, B5, C, and E.

MINERALS: Potassium and Zinc.

ALSO: Bee Pollen, Coenzyme Q10, Garlic capsules, Germanium, Protein, and Proteolytic enzymes.

HELPFUL FOODS: Apples, citrus fruit, celery, herring, oysters, and turnip greens.

JUICES: Lemon juice with a little horseradish.

<u>SKIN</u> (Bites, Stings, and Poisons)

SPECIFICS: More people die from bee stings than from poisonous bites. People with known allergies to bites or stings should carry vitamin C with them; if bitten take large amounts of C immediately and frequently thereafter.

(BeneficialRemedies,Treatments,andNutrients)

HERBAL COMBINATION: (EchinaGuard).

PHYSIOLOGIC ACTION: Echinacea was used by the Plains Indians to lessen the effects of poisonous bites. EchinaGuard would be very beneficial. Take large doses of vitamin C and Calcium. Use vitamin E topically to reduce pain.

SINGLE HERBS: Echinacea.

VITAMINS: Multi-vitamin complex.

MINERALS: Mineral complex.

HELPFUL FOODS: Broccoli, cauliflower, tomatoes, dark leafy vegetables, apples, black currants, citrus fruits, almonds, sesame seeds, sardines, and salmon.

<u>SKIN</u> (Acne, Pimples, etc.)

SPECIFICS: A disorder of the oil(sebaceous) glands in the skin. It is believed that stress is a significant factor in acne. Other factors that contribute to acne and pimples are allergies, heredity, oral contraceptives, overindulgence in carbohydrates, foods with high fat or sugar content, and androgens(male hormones) produced in increased amounts when the girl or boy reaches puberty.

(BeneficialRemedies,Treatments,andNutrients)

SINGLE HERBS: Hautex, and Yucca.

PHYSIOLOGIC ACTION: To work from within to encourage skin secretion, effective for acne, blackheads, pimples, itch, and rash.

VITAMINS: A, B complex, E, and C with Rosehips.

MINERALS: Calcium and Zinc.

ALSO: Yu-ccan herbal drink, Efamol, Whey Powder, and Acidophilus.

HELPFUL FOODS: Avocados, bananas, broccoli, lean beef, carrots, celery, fruits (citrus and other), green leafy vegetables, pumpkin, radish, and vegetable oils.

SKIN BLEMISHES

SPECIFICS: A small circumscribed alteration of the skin considered to be unesthetic but insignificant.

(Beneficial Remedies, Treatments, and Nutrients)

HERBAL COMBINATION: (AKN).

PHYSIOLOGIC ACTION: AKN helps cleanse the bloodstream. Pimples, blackheads, and other superficial skin eruptions, and more serious conditions such as boils, carbuncles, dermatitis, eczema, and pleuritis will be eliminated when the blood has been cleansed.

VITAMINS: A, B2, B3, B5, B6, C, F, P, Biotin, and Paba.

MINERALS: Iron, Silicon, and Sulfur.

ALSO: Whey Powder and Brewers Yeast.

HELPFUL FOODS: Almonds, apricots, avocados, citrus fruits, fish liver oils, carrots, radish, sweet potatoes, green leafy vegetables, vegetable oils, and flax seed.

SKIN CANCER
(refer to Melanoma)

SKIN PROBLEMS
(BeneficialRemedies,Treatments,andNutrients)

AgeSpots-B complex, B5, C, Lactobacillus bulgaricus.

Dry Skin — Chamomile, Dandelion, Lavender, Peppermint, Oat Extract, Evening Primrose Oil, Vitamin A, B complex, C, and Aloe Vera. Add Herbal oils to bath (Lavender oil is very nice).

ItchySkin — Chickweed, Calendula, Elder, Yarrow, vegetable oil daily, and apple cider vinegar to bath. X-Itch ointment is also very effective.

Oily Skin — Vitamin B complex, Liver, Lemon Grass, Licorice root, Rosemary, and Rose buds.

Scars — Vitamin E orally and topically.

Stretchmarks — Vitamin E, B complex, B5, C, Aloe Vera, Zinc, and Carnation oil.

Sunburn — B vitamins, Paba, C, E, Calcium, Zinc, and Aloe Vera.

Wrinkles — Vitamins A, B complex, E, Zinc, Selenium, and Almond oil.

SMOKING

SPECIFICS: Tobacco smoke contains over 3,700 compounds, most are toxic and many are carcinogenic. 90% of lung cancer is due to smoking and over 30% of all cancer deaths can be attributed to smoking. The risk of developing lung cancer begins to deminish as soon as smoking is stopped.

(BeneficialRemedies,Treatments,andNutrients)

HERBAL COMBINATIONS: (Milk thistle extract) or (Thisilyn).

PHYSIOLOGIC ACTION: The herbal combination decreases the desire for tobacco and protects the liver from the negative effects of smoking. Vitamins and minerals should be taken to rebuild the nutritional system after a juice fast. The juice fast cleanses the accumulated poisons from the body, thus eliminating the physiological dependence.

Note: Tobacco, alcohol, caffeine, and other drug "cravings" are brought about by a physiological body dependence on the poison which develops during prolonged use. The addicts blood poison level must remain at a certain level at all times. As the poison level drops, there is a "desire" to take in more of the drug, to bring the level back again.

(BeneficialRemedies,Treatments,andNutrients)

SINGLE HERBS: Catnip, Chaparral, Hops, Licorice, Lobelia, Skullcap, Slippery Elm, and Valerian.
VITAMINS AND MINERALS: All.
AMINO ACIDS: L- Cysteine, L- Cystine, and L- Methionine.
ALSO: Coenzyme Q10, Germanium, and Raw thymus.
Fasting: Drink juice only.

SNAKE BITE

SPECIFICS: All snake bite victims should remain as still as possible and should be seen by a doctor immediately. After seeing a doctor the following supplements will help alleviate pain and symptoms.

(BeneficialRemedies,Treatments,andNutrients)

SINGLE HERBS: Echinacea, and Yellow dock.
VITAMINS: B5, and C.
MINERALS: Calcium.
HELPFUL FOODS: Brewers yeast, egg yolk, liver, rosehips, strawberries, and wheat germ.

SPASTIC COLON
(refer to Colitis)

SPIDER AND SCORPION BITE

SPECIFICS: Rattlesnake and black widow venom are almost the same so should be treated similarly. Rid the body of as much poison as possible by encouraging bleeding and see your doctor immediately. After seeing a doctor the following supplements will help alleviate pain and symptoms.

(BeneficialRemedies,Treatments,andNutrients)

SINGLE HERBS: Echinacea and Yellow dock.
VITAMINS: B5 and C.
MINERALS: Calcium.
ALSO: Apply Comfrey or Plantain salve.
HELPFUL FOODS: Same as snake bite.

SPONDYLITIS

SPECIFICS: Inflammation of the joints between the vertebrae in the spine. usually caused by osteoasthritis or rheumatoid arthritis. In rare cases it is caused by a bacterial infection that has spread from another area of the body.

(BeneficialRemedies,Treatments,andNutrients)

HERBAL COMBINATION: (Rheum-Aid) or (Yucca -AR).

PHYSIOLOGIC ACTION: Relieves symptoms associated with bursitis, calcification, gout, rheumatoid arthritis, rheumatism, and osteoarthritis. Helps the body reduce or eliminate swelling and inflammation in the joints and connective tissue and helps to relieve stiffness and pain.

SINGLE HERBS: Alfalfa, Black Cohosh, Burdock, Cayenne, Celery seed, Chaparral, Devil's Claw, Valerian root, and Yucca.

HOMEOPATHIC COMBINATION: Arthritis Pain Formula.

VITAMINS: Niacin, B5, B6, B12, B complex, C, D, E, F, and P.

MINERALS: A strong Multi-mineral complex, plus Calcium, and Magnesium.

ALSO: Cod liver oil, Yu-ccan herbal drink, Green Magma, Aqua life, Seatone, and Bromelain.

HELPFUL FOODS: Almonds, apricots, beef, butter, broccoli, buckwheat, all fruits, cheese, sardines, soybeans, spinach, safflower, goats milk, and mung beans.

JUICES: Parsley and celery juice; cherry and pineapple juice.

SPRAIN

SPECIFICS: If a person stresses a muscle beyond its capability the ligament connecting the bone to the muscle may tear causing a sprain. A well-balanced diet that is high in protein and the following supplement program will help these injuries heal.

(BeneficialRemedies,Treatments,andNutrients)

HERBAL COMBINATION: (B F + C)

PHYSIOLOGIC ACTION: A special formula to aid in healing processes for torn cartilage's and ligaments.

SINGLE HERBS: White Oak Bark, Comfrey Root, Black Walnut Hulls, Lobelia, Skullcap and Yucca.

HOMEOPATHIC COMBINATION: Injury and Backache Formula.

VITAMINS: B complex, B5, B6, B12, C, and E.

MINERALS: A complete multi-mineral one a day, (time released).

ALSO: Bee pollen, Coenzyme Q10, Germanium, L-Arginine, L-Carnitine, L-Lysine, Green-Lipped Mussel, Liver, Protein, Proteolytic enzymes, Silica, and Unsaturated fatty acids.

HELPFUL FOODS: Beef, fruits, nuts, unpolished rice, soybeans, spinach, vegetable oils, liver, and whole wheat.

STASIS ULCER
(refer to Leg Ulcers)

STRETCH MARKS
(refer to Skin Problems)

STRESS

SPECIFICS: The body can handle some stress, but long term stress causes the body to break down. Long term stress occurs when the situation that causes anxiety is not relieved. Find the cause and handle it constructively. People experiencing stress should maintain a well-balanced diet and replace the nutrients depleted during stress.

(Beneficial Remedies, Treatments, and Nutrients)

HERBAL COMBINATIONS: (Calm aid) (Ex stress) (Kalmin extract).

PHYSIOLOGIC ACTION: Special formulas for insomnia and stress related conditions. Relieve nervous tension, rebuilds nerve sheaths. Soothing and calming effect on the whole nervous system.

SINGLE HERBS: Black Cohosh Root, Cayenne, Lady's Slipper, Skullcap, Valerian Root, and Yucca.

VITAMINS: A, all B's, C, D, E, Paba, Folic Acid, and Choline.

MINERALS: Calcium, Chromium, Copper, Iron, Selenium, and Zinc.

ALSO: L-Tyrosine and Protein.

HELPFUL FOODS: Dulse, flax seed, sea salt, fruit(citrus and other), bacon, beef, chicken, all dairy products, all vegetables, mushrooms, and whole rye.

JUICES: Carrot, celery, lettuce, tomato, and prune juice.

STROKE

SPECIFICS: When the blood supply is cut off to an area of brain cells, resulting in the death of the deprived cells. Emphasis should be placed on the reduction of being overweight, restricting sodium consumption, and reduce cholesterol intake. A sensible diet is of the upmost importance.

(BeneficialRemedies,Treatments,andNutrients)

HERBAL COMBINATION: (Garlicin HC).

PHYSIOLOGIC ACTION: A combination of herbs which supports the cardiovascular system. Helps to strengthen the heart, while building and cleansing the arteries and veins.

SPECIFICS: Recent animal studies suggest that vitamin C deficiency could be involved in the causation of stroke. E.F.A.s (essential fatty acids) play a fundamental role in keeping cell membranes fluid and flexible.

SINGLE HERBS: Cayenne, Comfrey, Evening Primrose Oil, Fish Oil, Garlic, Golden Seal, and Rose Hips.

VITAMINS: B complex, C, E, Niacin, Inositol, and Choline.

MINERALS: Multi-mineral plus Calcium and Magnesium.

ALSO: (E.F.A.s) — Fish oils and cold pressed vegetable oils.

HELPFUL FOODS: Fruits(citrus and other), green leafy vegetables, turnip greens, tuna, herring, sardines, salmon, oysters, and shellfish.

SUBSTANCE ABUSE
(refertoDrugDependency)

SUNBURN
(refertoSkinProblems)

SWOLLEN GLANDS

SPECIFICS: A term commonly used to describe the enlargement of any of the lymph glands. Swollen glands may indicate a localized infection or may be a symptom of a more serious disease such as cancer, chicken pox, leukemia, measles, mononucleosis, syphilis, or tuberculosis. Treatment includes a well-balanced diet with an increased intake of fluids, calories, and protein.

(BeneficialRemedies,Treatments,andNutrients)

HERBAL COMBINATION: (IGL).

PHYSIOLOGIC ACTION: Combats infection and reduces inflammation from the body, especially the lymphatic system, ears, throat, lungs, breasts, and organs of the body.

SINGLE HERBS: Propolis, Golden Seal, Pau d'Arco, Saw Palmetto, and Echinacea.

VITAMINS: A good multi-vitamin plus C.

MINERALS: Multi-mineral complex.

HELPFUL FOODS: Aloe Vera, apples, bananas, broccoli, oat bran, carrots, citrus fruits, green leafy vegetables, soybeans, sweet potatoes, turnip greens, vegetable oils, lean red meat, and fish liver oils.

JUICES: Celery juice.

SYPHILIS

SPECIFICS: Syphilis is caused by a bacterium called Treponema pallidum and is transmitted through physical contact such as kissing, as well as sexual intimacy. Complications of syphilis may result in blindness, brain damage, heart disease, hearing loss, and sterility. Penicillin or another antibiotic is the usual treatment. In addition to medical treatment, an afflicted person should maintain a high nutrient diet to help repair the tissue damage that has occurred.

(Beneficial Remedies, Treatments, and Nutrients)

SINGLE HERBS: Echinacea, Goldenseal, Pau d'Arco and Suma.

VITAMINS: B complex and K.

MINERALS: Zinc.

ALSO: Acidophilus, Coenzyme Q10, Germanium, and Protein.

HELPFUL FOODS: All red meats, fruits, aloe vera, kelp, herring, oysters, liver, nuts, and yogurt.

TAPEWORMS

SPECIFICS: Tapeworms live in the gastrointestinal tract. Early signs include diarrhea, loss of appetite, and rectal itching. If not eliminated they will result in the loss of weight, colon disorders, and anemia. Causes include ingestion of eggs or larvae from partially cooked meat and improper disposal of human waste.

(Beneficial Remedies, Treatments, and Nutrients)

HERBAL COMBINATIONS: (Para-X) (Para-VF).

PHYSIOLOGIC ACTION: Useful in destroying and eliminating parasites, such as worms. Also helps relieve many kinds of skin problems. The Para-VF is a liquid and is useful for children and the elderly who cannot swallow capsules.

Warning: Do not use during pregnancy!

SINGLE HERBS: Black Walnut, Garlic, Pumpkin Seeds, Sage, Swedish Bitters, and Wormwood.

VITAMINS: Folic Acid.

MINERALS: Iron and Zinc.

Children: Chamomile tea or raisins soaked in Senna tea for older children may be helpful.

HELPFUL FOODS: Asparagus, brewers yeast, broccoli, lettuce, lima beans, liver, mushrooms, nuts, and spinach.

TEETH and GUM DISORDERS

SPECIFICS: Although cavities are a major dental disease, Periodontitis(a gum disease) accounts for the loss of more teeth than cavities. Periodontitis is an inflammation of the bones and gums that surround and support the teeth, caused by improper cleaning of teeth and gums, poorly fitting dentures, loose fillings, or an inadequate diet. (Also refer to pyorrhea).

(Beneficial Remedies, Treatments, and Nutrients)

SINGLE HERBS: Chamomile, Echinacea, Lobelia, Myrrh Gum, and White Oak Bark.

VITAMINS: A, B complex, C, D, P, Niacin, and Folic Acid.

MINERALS: Calcium, Copper, Magnesium, Manganese, Phosphorus, Potassium, Silicon, Sodium, and Zinc.

ALSO: Protein and Unsaturated fatty acids.

269   Toothache — Primrose oil or oil of cloves.

270   Stained or yellow teeth — brush with fresh strawberries.

HELPFUL FOODS: All dairy products, red meat, chicken, tuna, salmon, sardines, all vegetables, and vegetable oils.

JUICES: Beet greens, celery, kale, and parsley juice.

TEETH GRINDING (Bruxism)

SPECIFICS: Bruxism can develop if the bite needs adjusting, the teeth are out of line, or the teeth become sensitive to heat and cold. However, the most common cause of bruxism is a deficiency of calcium or pantothenic acid.

(BeneficialRemedies,Treatments,andNutrients)

SINGLE HERBS: Chamomile and Skullcap.

VITAMINS: Multi-vitamins, pantothenic acid, B complex. Take tablets before bed for best results.

ALSO: Bonemeal or other Calcium supplement.

HELPFUL FOODS: Brewers yeast, cheese, milk, butter, egg yolk, almonds, walnuts, fish, wheat germ, and oat bran.

TEETHING

SPECIFICS: The following nutrients are to help your infant cope with the irritation and pain that is associated with teething.

(BeneficialRemedies,Treatments,andNutrients)

SINGLE HERBS: Lobelia Extract, Aloe Vera Gel, or Peppermint Oil can be rubbed on the gums.

HOMEOPATHIC COMBINATION: Teething Formula.

TISSUE SALTS: Combination "R."

ALSO: Teething Tablets from Hylands.

TEMPEROMANDIBULAR JOINT SYNDROME (TMJ)

SPECIFICS: TMJ syndrome is usually caused by spasm of the chewing muscles, as the result of clenching the teeth due to emotional stress. Symptoms include a dull aching facial pain, tenderness of the jaw, and headaches. A correct diet and proper supplements often solve the problem.

(BeneficialRemedies,Treatments,andNutrients)

SINGLE HERBS: Hops, Passionflower, Skullcap and Valerian Root.

VITAMINS: B complex, B5, B6, and C.

MINERALS: Calcium and Magnesium.

ALSO: Coenzyme Q10 and L- Tyrosine.

HELPFUL FOODS: Green leafy vegetables, fruit, brown rice, soybeans, and whole grains.

TENNIS ELBOW

SPECIFICS: Tennis elbow is caused by inflammation of the tendon that attaches the extensor muscles. This condition results from constant overuse of muscles.

(BeneficialRemedies,Treatments,andNutrients)

HERBAL COMBINATION: (B F + C)

PHYSIOLOGIC ACTION: A special formula to aid in healing processes for swelling and inflammation.

SINGLE HERBS: White Oak Bark, Comfrey Root, Black Walnut Hulls, Lobelia, Skullcap and Yucca.

HOMEOPATHIC COMBINATION: Injury and Backache Formula.

VITAMINS: B complex, B5, B6, B12, C, and E.

MINERALS: A complete multi-mineral one a day, (time released).

ALSO: Bee pollen, Coenzyme Q10, Germanium, L-Arginine, L-Carnitine, L-Lysine, Green-Lipped Mussel, Liver, Protein, Proteolytic enzymes, Silica, and Unsaturated fatty acids.

HELPFUL FOODS: Beef, fruits, nuts, unpolished rice, soybeans, spinach, vegetable oils, liver, and whole wheat.

TENSION

SPECIFICS: Tension is generally a direct result of stress. The body can handle some stress but long term stress causes the body to break down. Long term stress occurs when the situation that causes anxiety is not relieved. Find the cause and handle it constructively. People experiencing stress should maintain a well-balanced diet and replace the nutrients depleted during stress.

(BeneficialRemedies,Treatments,andNutrients)

HERBAL COMBINATIONS: (Calm-aid) or (Ex stress comb).

PHYSIOLOGIC ACTION: A proven formula that is soothing, strengthening, and healing to the whole nervous system to relieve nervous tension and rebuild the nerve sheaths. Excellent aid for insomnia, chronic nervousness, and stress-related conditions.

SINGLE HERBS: Evening Primrose Oil, Hops, Mistletoe, Skullcap, and Valerian.

VITAMINS: B complex, B1, B2, B3, B5, B6, and C.

MINERALS: Calcium, Iodine, Iron, Magnesium, Phosphorus, Potassium, Silicon, and Sodium.

HELPFUL FOODS: Dulse, flax seed, sea salt, fruit(citrus and other), bacon, beef, chicken, all dairy products, all vegetables, mushrooms, and whole rye.

JUICES: Carrot, celery, and prune juice.

THREADWORMS

SPECIFICS: Thread worms live in the gastrointestinal tract. Early signs include diarrhea, loss of appetite, and rectal itching. If not eliminated they will result in the loss of weight, colon disorders, and anemia. Causes include ingestion of eggs or larvae from partially cooked meat, improper disposal of human waste, and walking barefoot on contaminated soil.

(BeneficialRemedies,Treatments,andNutrients)

HERBAL COMBINATIONS: (Para-X) (Para-VF).

PHYSIOLOGIC ACTION: Useful in destroying and eliminating parasites, such as thread worms. Also helps relieve many kinds of skin problems. The Para-VF is liquid and is useful for children and the elderly who cannot swallow capsules.

Warning: Do not use during pregnancy!

SINGLE HERBS: Black Walnut, Garlic, Pumpkin Seeds, Sage, Swedish Bitters, and Wormwood.

VITAMINS: Folic Acid.

MINERALS: A multi-mineral complex.

Children: Chamomile tea or raisins soaked in Senna tea for older children may be helpful.

HELPFUL FOODS: Asparagus, brewers yeast, broccoli, lettuce, lima beans, liver, mushrooms, nuts, and spinach.

THROMBOPHLEBITIS

SPECIFICS: An Inflammation of the vein, often accompanied by clot formation (usually found in the legs) and can be a complication of varicose veins. Prevention and treatment require a diet rich in vitamins B, C, and E, plus regular exercise.

(BeneficialRemedies,Treatments,andNutrients)

HERBAL COMBINATIONS: (H Formula) (Garlicin HC).

PHYSIOLOGIC ACTION: The herbs in these combinations are known to strengthen and support the cardiovascular system. Supplementing the body with niacin (B3) may be useful to help prevent clot formation. Vitamin C can help strengthen the blood vessel walls. Some research indicates that vitamin E may dilate the blood vessels, thus discouraging the formation of varicose veins and phlebitis.

SINGLE HERBS: Ginkgo, Horse Chestnut, and Yarrow.

VITAMINS: B complex, Niacin, Pantothenic acid, C, and E.

MINERALS: A multi-mineral complex.

HELPFUL FOODS: Beef, broccoli, fruit(citrus and other), nuts, green leafy vegetables, turnip greens, vegetable oils, and unpolished rice.

THROMBOSIS

SPECIFICS: Thrombosis is due to the gradual build-up of calcium and cholesterol-containing masses known as plaques on the inside of the artery walls. The clot will slow or restrict the circulation of the blood causing high blood pressure. Symptoms of this disease are cramping of muscles, chest pains and pressure, and hypertension. The main causes are poor diet, drug abuse, alcoholism, smoking, heredity, obesity, and stress.

(Beneficial Remedies, Treatments, and Nutrients)

HERBAL COMBINATION: (Garlicin HC).

PHYSIOLOGIC ACTION: A combination of herbs which supports the cardiovascular system. Helps to strengthen the heart, while building and cleansing the arteries and veins.

SPECIFICS: Recent animal studies suggest that vitamin C deficiency could be involved in the causation of thrombosis. E.F.A.s (essential fatty acids) play a fundamental role in keeping cell membranes fluid and flexible.

SINGLE HERBS: Cayenne, Comfrey, Evening Primrose Oil, Fish Oil, Garlic, Golden Seal, and Rose Hips.

VITAMINS: B complex, C, E, Niacin, Inositol, and Choline.

MINERALS: Calcium, Magnesium, and Selenium.

ALSO: (E.F.A.s) — Fish oils and cold pressed vegetable oils.

HELPFUL FOODS: Fish and fish liver oils, vegetable oils, oat bran, high fiber fruits, kelp, green tea, yogurt, and legumes.

JUICES: Alfalfa, beet, blackberry, grape, parsley, and pineapple juice.

THRUSH

SPECIFICS: Thrush is a yeast-like fungus that inhabits the oral cavity. White sores form on the tongue, gums, and inside the cheeks. Diabetics are at great risk of contracting the fungus, so if a person is diagnosed with yeast infection, he or she should be checked for diabetes.

(BeneficialRemedies,Treatments,andNutrients)

HERBAL COMBINATION: (Cantrol).

PHYSIOLOGIC ACTION: An excellent, well-balanced, formula of herbs and supplements which balance the system while killing yeast. It includes caprylic acid and anti-oxidants for the control and eventual elimination of the yeast infection.

SINGLE HERBS: Black Walnut, Caprinex, Garlicin, and Pau d'Arco.

VITAMINS: Biotin and B complex.

ALSO: Caprilic Acid, Coenzyme Q10, L-Cysteine, Primadophilus, Primrose oil, and Salmon oil.

HELPFUL FOODS: Egg yolk, apricot, citrus fruits, beef kidney, beef liver, and vegetable and fish oils.

THYROID DISORDERS

SPECIFICS: Most thyroid disorders occur when there is an over or underproduction of hormones by the thyroid gland, resulting in lowered cellular metabolism. In most thyroid disorders, the brain cells are effected and intellectual capacity is impaired. Problems with the thyroid gland can be the cause of many recurring illnesses, infections, and chronic fatigue.

(BeneficialRemedies,Treatments,andNutrients)

HERBAL COMBINATION: (T).

PHYSIOLOGIC ACTION: Rich in natural vitamins and minerals, this excellent formula helps revitalize and promote healing of the thyroid glands, thus restoring metabolism balance. Helps the body store up needed vitality and energy.

SINGLE HERBS: Black Walnut, Irish Moss, Kelp, Mullein, and Parsley.

VITAMINS: B1, B5, C, D, E, and F.

MINERALS: Chlorine, Iodine, Potassium, and Zinc.

ALSO: Thyroid glandular.

HELPFUL FOODS: All fruits(citrus and other), black molasses, butter, cheese, beef, tuna, sardines, fish liver oils, beets, broccoli, carrots, vegetable oils, green leafy vegetables, soybeans, and sunflower seeds.

JUICES: Clam and celery juice.

TICK BITE
(refer to Lyme disease)

TMJ SYNDROME
(refer to Temporomandibular Joint Syndrome)

TINNITUS

SPECIFICS: This ailment is characterized by a buzzing, hissing, or ringing in one or both ears. ringing in the ears. Tinnitus is most often caused by impaired blood flow to the brain from clogged arteries and poor circulation.

(Beneficial Remedies, Treatments, and Nutrients)

HERBAL COMBINATIONS: (H Formula) (Ginkgold).

PHYSIOLOGIC ACTION: Contains herbs which strengthen the heart and builds the vascular system. When taken with Cayenne, it improves circulation and pulse rate, giving a warming and calming sensation to the ears.

SINGLE HERBS: Cayenne, Black Cohosh, Bayberry, Butchers Broom, Ginkgo, and Yarrow

VITAMINS: A, B complex, B3, B6, C, and E.

MINERALS: Calcium, Magnesium, Manganese, and Potassium.

ALSO: Bio-Strath, Coenzyme Q10, and Lecithin.

HELPFUL FOODS: All vegetables and vegetable oils, apples, bananas, citrus fruits, beets, broccoli, carrots, oat bran, soya beans, and whole wheat

TIREDNESS
(refer to Fatigue "General")

TONSILITIS

SPECIFICS: Inflammation of the tonsils; the glands of lymph tissue located on either side of the entrance to the throat. The most effective prevention and treatment for tonsillitis is a proper diet, high in vitamins, minerals, and protein.

(BeneficialRemedies,Treatments,andNutrients)

HERBAL COMBINATION: (IF) (IGL).

PHYSIOLOGIC ACTION: Effective formulas that help cleanse toxins, combat infections, and reduce infection. Especially effective for healing the lymphatic system.

SINGLEHERBS: Bayberry Root, Echina Guard, Echinacea, Ginger Root and Pau d'Arco.

VITAMINS AND MINERALS: A complete, one a day multi complex.

ALSO: Canaid herbal drink.

HELPFUL FOODS: Beef, broccoli, fruit(citrus and other), nuts, soybeans, spinach, sweet potatoes, turnip greens, unpolished rice, and whole grains.

TOOTHACHE
(refer to "Teeth and Gums" Page)

TOXOCARIASIS

SPECIFICS: An infestation of humans, with the larvae of toxocara canis, a threadlike worm that lives in the intestines of dogs. Early signs include diarrhea, loss of appetite, and rectal itching.
If not eliminated they will result in the loss of weight, colon disorders, and anemia.

(BeneficialRemedies,Treatments,andNutrients)

HERBAL COMBINATIONS: (Para-X) (Para-VF).

PHYSIOLOGIC ACTION: Useful in destroying and eliminating parasites, such as worms. Also helps relieve many kinds of skin problems. The Para-VF is liquid and is useful for children and the elderly who cannot swallow capsules.

Warning: Do not use during pregnancy!

SINGLE HERBS: Black Walnut, Garlic, Pumpkin Seeds, Sage, Swedish Bitters, and Wormwood.

VITAMINS: Folic Acid.

MINERALS: A multi-mineral complex.

Children: Chamomile tea or raisins soaked in Senna tea for older children may be helpful.

TREMORS and TWITCHES

SPECIFICS: The most common cause of tremors and twitches is a deficiency of potassium, magnesium, and B vitamins. These nutrients are essential for the nerve impulses that pass to a muscle and control its movement.

(BeneficialRemedies,Treatments,andNutrients)

VITAMINS: B6, B12, Niacin, and B complex.

MINERALS: Magnesium and Potassium.

HELPFUL FOODS: All vegetables, brewers yeast, apples, bananas, dates, figs, fish, liver, kidney, oat bran, wheat germ, and whole wheat products.

TRENCH MOUTH
(refer to Gingivitis)

TUBERCULOSIS (TB)

SPECIFICS: A highly contagious disease caused by the bacteria, Mycobacterium Tuberculosis. It usually affects the lungs, but it may also involve other organs and tissues. The risk of contracting TB increases with an impaired immune system, an unbalanced diet, and close contact with someone infected. A diet high in protein and the essential vitamins and minerals will help prevent tuberculosis from recurring.

(BeneficialRemedies,Treatments,andNutrients)

SINGLE HERBS: Echinacea and Pau d'Arco.

VITAMINS: A, B complex, B2, B6, Folic acid, Pantothenic acid, C, D, and E.

MINERALS: Zinc.

ALSO: L-Cysteine, L-Methionine, Germanium, and Protein.

HELPFUL FOODS: Apples, bananas, lean beef, black molasses, tuna, fish liver oils, cheese, non citrus fruit, mushrooms, and sweet potatoes.

TUMORS

SPECIFICS: Benign tumors are an abnormal growth of tissues that can occur anywhere in the body. These tumors do not spread and generally do not return after being removed. For information on malignant tumors, refer to "cancer" in this manual.

(BeneficialRemedies,Treatments,andNutrients)

SINGLE HERBS: Dandelion, Kelp, Pau d'Arco, and Red Clover.

VITAMINS: A, B5, B6, B complex, C, and E.

MINERALS: A high potency multi-mineral.

ALSO: Coenzyme Q10, Germanium, Lecithin, Proteolytic enzymes, and Sheep Sorrel is an excellent poultice for external tumors.

HELPFUL FOODS: Aloe Vera, apples, bananas, broccoli, bran, carrots, citrus fruits, green leafy vegetables, soybeans, sweet potatoes, turnip greens, vegetable oils, lean red meat, and fish liver oils.

ULCERATIVE COLITIS

SPECIFICS: Ulcerative Colitis is often associated with, and made worse by psychological stress. Emotional upset should be avoided. Various herbs with multiple properties must be used to address the complexity of this situation.

Note: Avoid citrus juices. Bananas are very soothing and healing in ulcerative colitis. Primadophilus is effective in stabilizing flora in lower bowel.

(BeneficialRemedies,Treatments,andNutrients)

SINGLE HERBS: Alfalfa, Bayberry, Chamomile, Caraway, Garlic, Reshi Mushroom, Plantain, Valerian, Wild Yam, and Yucca.

VITAMINS: A, B6, Folic acid, Pantothenic acid, B complex, C, and E.

MINERALS: Calcium, Iron, Magnesium, and Potassium.

ALSO: Multi-digestive and Proteolytic enzymes, Raw thymus glandular, and unsaturated fatty acids.

HELPFUL FOODS: Apples, bananas, lean beef, black molasses, tuna, fish liver oils, cheese, non citrus fruit, mushrooms, and sweet potatoes.

ULCERS – SKIN

SPECIFICS: Skin ulcers are open sores on the skin that are generally caused as result of inadequate blood supply. Skin ulcers can be deep or shallow and are nearly always inflamed and painful.

(BeneficialRemedies,Treatments,andNutrients)

HERBAL COMBINATION: (Myrrh – Golden seal).

PHYSIOLOGIC ACTION: Ingredients needed by the body to heal ulcers, cuts, wounds, bruises, sprains, and burns. Also good as a poultice for external wounds.

VITAMINS: Folic acid, Pantothenic acid, C, and E.

MINERALS: Multi-mineral complex.

ALSO: Aloe Vera and Unsaturated fatty acids.

Skin ulcers that do not heal – Vitamin E, topical application of comfrey root and/or tea leaf. Dress with a paste made of raw garlic on gauze for 8-10 hours. Take Vitamin A, C, Zinc and Calcium orally.

HELPFUL FOODS: Beef, fruits, nuts, unpolished rice, soybeans, spinach, vegetable oils, liver, and whole wheat.

ULCERS – STOMACH

SPECIFICS: Stomach ulcers occur along the gastrointestinal tract and result when, during stress, the stomach is unable to secrete sufficient mucus, to protect against the strong acid essential for digestion. Symptoms of an ulcer are choking sensations, lower back pain, and stomach pain. Most ulcers are aggravated by the level of anxiety of the individual before eating.

(BeneficialRemedies,Treatments,andNutrients)

HERBAL COMBINATION: (Myrrh – Gold Seal Plus).

SINGLE HERBS: Cayenne (stomach ulcers only), Golden Seal, Myrrh, Pau d'Arco, Red Raspberry, Slippery Elm Bark, Valerian, and White Oak Bark.

VITAMINS: A, B complex, B2, B5, B6, B12, C, D, E, P, Choline, and Folic acid.

MINERALS: Calcium, Manganese, and Zinc,

ALSO: Acidophilus, Chlorophyll, Raw Cabbage, Goat's milk, Brewer's yeast, and Halibut oil.

Refer to "Digestive Disorders" in this manual.

HELPFUL FOODS: Avocados, bananas, green leafy vegetables, red meat, bacon, chicken, cheese, fish liver oils, vegetable oils, oat bran, and whole grains.

JUICES: Aloe Vera, celery, grapefruit, potato, and spinach juice.

UNDERWEIGHT

SPECIFICS: Treating undernourished people requires, first, stimulating the appetite. Consideration should be given to the eating environment, as well as the appearance and smell of food. People who have increased nutrient requirements would include victims of anorexia, burns, cancer treatments, hepatitis, and trauma.

(BeneficialRemedies,Treatments,andNutrients)

SINGLE HERBS: Catnip, Fenugreek, Ginger root, Ginseng, Gota Kola, Saw Palmetto berries, Yucca, and bitter herbs such as those found in Swedish Bitters will stimulate appetite.

VITAMINS: Multi-vitamins plus A and B complex.

MINERALS: Multi-minerals plus Calcium, Copper, Magnesium, and Zinc.

ALSO: Brewers yeast, Bio-Strath, Digestive enzymes, Protein, and Unsaturated fatty acids.

HELPFUL FOODS: All dairy products, brewers yeast, beef, chicken, beer, fish and vegetable oils, potatoes, whole grain products, and nuts.

URINARY TRACT (Infections)

SPECIFICS: There are many problems that may occur in the urinary tract, however most of the problems are caused by infection. The symptoms of urinary tract infections are loss of appetite, chills, fever, frequency of urination, back pain, nausea, and vomiting.

(BeneficialRemedies,Treatments,andNutrients)

HERBAL COMBINATION: (KB).

PHYSIOLOGIC ACTION: Extremely valuable in healing and strengthening the kidneys, bladder, and genito-urinary area. Useful to stop bed-wetting, but is a diuretic when congestion of the kidneys is indicated. Helps remove bladder, uterine, and urethral toxins.

Warning: Intended for occasional use only. May cause green-yellow discoloration of urine.

SINGLE HERBS: Alfalfa, Barberry root, Catnip, Dandelion, Fennel, Ginger root, Goldenrod, Horsetail, Uva Ursi, and Wild Yam.

VITAMINS: A, B complex, C, D, E, and Choline.

MINERALS: Calcium, Magnesium, and Potassium.

ALSO: Digestive enzymes, Lecithin, L-Arginine, L-Methionine, Propolis, Uratonic, Watermelon, 3-way herb teas, and other Diuretic tablets.

HELPFUL FOODS: All vegetables, apples, bananas, broccoli, carrots, cheese and other dairy products, tuna, and fish liver oils, red meat, and sprouted seeds.

JUICES: Asparagus, black currant, cranberry, celery, juniper berry, parsley, and pomegranate juice.

URTICARIA

SPECIFICS: This ailment is caused when the sap of the poison ivy or nettles touches the skin, it can cause persistent itching, rash, swelling, and blistering in sensitive people. The following nutrients will help alleviate the symptoms.

(BeneficialRemedies,Treatments,andNutrients)

SINGLE HERBS: Echinacea, Goldenseal, and Lobelia.

VITAMINS: A, C, and E.

MINERALS: Zinc.

HELPFUL FOODS: Broccoli, carrots, citrus fruits, melon, fish liver oils, and vegetable oils.

VAGINAL PROBLEMS
(GYNECOLOGICAL PROBLEMS)

(BeneficialRemedies,Treatments,andNutrients)

HERBAL COMBINATION: (Fem-Mend).

PHYSIOLOGIC ACTION: Menstrual regulator, tonic for genito-urinary system. Helpful for severe menstrual discomforts. Acts as an aid in rebuilding a malfunctioning reproductive system (Uterus, ovaries, fallopian tubes, etc.).

SINGLE HERBS: Aloe Vera, Blessed Thistle, Comfrey Root, Garlic, Ginger, Golden Seal Root, Red Raspberry, Slippery Elm Bark, Uva Ursi, and Yellow Dock Root.

VITAMINS: A, B complex, C, and E.

MINERALS: A complete multi-mineral complex.

HELPFUL FOODS: Dulse, pineapples, citrus fruits, broccoli, soybeans, spinach, sweet potatoes, turnip greens, vegetable oils, nuts, unpolished rice, and whole wheat.

VAGINITIS

SPECIFICS: An inflammation of the vagina, causing a white or yellow vaginal discharge, and a burning or itching sensation. The most common causes of vaginitis is diabetes, taking antibiotics, oral contraceptives, pregnancy, vitamin B deficiency, or a yeast infection.

(BeneficialRemedies,Treatments,andNutrients)

SINGLE HERBS: Garlic, and Pau d'Arco.

HOMEOPATHIC COMBINATION: Vaginitis Formula.

VITAMINS: A, B complex, B6, C, and D.

MINERALS: Calcium and Magnesium.

ALSO: Acidophilus, Protein, and Unsaturated fatty acids.

HELPFUL FOODS: Egg yolk, apricot, citrus fruits, beef kidney, beef liver, and vegetable and fish liver oils.

VARICELLA
(refer to Chicken Pox)

VARICOSE VEINS

SPECIFICS: Age, lack of exercise, and chronic constipation are contributing factors to varicose veins. B and C vitamins are necessary for the maintenance of strong blood vessels. Research has indicated vitamin E improves circulation by dilating blood vessels.

(BeneficialRemedies,Treatments,andNutrients)

SINGLE HERBS: Butchers Broom, Collinsonia, Hawthorn, Parsley, Horse chestnut, Marigold, Mistletoe, Witch Hazel, White Oak Bark, Uva Ursi, and Yarrow.

VITAMINS: Multi-vitamin, plus B6, B12, B complex, C, and E.

MINERALS: Potassium and Zinc.

ALSO: Brewer's yeast, Lecithin, Protein, and Unsaturated fatty acids.

HELPFUL FOODS: Apples, lean beef, broccoli, fruits(citrus and other),sprouted seeds, sunflower seeds, sweet potatoes, sardines, tuna, turnip greens, and yellow corn.

VENEREAL DISEASE

SPECIFICS: Gonorrhea is transmitted through sexual intimacy or from the mother to the newborn infant as it passes through the infected birth canal. Complications of gonorrhea may result in sterility in both sexes. Penicillin or another antibiotic is the usual treatment. In addition to medical treatment, an afflicted person should maintain a high nutrient diet to help repair the tissue damage that has occurred.

(BeneficialRemedies,Treatments,andNutrients)

SINGLE HERBS: Echinacea, Goldenseal, Pau d'Arco and Suma.

VITAMINS: B complex and K.

MINERALS: Zinc.

ALSO: Acidophilus, Coenzyme Q10, Germanium, and Protein.

HELPFUL FOODS: All red meats, fruits, aloe vera, kelp, herring, oysters, liver, nuts, and yogurt.

VERTIGO

SPECIFICS: Vertigo occurs when the central nervous system receives conflicting messages from the inner ear, causing a sensation of lightheadedness or dizziness. The main causes are allergies, anemia, high or low blood pressure, lack of oxygen to the brain, stress, and nutritional deficiencies.

(BeneficialRemedies,Treatments,andNutrients)

HERBAL COMBINATIONS: (ImmunAid) (B&B Extract) and (EchinaGuard).

PHYSIOLOGIC ACTION: Vertigo is generally caused by infections to the inner ear. ImmunAid boosts immunity, thereby helping with ear infections. EchinaGuard is a liquid. Echinacea extract is excellent for small children with ear infections. B&B Extract can be placed in the ear or taken internally and is used to aid poor equilibrium and nervous conditions.

SINGLE HERBS: Blue Cohosh, Echinacea, Garlic Oil, Garlic, Mullein Oil, Mullein, Skullcap, and St. Johns Wort.

VITAMINS: A, B3, B6, B12, B complex, C, and E.

MINERALS: Calcium and Magnesium.

ALSO: Canaid herbal drink, Coenzyme Q10, Germanium, Lecithin, Propolis, and Primadophilus.

HELPFUL FOODS: Lean red meat, carrots, green vegetables, citrus fruits, fish liver oils, herring, oysters, sardines, nuts, sprouted seeds, and sunflower seeds.

ALSO: When combating ear infections, it is imperative to exclude allergen foods from the diet. This is particularly true of all dairy products.

VINCENT'S DISEASE
(refer to Gingivitis)

VIRAL INFECTIONS

SPECIFICS: Viruses are smaller than bacteria and live on the body's cell enzymes. Most viral infections cause chills, fever, headache, and muscular aches and pains.

(Beneficial Remedies, Treatments, and Nutrients)

SINGLE HERBS: Catnip, Echinacea, Garlic, Kelp, and Pau d'Arco.

VITAMINS: A, B complex, B5, and C.

MINERALS: A high potency multi-mineral plus Zinc.

ALSO: Germanium, L-Cysteine, Proteolytic enzymes, Canaid herbal drink, and Raw thymus.

HELPFUL FOODS: Apricots, bananas, citrus fruits, broccoli, carrots, celery, corn, green leafy vegetables, bacon, beef, chicken, and fish liver oils.

JUICES: Celery, grapefruit, lemon, and parsley juice.

VITILIGO

SPECIFICS: A skin condition characterized by white patches surrounded by a dark border. Often thyroid malfunction is behind this disorder.

(Beneficial Remedies, Treatments, and Nutrients)

HERBAL COMBINATION: (T).

PHYSIOLOGIC ACTION: Rich in natural vitamins and minerals, this excellent formula helps revitalize and promote healing of the thyroid glands, thus restoring metabolism balance. Helps the body store up needed vitality and energy.

SINGLE HERBS: Black Walnut, Irish Moss, Kelp, Mullein, and Parsley.

VITAMINS: B1, B5, C, D, E, and F.

MINERALS: Chlorine, Iodine, Potassium, and Zinc.

ALSO: Thyroid glandular, and Essential fatty acids.

HELPFUL FOODS: All fruits(citrus and other), black molasses, butter, cheese, beef, tuna, sardines, fish liver oils, beets, broccoli, carrots, vegetable oils, green leafy vegetables, soybeans, and sunflower seeds.

JUICES: Clam and celery juice.

WARS (Common)

SPECIFICS: Warts are highly contagious, rough, irregular skin growths. They can be spread by trimming, picking, touching, or shaving. Typically they do not cause pain or itching. Proper nutrition and the supplements listed below will control or eliminate common warts.

(BeneficialRemedies,Treatments,andNutrients)

SINGLE HERBS: Echinacea, Garlic, Golden Seal, and Pau d' Arco.

VITAMINS: A, B complex, C, and E.

MINERALS: Zinc.

ALSO: L-Cysteine, and 28000 IU vitamin E oil applied twice a day is an effective treatment.

HELPFUL FOODS: Fish and fish liver oils, all vegetables and vegetable oils, mushrooms, unpolished rice, fruit, and whole wheat.

WATER RETENTION

SPECIFICS: Disorders that cause water retention are sodium retention, congestive heart failure, weak kidneys, varicose veins, and protein and thiamine deficiencies.

(BeneficialRemedies,Treatments,andNutrients)

HERBAL COMBINATION: (KB).

PHYSIOLOGIC ACTION: KB acts as a mild diuretic to rid the body of excessive water.

SINGLE HERBS: Buchu, Cranberry, Dandelion, Juniper, Parsley, and Uva Ursi.

VITAMINS: B6 and C.

MINERALS: Calcium and Potassium.

ALSO: Limited consumption of common table salt.

HELPFUL FOODS: Bananas, citrus fruits, cheese, nuts, oat bran, sweet potatoes, and turnip greens.

WEIGHT CONTROL (Overweight)

SPECIFICS: A person who has twenty percent excess body fat over the norm for their age, build, and height is considered overweight. Losing weight is a matter of consciously regulating the types and amount of food eaten and increasing daily activity.

(BeneficialRemedies,Treatments,andNutrients)

HERBAL COMBINATIONS: (SKC) or (Herbal Slim).

PHYSIOLOGIC ACTION: A special, well-balanced, combination that helps control your appetite, dissolve excess fat, ease stress and anxiety, gently cleanse the bowels, eliminate excess water, and in conjunction with your diet and exercise program, helps you lose weight naturally. Safe and effective.

SINGLE HERBS: Guar Gum, Konjac Root, and Yucca.

VITAMINS: A, C, and E.

MINERALS: A complete multi-mineral complex.

ALSO: Super D's tea, Slim tea, Spirulina diet, Bee Pollen, and Grapefruit Plus.

HELPFUL FOODS: Citrus fruits, melon, fish liver oils, green leafy vegetables, and oat bran.

WEIGHT GAIN

SPECIFICS: Treating undernourished people requires, first, stimulating the appetite. Consideration should be given to the eating environment, as well as the appearance and smell of food. People who have increased nutrient requirements would include victims of anorexia, burns, cancer treatments, hepatitis, and trauma.

(BeneficialRemedies,Treatments,andNutrients)

SINGLE HERBS: Catnip, Fenugreek, Ginger root, Ginseng, Gota Kola, Saw Palmetto berries, and bitter herbs such as those found in Swedish Bitters will stimulate appetite.

VITAMINS: Multi-vitamins plus A and B complex.

MINERALS: Multi-minerals plus Calcium, Copper, Magnesium, and Zinc.

ALSO: Brewers yeast, Bio-Strath, Digestive enzymes, Protein, and Unsaturated fatty acids.

HELPFUL FOODS: All dairy products, brewers yeast, beef, chicken, beer, fish and vegetable oils, potatoes, whole grain products, and nuts.

WHOOPING COUGH

SPECIFICS: A distressing infectious disease, also known as pertussis which mainly affects young children and infants. The main features of the illness are paroxysms of coughing often ending in a characteristic "whoop".

(BeneficialRemedies,Treatments,andNutrients)

HERBAL COMBINATION: (A-P).

PHYSIOLOGIC ACTION: A natural way to ease chronic pain associated with nervous tension, spasms, and whooping cough.

SINGLE HERBS: Elecampane, Horehound, Kalmin, Mouse Ear, Sundew, Valerian Root, Wild Cherry Bark, and Wild Lettuce.

VITAMINS: Multi-vitamin complex.

MINERALS: Multi-mineral complex plus Zinc.

HELPFUL FOODS: Apples, citrus fruit, celery, herring, oysters, and turnip greens.

JUICES: Apple, celery, and watercress.

WORMS

SPECIFICS: Worms live in the gastrointestinal tract. Early signs include diarrhea, loss of appetite, and rectal itching.
If not eliminated they will result in the loss of weight, colon disorders, and anemia. Causes include ingestion of eggs or larvae from partially cooked meat, improper disposal of human waste, and walking barefoot on contaminated soil.

(BeneficialRemedies,Treatments,andNutrients)

HERBAL COMBINATIONS: (Para-X) (Para-VF).

PHYSIOLOGIC ACTION: Useful in destroying and eliminating parasites, such as worms. Also helps relieve many kinds of skin problems. The Para-VF is liquid and is useful for children and the elderly who cannot swallow capsules.

Warning: Do not use during pregnancy!

SINGLE HERBS: Black Walnut, Garlic, Pumpkin Seeds, Sage, Swedish Bitters, and Wormwood.

VITAMINS: Folic Acid.

MINERALS: A multi-mineral complex.

Children: Chamomile tea or raisins soaked in Senna tea for older children may be helpful.

HELPFUL FOODS: Asparagus, brewers yeast, broccoli, lettuce, lima beans, liver, mushrooms, nuts, and spinach.

WRINKLES
(refer to Skin Problems)

YEAST INFECTION

SPECIFICS: A fungus such as candida albicans inhabits the genital tract, intestines, mouth and throat. Yeast infections affect both men and women; when the fungus infects the vagina it results in vaginitis; when it infects the oral cavity, it is called thrush. Diabetics are at great risk of contracting the fungus, so if a person is diagnosed with yeast infection, he or she should be checked for diabetes.

(Beneficial Remedies, Treatments, and Nutrients)

HERBAL COMBINATIONS: (Garlicin) (Control, Caprinex).

PHYSIOLOGIC ACTION: Excellent well-balanced formulas for control and eventual elimination of candida overgrowth.

SINGLE HERBS: Black Walnut, Garlic, and Pau d'Arco.

VITAMINS: A, C, E, and Biotin.

MINERALS: Calcium and Magnesium.

ALSO: Primrose oil, Protein, and Primadophilus.

DOSAGES

VITAMINS & MINERALS

Continual debate rages over what is an (adequate) daily intake of vitamins and minerals. The guide below is just that — a guide only. RDA and Margin of Allowances, are based on the minimum needs of an average adult 23 to 50 years of age, with no special health problems.

VITAMINS		RDA for adult, 23-50 *	Margin of Allowance**
Vitamin A	Adults	4,000 IU	5-10 times RDA **
	Children	2,000 IU	4,000 IU
	Infants	1,400 IU	2,000 IU
Beta-carotene	Adults	7,500 IU	5-10 times RDA ***
B complex	See individual B vitamins - Relatively non-toxic		
(B1)	Men	1.4 mg	200 times RDA **
Thiamin	Women	1.0 mg	200 times RDA **
	Children	.7 to 1.2 mg	n/a
	Infants	.3 to .5 mg	n/a
(B2)	Men	1.6 mg	588 times RDA **
Riboflavin	Women	1.2 mg	588 times RDA **
	Children	.8 to 1.4 mg	n/a
	Infants	.4 to .6 mg	n/a
(B3)	Men	16 mg	50 times RDA **
Niacin	Women	13 mg	50 times RDA **
	Children	9 mg	n/a
	Infants	6 mg	n/a

VITAMINS		RDA for adult, 23-50 *	Margin of Allowance**
(B5) Pantothenic acid	Adults	10 mg	100 times RDA **
	Children	3 to 7 mg	n/a
	Infants	2 to 3 mg	n/a
(B6) Pyridoxine	Men	2.2 mg	900 times RDA **
	Women	2 mg	900 times RDA **
	Children	.9 to 1.8 mg	n/a
	Infants	.3 to .6 mg	n/a
(B9) Folic acid	Adults	180 to 200 mcg	1000 times RDA **
	Children	100 mcg	n/a
	Infants	10 to 40 mcg	n/a
(B12) Cobalamin	Adults	6 mcg	25 to 100 mg ****
(B13) Orotic acid		Not available in the U.S.A. Available as calcium orotate outside of the U.S.A.	
(B15) Calc. Pangamate	Adults	50 mg ***	100 mg ****
(B17) Laetrile	Adults	.25 g ***	1g ****
Choline	Adults	900 mg ***	1 to 5g ****
Inositol	Adults	250 mg ***	500-1000 mg ****
PABA Para-amino benzoic Acid	Adults	100 mg ***	1000 mg ****
Vitamin C	Adults	60 mg	33-83 times RDA **
	Children	45 to 50 mg	n/a
	Infants	35 mg	n/a

VITAMINS		RDA for adult, 23-50 *	Margin of Allowance**	
Vitamin D	Adults	400 IU	2.5 to 5 times RDA	**
	Children	400 IU	2.5 times RDA	***
	Infants	200 IU	2.5 times RDA	***
Vitamin E	Men	15 IU	40 times RDA	**
	Women	12 IU	40 times RDA	**
	Children	7 to 12 IU	20 times RDA	***
	Infants	4 to 6 IU	15 times RDA	***
Vitamin F Unsaturated fatty acids	Adults	100 mg	1,000 mg	***
Vitamin H Biotin	Adults	250 mcg	1,000 mcg	***
	Children	100 mcg	200 mcg	***
	Infants	35 to 50 mcg	n/a	
Vitamin K - 1	Adults	65 to 80 mcg	10 to 15 times RDA	***
Vitamin K - 2	Children	20 to 50 mcg	5 to 10 times RDA	***
	Infants	10 to 20 mcg	3 to 5 times RDA	***
Vitamin K - 3 Menadione	Adults	65-80 mcg	500 mcg	***
Vitamin P Bioflavonoids	Adults	12 mg	33-83 times RDA	**
Vitamin T Sesame seeds		n/a	n/a	
Vitamin U Raw cabbage		n/a	n/a	

DOSAGES

MINERALS		RDA for adult, 23-50 *		Margin of Allowance**	
Boron	Adults	2 mg		3 to 6 mg	***
Calcium	Adults	800 mg		10 times RDA	**
	Children	800 to 1200 mg		10 times RDA	**
	Infants	360 to 540 mg		n/a	
Chlorine	Adults	500 mg		1500 mg	****
Chromium	Adults	.05 to .2 mg	***	.2 to .6 mg	***
	Children	.02 to .2 mg	***	n/a	
	Infants	.01 to .06 mg	***	n/a	
Cobalt	Adults	5 to 8 mcg	***	n/a	
Copper	Adults	2 to 3 mg		5.5 times RDA	**
	Children	1 to 3 mg		n/a	
	Infants	.5 to 1 mg		n/a	
Fluorine	Adults	1.5 mg	***	4 mg	****
	Children	.5 mg	***	2.5 mg	****
	Infants	.1 mg	***	1 mg	****
Iodine	Adults	150 mcg		1000 mcg	***
	Children	70 to 150 mcg		300 mcg	***
	Infants	40 to 50 mcg		100 mcg	***
Iron	Men	10 mg		5.5 times RDA	**
	Women	18 mg		5.5 times RDA	**
	Children	15 to 18 mg		n/a	
	Infants	10 to 15 mg		n/a	
Lithium		n/a		n/a	

MINERALS		RDA for adult, 23-50 *		Margin of Allowance**	
Magnesium	Men	350 mg		15 times RDA	**
	Women	300 mg		15 times RDA	**
	Children	150 to 300 mg		5 times RDA	***
	Infants	50 to 70 mg		n/a	
Manganese	Adults	2.5 to 5 mg		15 to 30 mg	****
	Children	1 to 5 mg		n/a	
	Infants	.5 to 1 mg		n/a	
Molybdenum	Adults	.15 to .25 mg	***	.5 mg	****
	Children	.05 to .25 mg	***	.5 mg	****
	Infants	.03 to .05 mg	***	.08 mg	****
Nickel		n/a		Excessive intake may be toxic.	
Phosphorus	Adults	1000 mg		10 times RDA	**
	Children	800 to 1200 mg		5 times RDA	***
	Infants	240 to 360 mg		n/a	
Potassium	Adults	1875 to 5625 mg		No known toxicity.	
	Children	550 to 4575 mg		n/a	
	Infants	350 to 1275 mg		n/a	
Selenium	Men	.07 mg		.2 mg	***
	Women	.05 mg		.15 mg	***
	Children	.02 mg		.1 mg	***
	Infants	.01 mg		.06 mg	***
Silicon	Adults	n/a		No side effects have been found to date.	
Sodium	Adults	1100 to 3300 mg		8 grams	****
	Children	325 to 2700 mg		2 to 6 grams	****
	Infants	115 to 750 mg		1 to 2 grams	****

MINERALS		RDA for adult, 23-50 *	Margin of Allowance**
Sulfur	Adults	n/a	Inorganic sulfur can be toxic.
Vanadium	Adults	n/a	Can be toxic in synthetic form.
Zinc	Adults	15 mg	33 times RDA **
	Children	10 to 15 mg	15 times RDA ***
	Infants	3 to 5 mg	5 times RDA ***

* U.S.A. (Recommended Daily Allowances) are based on estimates by the National Academy of Sciences and National Research Council.

** Adapted from John Hathcock's "Quantitative Evaluation of Vitamin Safety," Pharmacy Times, May 1985.

*** Estimate only — from Global Health Research on data available.

**** Usual therapeutic dose.

RDAs and Margin of Allowances courtesy of the "Natural Life Magazine" Burnaby, B.C., Canada.

Vitamins

Vitamin	NaturalSources	AffectedComponents
A (Fat soluble) RDA 5000 IU	Fish liver oils, liver, carrots, green leafy vegetables (kale, turnip greens, spinach), Colorado fruits, melon, squash, yams, tomatoes, margarine, eggs, milk and dairy products.	Bones, eyes, hair, mucous linings, membranes, nails, skin, and teeth.
B1 **Thiamine** (Water soluble) RDA 1.4 mg	Brewers yeast, wheat germ, rice polishings, all seeds, nuts and nut butters, soy beans, beets, potatoes, leafy green vegetables, milk and dairy products.	Brain, ears, eyes, hair, heart, nervous system, and muscles.
B2 **Riboflavin** (Water soluble) RDA 1.6 mg	Milk, liver, kidney, cheese, fish, eggs, whole grains, brewers yeast, torula yeast, wheat germ, almonds, sunflower seeds, and cooked leafy vegetables.	Eyes, skin, nails, and hair

Functions

Visual purple production (necessary for night vision), promotes growth and vitality, resists infection, repairs and maintains body tissue, helps prevent premature aging and senility.

Deficiency Symptoms

Allergies, appetite loss, blemishes, dry hair, fatigue, itching/burning eyes, loss of smell, night blindness, rough dry skin, sinus trouble, soft tooth enamel, and susceptibility to infections.

TherapeuticUses

Acne, alcoholism, allergies, arthritis, asthma, athletes foot, boils, bronchitis, colds, cystitis, diabetes, carbuncles, eczema, heart disease, peptitis, migraine headaches, hy-perthyroidism, psoriasis, sinusitis, stress, tooth and gum disorders.

Appetite, blood building, carbohydrate metabolism, circulation, aids digestion, energy, growth, learning capacity, prevents liquid retention, prevents constipation, muscle tone maintenance (intestine, stomach, heart).

Appetite loss, beriberi, digestive disturbances, fatigue, irritability, muscular weakness, nervousness, numbness of hands and feet, mental depression, pains around heart, and shortness of breath.

Alcoholism, anemia, congestive heart failure, fluid retention, constipation, diarrhea, diabetes, indigestion, lead poisoning, nausea, mental illness, pain, rapid heart rate, and stress.

Aids growth and reproduction, alleviates eye fatigue, antibody & red blood cell formation, promotes healthy skin, nails and hair, metabolism (carbohydrate, fat protein).

Bloodshot and burning eyes, cataracts, corner of mouth cracks & sores, dizziness, poor digestion, premature wrinkles, retarded growth, and red sore tongue.

Arteriosclerosis, baldness, cholesterol (high), cystitis, facial oiliness, hypoglycemia, light sensitivity, mental retardation, muscular disorders, nervous disorders, nausea in pregnancy, overweight, premature wrinkles, and stress.

Vitamins continued

Vitamin	Natural Sources	Affected Components
B3 **Niacin** (Water soluble) RDA 20 mg	Liver, lean meat, white meat of poultry, kidney, fish, eggs, roasted peanuts, avocadoes, dates, figs, prunes, green vegetables, whole wheat products, brewers yeast, torula yeast, wheat germ, rice bran, rice polishings, and sunflower seeds.	Brain, gastro-intestinal tract, nervous system, liver, and skin.
B6 **Pyridoxine** (Water soluble) RDA 2 mg	Brewers yeast, bananas, avocadoes, wheat germ, wheat bran, cantaloupe, milk, eggs, beef, liver, kidney, heart, blackstrap molasses, soybeans, walnuts, peanuts, pecans, green leafy vegetables, green peppers and carrots.	Blood, muscles, nerves, and skin.
B9 **Folic Acid** (Water soluble) RDA 4 mcg	brewers yeast, wheat germ, mushrooms, nuts, liver, broccoli, asparagus, lima beans, lettuce, spinach and deep green leafy vegetables.	Blood, glands, hair, liver and skin.
B12 **Cobalamin** (Water soluble) RDA 6 mcg	Comfrey leaves, kelp, bananas, peanuts, concord grapes, sunflower seeds, brewers yeast, wheat germ, bee pollen, liver, beef, eggs, pork, milk, cheese, and kidney.	Red blood cells, nerves, and brain.

Functions	Deficiency Symptoms	Therapeutic Uses
Circulation, cholesterol level, dilates blood vessels, hydrochloric acid production, metabolism (protein, fat carbohydrate), tones nervous system, and sex hormone production.	Appetite loss, canker sores, cold feet and hands, depression, fatigue, halitosis, headaches, indigestion, insomnia, muscular weakness, nausea, nervous disorders, pellagra, and skin eruptions.	Acne, baldness, canker sores, diarrhea, halitosis, high blood pressure, leg cramps, migraine headaches, schizophrenia, poor circulation, stress, and tooth decay.
Alleviates nausea, antibody formation, digestion (hydrochloric acid production), fat and protein utilization (weight control), and maintains sodium/poassium balance (nerves).	Acne, anemia, arthritis, convulsions in babies, depression, dizziness, nervous disorders, hair loss, irritability, learning disabilities, muscle spasms, urination problems, and weakness.	Alcoholism, allergies, anemia, arthritis, bronchial asthma, bursitis, epilepsy, fatigue, glossitis, hypoglycemia, insomnia, premenstrual edema, neuritis, overweight, shingles, stress, and seborrheic.
Analgesic for pain, appetite, body growth & reproduction, division of body cells, hydrochloric acid production, improves lactation, protein metabolism, and red blood cell formation.	Anemia, canker sores, digestive disturbances, graying hair, growth problems, impaired circulation, fatigue, and mental depression.	Anemia, arteriosclerosis, baldness, cholesterol (high), constipation, heart disease, loss of libido, overweight, and macro-cytic anemia.
Appetite, blood cell formation, cell longevity, increases energy and memory, nervous system, metabolism (carbohydrate, fat, protein), and promotes growth.	Chronic fatigue, general weakness, nervousness, pernicious anemia, poor appetite, walking and speaking difficulties.	Baldness, brain damage, dermatitis, eczema, leg cramps, and pernicious anemia.

Vitamins continued

Vitamin	Natural Sources	Affected Components
B13 **Orotic Acid** (Calcium orotate) RDA N/A	Root vegetables, whey, the liquid portion of soured or curdled milk.	Cells, and liver.
B17 **Laetrile** **Nitrilosides** RDA N/A	Whole seeds — apricot, peach and plum pits, mung beans, lima beans, garbanzos, blackberries, blueberries, cranberries, raspberries, millet and flaxseed.	Not known.
Biotin *B* **Complex** (Water soluble) also Vit-H RDA 3 mcg	Brewers yeast, fruits, nuts, soybeans, unpolished rice, beef, liver, egg yolk, milk, and kidney.	Hair, skin, and muscles.
Choline *B* **Complex** (Water soluble) RDA N/A	Granular or liquid lecithin, brewers yeast, wheat germ, egg yolk, liver, and green leafy vegetables.	Brain, hair, gallbladder, kidneys, liver, thymus gland, and controls cholesterol buildup.

Functions	Deficiency Symptoms	Therapeutic Uses
Essential for the biosynthesis of nucleic acid, regenerative processes in cells.	Not known.	Multiple sclerosis.
Purported to have cancer controlling and preventive properties.	May lead to diminished resistance to malignancies.	Cancer.
Antiseptic, cell growth, fatty acid production, hair growth, metabolism (carbohydrate, fat, protein), and vitamin B utilization.	Dandruff, depression, dry skin, fatigue, grayish skin, heart abnormalities, color, insomnia, muscular pain, and poor appetite.	Alcoholism, arteriosclerosis, baldness, cholesterol (high), constipation, dizziness, eczema, ear noises, dermatitis, hardening of the arteries, headaches, heart trouble, high blood pressure, hypoglycemia, insomnia, and seborrhea.
Controls cholesterol buildup, lecithin formation, liver & gall bladder regulation, lowers blood pressure, metabolism (fats, cholesterol), and nerve transmission.	Bleeding stomach ulcers, cirrhosis, growth problems, heart trouble, high blood pressure, impaired liver & kidney function, and intolerance to fats.	Alcoholism, anemia, arteriosclerosis, Alzheimer's disease, baldness, cirrhosis, diarrhea, fatigue, menstrual problems, mental illness, stomach ulcers, and stress.

Vitamins continued

Vitamin	Natural Sources	Affected Components
Inositol **B Complex** (Water soluble) RDA N/A	Liver, brewers yeast, beef brains and heart, cabbage, citrus fruits, cantaloupe, raisins, wheat germ, whole grains, peanuts, lecithin, milk, and unrefined molasses.	Brain, heart, kidneys, liver muscles, hair and skin.
C **Ascorbic Acid** (Water soluble) RDA 60 mg	Rose hips, citrus fruits, apples, black currants, strawberries, cabbage, broccoli, cauliflower, persimmons, guavas, tomatoes, sweet potatoes, turnip greens, and green bell peppers.	Ligaments, bones, skin, gums, heart, teeth, blood, adrenal glands, and capillary walls.
D **Ergosterol** (Water soluble) RDA 400 IU	Egg yolks, milk, butter, fish liver oils, sardines, herring, salmon, tuna, sprouted seeds, mushrooms, sunflower seeds	Bones, heart, nerves, skin, teeth, and thyroid gland.

Functions	**Deficiency Symptoms**	**Therapeutic Uses**
Artery hardening retardation, calming effect, cholesterol reduction, hair growth, lecithin formation, metabolism (fat & cholesterol), preventing eczema.	Cholesterol (high), constipation, eczema, eye abnormalities, and hair loss.	Eczema, obesity, schizophrenia baldness, high blood pressure, and poor circulation.
Accelerates healing after surgery, bone & tooth formation, collagen production, common cold prevention, digestion, heals wounds, burns, and bleeding gums, iodine conservation, red blood cell formation, shock and infection resistance, protection against cancer-producing agents.	Anemia, hemorrhages, capillary wall ruptures, bruise easily, dental cavities, low infection resistance (colds), premature aging, poor digestion, soft and bleeding gums, and thyroid insufficiency.	Alcoholism, asthma, arteriosclerosis, arthritis, cholesterol (high), colds, cystitis, hypoglycemia, heart disease, hepatitis, insect bites, pyorrhea, prickly heat, scurvy, sinusitis, stress, and tooth decay.
Aids in assimilating vitamin A, calcium & phosphorus metabolism (bone, teeth, heart action, nervous system maintenance, normal blood clotting, skin respiration.	Diarrhea, insomnia, myopia, muscular weakness, nervousness, premature aging, poor metabolism, softening bones & teeth, and tooth decay.	Acne alcoholism, allergies, arthritis, cystitis, pyorrhea, psoriasis, osteomalacia, osteoporosis, and rickets.

Vitamins continued

Vitamin	Natural Sources	Affected Components
E **Tocopherol** (Fat soluble) RDA 10 mg	Wheat germ, brussel sprouts, leafy greens, spinach, whole wheat, whole grain cereals, vegetable oils, soybeans, and eggs.	Blood vessels, heart, liver, lungs, adrenal and pituitary glands, testes, uterus and fatty tissues.
H **Biotin** RDA 3 mcg	Also a B Complex. See Page 200.	
K **Menadione** (Fat soluble) RDA N/A	Kelp, alfalfa, liver, yogurt, egg yolk, safflower and soybean oil, fish liver oil, and leafy green vegetables.	Blood, and liver.
P **Rutin** **Bioflavonoids** (Water soluble) RDA N/A	Apricots, blackberries, cherries, buck wheat and the white skins and segment part of all citrus fruit.	Blood, bones, capillary walls, gums, ligaments, skin, and teeth.

Functions

Deficiency Symptoms

Therapeutic Uses

Anti-coagulant, alleviates fatigue, dilates blood vessels, blood cholesterol reduction, improves circulation, capillary wall strengthening, fertility, male potency, lung protection (antipollution), muscle & nerve maintenance, prevents and dissolves blood clots.

Anemias, dry, dull or falling hair, enlarged prostrate gland, gastrointestinal disease, heart disease, impotency, premature aging, miscarriages, muscular wasting, sterility, and tooth decay.

Allergies, arteriosclerosis, baldness, blood clots, cholesterol (high), cystiotos, diabetes, menopausal and menstrual disorders, migraine headaches, myopia, phlebitis, sinusitis, stress, sterility, thrombosis, varicose veins. External: burns, scars, warts, wrinkles, and wounds.

Activates energy producing tissues, blood clotting (coagulation), important for normal liver function.

Bleeding ulcers, diarrhea, increased tendency to hemorrhage and miscarriages, lowered vitality, and nose bleeds.

Bruising, eye hemorrhages, celiac disease, colitis, gall stones, hemorrhaging, menstrual problems, preparing women for childbirth, and ulcers.

Aids in healing bleeding gums, blood vessel wall maintenance, bruising minimization, cold and flu prevention, strong capillary maintenance.

Bleeding gums, cirrhosis of the liver, eczema, hemorrhaging, hardening of arteries, and respiratory infections.

Asthma, bleeding gums, colds, eczema, edema, dizziness (caused by inner ear hemorrhoids, high blood pressure, hypertension, miscarriages, rheumatic fever, rheumatism, ulcers, and varicose veins.

Vitamins continued

Vitamin	Natural Sources	Affected Components
T Sesame Seed Factor	Sesame seeds, sesame butter, and egg yolks.	Blood.
U (Fat soluble) RDA N/A	Raw cabbage juice, fresh cabbage, and sauerkraut.	Stomach.

Functions	Deficiency Symptoms	Therapeutic Uses
Combats anemia and hemophilia, improves memory.	Not known.	Anemia and hemophilia.
Promotes healing in peptic ulcers.	Not known.	Peptic ulcers and duodenal ulcers.

Minerals

Mineral	Natural Sources	Affected Components
Calcium RDA 800 to 1200 mg	Milk, cheese, sardines, salmon, soybeans, dark leafy vegetables, sesame seeds, oats, navy beans, almonds, millet, walnuts, sunflower seeds, and tortillas.	Bones, teeth, nails, blood, heart, skin, and soft tissue.
Chlorine RDA 500 mg	Kelp. watercress, avocado, chard, cabbage, kale, celery, asparagus, cucumber, olives, tomatoes, turnip, saltwater fish.	Blood, liver, and stomach.
Chromium RDA N/A	Brewers yeast, cane sugar, meat, shell fish, chicken, clams, and corn oil.	Arteries, and blood.
Cobalt RDA N/A	All green leafy vegetables, clams, kidney, liver, oysters, milk, and red meat.	Blood.
Copper RDA 2 mg	Beef liver, seafood, almonds, beans, peas, prunes, raisins, whole grain products, and green leafy vegetables.	Blood, bones, brain, connective tissues, and nerves.
Fluorine RDA N/A	Milk, cheese, carrots, garlic, sunflower seeds, seafood, and fluoridated drinking water.	Bones and teeth.

Functions	Deficiency Symptoms	Therapeutic Uses
Bone/tooth formation, blood clotting, heart rhy-thm, nerve tranquilization, nerve transmission, mus-cle growth and contraction.	Heart palpitations, insomnia, muscle cramps, nervousness, arm & leg numbness , and tooth decay.	Arthritis, aging symptoms (backache, bone pain, finger tremors, foot/leg cramps, insomnia, menstrual cramps, menopause problems, nervousness, over- weight, premenstrual tension, and rheumat- ism.
Maintains fluid and electrolyte balance, helps liver, and the production of hy- drochloric acid.	Impaired digestion, loss of hair and teeth, derangement of fluid levels in the body.	Digestion, stomach acidity, and stiffness of joints.
Blood sugar level, glucose metabolism (energy).	Arteriosclerosis, glucose intolerance in diabetics.	Diabetes and hypogly- cemia.
Aids in hemoglobin formation.	Development of pernicious anemia.	Anemia.
Development of bones, brain, nerves and connective tissues, hair & skin color, healing processes of body, hemoglobin and red blood cell formation.	General weakness, im- paired respiration, and skin sores.	Anemia and baldness.
Strengthens bones and reduces tooth decay	Not known.	Tooth decay.

Minerals

Mineral	Natural Sources	Affected Components
Germanium RDA N/A	Garlic, aloe, comfrey, chorella, ginseng, and water cress.	All cells.
Iodine RDA 150 mcg	Kelp, dulse and other seaweed, seafoods and fish liver oils, egg yolks, citrus fruits, artichokes, garlic, turnip greens, watercress, pineapples, and pears.	Hair, nails, thyroid gland, brain, skin, and teeth.
Iron RDA 10 mg. males 18 mg. females	Apricots, peaches, bananas, black molasses, prunes, raisins, whole rye, walnuts, brewers yeast, kelp, dulse, dry beans and lentils, liver, kidney, heart, egg yolks, red meat, oysters, and raw clams.	Blood, bones, nails, skin, and teeth.
Lithium RDA N/A	Kelp, dulse, and seafood.	Nerves, muscles, and brain.
Magnesium RDA 350 mg	Apples, figs, lemons, peaches, kale, endive, chard, celery, alfalfa, beet tops, whole grains, brown rice, sesame seeds, sunflower seeds, almonds, and yellow corn.	Arteries, bones, heart, muscles, nerves, and teeth.
Manganese RDA N/A	Nuts and grains, spinach, beets, brussel sprouts, peas, kelp, wheat germ, apricots, blueberries, egg yolks, and citrus fruits.	Brain, thyroid and mammary glands, muscles, and nerves.

Functions	Deficiency Symptoms	Therapeutic Uses
A relatively new mineral. builds immune cells, gives energy, and has rejuvenative properties.	Not known.	Anemia.
Energy production, metabolism (excess fat), physical & mental development.	Cold hands and feet, dry hair, irritability, nervous-ness, and obesity.	Arteriosclerosis, hair problems, goiter, and hyperthyroidism.
Hemoglobin production, stress and disease resistance.	Breathing difficulties, brittle nails, iron deficiency, anemia (pale skin, fatigue), and constipation.	Alcoholism, anemia, col-itis, and menstrual problems.
Helps transport sodium metabolism to brain nerves and muscles.	Nervous and mental disorders.	Paranoid schizophrenic.
Acid/alkaline balance, blood sugar metabolism (energy), and metabolism (calcium & vitamin C).	Confusion, disorientation, easily aroused anger, nervousness, rapid pulse, and tremors.	Alcoholism, cholesterol (high), depression, heart conditions, kidney stones, nervousness, prostrate troubles, sensitivity to noise, stomach acidity, tooth decay, overweight.
Enzyme activation, reproduction & growth, sex hormone production, tissue respiration, vitamin B1 metabolism, and vitamin E utilization.	Ataxia (muscle coordination failure), dizziness, ear noises, and loss of hearing.	Allergies, asthma, diabetes, and fatigue.

Minerals continued

Mineral	Natural Sources	Affected Components
Molybdenu m RDA N/A	Brown rice, millet, buck wheat, legumes, leafy vegetables, brewers yeast, whole cereals	Blood.
Phosphorus RDA 800 to 1200 mg	Dairy products, whole grains, seeds and nuts, egg, fish, poultry, meat, dried fruits, legumes and corn.	Bones, brain, heart, kidneys, nerves, and teeth.
Potassium RDA 2000 to 2500 mg	All vegetables, bananas, citrus fruits, cantaloupe, tomatoes, water cress, sunflower seeds, whole grains, potatoes, milk, and mint leaves.	Blood, heart, kidneys, muscles, nerves, and skin.
Selenium RDA N/A	Wheat germ, brewers yeast, kelp, garlic, mushrooms, onions, tomatoes, broccoli, seafoods, milk, eggs, and bran.	Blood, prostrate gland, liver, and testicles.
Silicon RDA N/A	Flaxseed, steel cut oats, almonds, peanuts, sunflower seeds, apples, strawberries, grapes, kelp, beets, onions, and parsnips.	Bones, hair, nails, and teeth.
Sodium RDA 200 to 600 mg	Sea salt, kelp, shellfish, carrots, celery, asparagus, romaine lettuce, beets, dried beef, brains, kidney, bacon and watermelon.	Blood, lymph system, stomach, muscles, and nerves.

Functions	Deficiency Symptoms	Therapeutic Uses
Integral part of enzymes involved in oxidation processes.	Unknown.	Copper poisoning and improper carbohydrate metabolism.
Bone/tooth formation, cell growth & repair, energy production, heart muscle contraction, kidney function, metabolism (calcium, sugar), nerve & muscle activity, vitamin utilization.	Appetite loss, fatigue, irregular breathing, nervous disorders, overweight, and weight loss.	Arthritis, stunted growth in children, stress, tooth and gum disorders.
Heartbeat, rapid growth, muscle contraction, and nerve tranquilization.	Acne, continuous thirst, dry skin, constipation, general weakness, insomnia, muscle damage, nervousness, slow irregular heartbeat, and weak reflexes.	Acne, alcoholism, aller-gies, burns, colic in infants, diabetes, high blood pressure, heart disease (angina pectoris, congestive heart failure, myocardinal infraction).
Antioxdant, slows aging process and hardening of tissues through oxidation.	Premature stamina loss.	Degenerated liver, impotence, and mercury poisoning.
Building of strong bones, helps healing process and builds immune system, normal growth of hair, nails and teeth.	Aging symptoms of skin (wrinkles), thinning or loss of hair, poor bone development, soft or brittle nails.	Hair loss, irritations in mucous membranes, skin disorders, and insomnia.
Helps nerves and muscles function properly and normalizes glandular secretions.	Excessive sweating, chroic diarrhea, nausea, respiratory failure, heat exhaustion, and impaired carbohydrate digestion.	Sun stroke, heat prostration, muscular weakness, and mental apathy.

Minerals continued

Mineral	Natural Sources	Affected Components
Sulfur RDA N/A	Radish, turnip, onions, celery, horseradish, kale, soybeans, water cress, eggs, fish, lean and beef.	Hair, skin, nails, and nerves.
Vanadium RDA N/A	Fish	Heart and blood vessels.
Zinc RDA 15 mg	Sprouted seeds, wheat bran and germ, pumpkin seeds, sunflower seeds, brewers yeast, onions, nuts, green leafy vegetables, lean beef, lamb chops, pork loin, eggs, oysters, and herring.	Blood, brain, heart, and prostrate gland.

Functions	Deficiency Symptoms	Therapeutic Uses
Collagen synthesis and body tissue formation.	Not known.	Arthritis. External: skin disorders (eczema, dermatitis, psoriasis).
Inhibits formation of cholesterol in blood vessels.	High blood pressure, hardening of arteries.	Aids in preventing heart attacks and high blood pressure
Burn and wound healing, carbohydrate digestion, prostrate gland function, reproductive organ growth & development, sex organ growth and maturity, vitamin B1, and phos-phorus and protein metabolism.	Delayed sexual maturity, fatigue, loss of taste, poor appetite, prolonged wound healing, retarded growth, and sterility.	Alcoholism, arteriosclerosis, baldness, cirrhosis, diabetes, internal & external wound and injury healing, high cholesterol (eliminates deposits), and infertility.

VITAMINS

NATURAL OR SYNTHETIC?

It is a Global opinion that vitamins in their natural, balanced state are essential for better assimilation, synergistic action, and maximum biological effect. As a rule of thumb — if the source is not given, the product is synthetic. There are however, a growing number of natural supplement manufacturers that use synthetic vitamins, but use the words natural and/or organic on their labels, in order to mislead the public. The guide below will help you break through the deliberate labeling confusion used by some companies. Don't be misled; be an expert label reader even in a health food store.

Vitamin	Source	Form
Vitamin A	(Natural)	Carrot powder, carrot oil, fish liver oils, lemon grass.
	(Synthetic)	Acetate or palmitate.
Vitamin B1	(Natural)	Rice bran or yeast.
	(Synthetic)	Thiamine hydrochloride, thiamine chloride, thiamine mononitrate.
Vitamin B2	(Natural)	Rice bran or yeast.
	(Synthetic)	Riboflavin.
Vitamin B3	(Natural)	Rice bran or yeast.
	(Synthetic)	Nicotinic acid, niacinamide, or if source not given.
Vitamin B5	(Natural)	Yeast, rice bran, or royal bee jelly.
	(Synthetic)	Calcium pantothenate.
Vitamin B6	(Natural)	Yeast or bran.
	(Synthetic)	Pyridoxine hydrochloride.
Vitamin B9	(Natural)	Yeast or liver.
	(Synthetic)	Pteroylglutamic acid.

Vitamin Source Form

Vitamin B12 (Natural) Cobalamin, cyanocobalamin, liver, or yeast.

Biotin (Natural) Biotin, liver, or yeast.
(Synthetic) D-biotin.

Choline (Natural) Egg yolk, soy oil, lecithin, liver, or yeast.
(Synthetic) Chloine bitartrate, choline chloride, choline citrate.

Inositol (Natural) Corn, liver, soybeans, or yeast.

PABA (Natural) Liver or yeast.
(Synthetic) Para-aminobenzoic acid.

Vitamin B13 (Natural) Calcium orotate or orotic acid.

Vitamin B15 (Natural) Apricot kernels, rice bran, or calcium pangamate.
(Synthetic) Pangamic acid.

Vitamin B17 (Natural) Apricot, peach, and/or plum pits.

B Complex (Natural) Brewer's yeast or soy beans.
(Synthetic) Choline bitartrate, d-biotin, or if source not given.

Vitamin C (Natural) Rose hips, acerola, citrus fruits, green peppers.
(Synthetic) Ascorbic acid, calcium ascorbate, or sodium ascorbate.

Vitamin D (Natural) Fish oils.
(Synthetic) Calciferol or irradiated ergosterol.

Vitamin	Source	Form
Vitamin E	(Natural)	Tocopherol acetate, mixed tocopherols, wheat germ or vegetable oils.
	(Synthetic)	Dl-Alpha tocopherol acetate, dl-alpha tocopherol, or dl-alpha tocopheryl succinate.
Vitamin F	(Natural)	Linseed oil or vegetable oils.
Vitamin H	(Natural)	Yeast.
	(Synthetic)	D-biotin.
Vitamin K-1	(Natural)	From chlorophyll of green plants.
Vitamin K-2	(Natural)	Fish meal, or microorganism cultures.
Vitamin K-3	(Synthetic)	Menadione.
Vitamin P	(Natural)	Citrus bioflavonoids, citrin, hesperidin, rutin.
Vitamin T	(Natural)	Sesame seed.
Vitamin U	(Natural)	Cabbage extract.

MINERALS

NATURAL OR SYNTHETIC?

Mineral   Source   Form

Calcium   (Natural)   Calcium carbonate, calcium lactate, calcium gluconate, calcium oxide, Bone meal, dolomite, eggshell calcium, oyster-shell calcium.

            (Synthetic)   Di-cal phosphate.

Cobalt   (- - - -)   Available only in vitamin B12

Copper   (Natural)   Hemoglobin, chlorophyll, or copper carbonate.

            (Synthetic)   Copper gluconate or copper sulfate.

Chromium   (Natural)   Chromium carbonate or yeast.

Fluorine   (- - - -)   Available only in some complete multi-mineral supplements.

Iodine   (Natural)   Sea kelp, seaweed, or seasalt.
            (Synthetic)   Potassium iodide.

Iron   (Natural)   Bone marrow, desiccated liver, molasses, yeast, iron oxide.

            (Synthetic)   Ferrous fumerate, ferrous gluconate, ferrous sulfate, iron lactate, or iron peptonate.

Magnesium   (Natural)   Yeast, liver, dolomite, or magnesium oxide.

            (Synthetic)   magnesium gluconate, magnesium palmitate, or magnesium sulfate.

Manganese   (Natural)   Manganese carbonate, liver, or yeast.

            (Synthetic)   Manganese gluconate.

Mineral	Source	Form
Phosphorus	(Natural)	**Bone meal.**
	(Synthetic)	Calcium phosphate.
Potassium	(Natural)	**Potassium citrate.**
	(Synthetic)	Potassium gluconate or potassium chloride.
Selenium	(Natural)	**Yeast.**
	(Synthetic)	Sodium selenite.
Silicon	(Natural)	**Silica.**
Sodium	(Synthetic)	Sodium chloride.
Sulfur	(- - - -)	**Available in some complete multi-mineral supplements, and in ointment form.**
Zinc	(Natural)	**Zinc oxide, liver, or yeast.**
	(Synthetic)	Zinc citrate, zinc gluconate, or zinc sulfate.

A WORD ABOUT HERBS

HERBAL DOSAGES

You should only use the dosages recommended by the manufacturer as the strengths can vary. The quantities and frequencies written on the labels are for adults weighing approximately 150 lbs. When using herbal remedies for children or the elderly, the use should be decreased. Herbal capsules may be prepared as a tea. To make sure that the herbs are properly assimilated, they should be taken with a full glass of water.

HERBAL PREPARATIONS

SINGLE HERBS

A herb with medical properties used by Herbalists for the prevention and correction of disease. All herbs in this book are presented for the express purpose of making it easy for the layman to use.

DRIED HERBS

Dried herbs should be as fresh as possible and stored out of direct sunlight in an airtight container. These herbs may be brewed into a tea or put into capsules

FRESH HERBS

The beneficial properties of herbs as medicines will often depend upon the greenness and ripeness of the plant. Store out of direct sunlight in a refrigerated environment.

POWDERED HERBS

The useful part of a herb is ground into powder. The required dose may be mixed in water, juice, or prepared as a tea. Powders are also used in capsule or tablet form.

HERBAL COMBINATIONS

Herbal combinations consist of two or more herbs selected and compounded to cover symptoms of specific diseases. A single herb often does not have all of the therapeutic qualities that are required. Combinations are available in capsules, tablets, extracts, teas, ointments, and salves.

HERBAL TEAS

Herbal teas are made up of single herbs, or a combination of herbs that are especially designed to maintain balance and restore tone to a particular area. Herbal teas are sold in bulk or tea bag form. Use only as directed.

CREAMS, OINTMENTS, and SALVES.

The above preparations are for external use only and generally used on bruises, sores, and inflammations. Use only as directed, as some of the combinations can have potent ingredients.

EXTRACTS, SYRUPS and TINCTURES

When immediate results are needed, the liquid extracts are suitable because of their rapid absorption. They can be added to small amounts of juice, water, and herb teas to make them more palatable.

ESSENTIAL OILS

Essential oils are for external use only. Primarily used for aroma therapy, the practice of using fragrances to promote health and relaxation. Essential oils are found in bath oils, massage oils, and perfumes.

HERBAL COSMETICS

These are excellent alternatives to the chemical laden cosmetic lines found in supermarkets. Health food stores carry natural herbal cosmetics, shampoos and conditioners, moisturizers, facial cleansers, deodorants, perfumes, mouthwash, and toothpaste.

COMMON WESTERN HERBS

AGAR AGAR *(Gelidiumamansii)*

Medicinal Parts: Algae.

Actions and Uses: Absorbs moisture and putrifactive material in the intestinal tract. Used as a mechanical laxative for constipation (it swells into a soft mass) a good remedy when feces are hard and the intestines are dry. This herb is used in many formulas for intestinal lubrication and bulk.

Bodily Influence: Demulcent, Laxative, and Nutritive.

AGRIMONY *(Agrimoniaeupatoria)*

Medicinal Parts: Leaves, Root, Whole Herb.

Actions and Uses: A blood cleanser, opens the obstructions of the liver, and loosens the hardness of the spleen. It is healing to all inward wounds, bruises, pains, and other distempers. Useful for asthma, colds, fevers, diarrhea, bowel complaints, relaxed bowels, chronic mucous diseases, and is used as a douche for vaginal problems.

External Use: Tincture applied to draw out foreign objects such as thorns and splinters of wood.

Bodily Influence: Deobstruent, Diuretic, Hepatic, Stomachic, Mild Astringent, and Tonic.

ALE HOOF *(Glecoma hederacea)*

Medicinal Part: Leaves.

Actions and Uses: Ale Hoof will ease all gripping pains, gas, and choleric conditions of the stomach and spleen. A herb for all inward wounds, ulcerated lungs, or other parts indicating the same condition. It also opens the stoppage of the liver and gall-bladder, so is useful in treating Yellow Jaundice.

Bodily Influence: Pectoral, Stimulant, and Tonic.

ALFALFA *(Medicago sativia)*

Medicinal Parts: Flowers, Leaves, Petals, and Sprouts.

Actions and Uses: Very high in vitamins and minerals thus nourishes the entire system. Excellent for pregnant women and nursing mothers. Good for the pituitary gland. It alkalizes the body rapidly and helps detoxify the liver. Helps rebuild decayed teeth, relieves fluid retention, dissolves kidney stones, and relieves arthritic and rheumatic pain. Also aids in the assimilation of protein, fats, and carbohydrates. Contains an anti fungus agent.

Bodily Influence: Alterative, Nutrient, and Tonic.

ALFA-MAX *(Medicago sativa)*

Medicinal Part: Leaves.

Actions and Uses: A concentrated alfalfa extract made from the leaves of alfalfa. Alfalfa surpasses all other natural, unprocessed foods in vitamin and mineral content. Approximately one ton of green alfalfa makes 80 lbs. of Alfa-Max.

Warning: If you have an auto-immune problem, such as lupus, avoid Alfa-Max.

Bodily Influence: Nutrient, and Tonic.

ALLIUM *(Allium liliaceae)*

Medicinal Part: Bulb.

Actions and Uses: Natural antibiotic, stimulates activity of the digestive organs, therefore relieves problems associated with poor digestion. It is used to emulsify the cholesterol and loosen it from the arterial walls. Proven useful in asthma and whooping cough. Its anti fungal properties make it a good adjunct in treating vaginal yeast infections *(candida albicans)*. Valuable in intestinal infections and effective in reducing high blood pressure. Recent studies show that Aullium has cancer-inhibiting properties (Aullium is toxic to some tumor cells).

External Use: Apply directly on affected parts for aches, sprains and skin disorders. Drops in ear relieves earache.

Bodily Influence: Alterative, Antibiotic, and Esculent.

ALMOND *(Prunus amygdalus)*

Medicinal Part: Seed.

Actions and Uses: The Chinese have used almond oil for over two thousand years as a muscle relaxer and a local anesthetic. According to a study at the Health Research and Studies Center in Los Altos, California, almond oil was a more effective cholesterol-reducing agent than olive oil, so it may also help prevent heart disease.

External Use: Almond oil can moisturize and soften the skin.

Bodily Influence: Antibiotic, Emollient, and Nervine.

ALOE VERA *(Aloe barbadenis)*

Medicinal Part: Leaves.

Actions and Uses: Aloe Vera is a potent medicine and healer. An excellent colon cleanser. Healing and soothing to the stomach as well as liver, kidneys, spleen, and bladder. Works with your immune system to keep you healthy, strong, and vibrant.

External use: An excellent remedy for piles and hemorrhoids. Keeps skin soft and supple, useful for minor burns, mild skin irritations, and insect bites.

Warning: Aloe is an effective laxative, and should not be taken internally during pregnancy.

Bodily Influence: Anthelmintic, Emmenagogue, Purgative, and Tonic.

ALUM ROOT *(Heuchera americana)*

Medicinal Parts: Root.

Actions and Uses: A pure and powerful astringent used in hemorrhage of surface capillaries and small bleeding vessels of the nose. Good for diarrhea and dysentery. Also used as an injection for bleeding piles, and leukorrhea.

Bodily Influence: Astringent, and Styptic.

AMERICAN SLOE *(Viburnum punifolium)*

Medicinal Part: Root bark.

Actions and Uses: Black haw is commonly used to ease contractions and cramps in the pelvic organs. An excellent treatment for painful menstruation, whether due to congested tissue or nerve disability. Used as a sedative to the female reproductive organs and has a tonic effect during pregnancy. Also a valuable remedy in chronic uterine inflammation, congested uterus, and leukorrhea.

Bodily Influence: Antispasmodic, Emmenagogue, and Sedative, and Tonic.

ANGELICA *(Angelicaarchangelica)*

Medicinal Parts: Herb, Root, and Seed.

Actions and Uses: Resists poisons, aids in expulsion of gas from the stomach and intestines, also good for colic, gripe and heartburn. Antispasmodic action relieves menstrual cramps. Reduces buildup of phlegm due to bronchitis and asthma. Promotes secretion of fluid from respiratory track. Tea taken hot, will quickly break up a cold and one to three capsules can be taken each day for a tonic.

Warning: Diabetics should avoid using angelica as it may cause weakness. This herb is a strong emmenagogue and should not be taken by pregnant women.

External use: Liniment or poultice used to treat chest congestion, rheumatic pains, and muscle spasms.

Bodily Influence: Aromatic, Carminative, Diaphoretic, Diuretic, Emmenagogue, Expectorant, and Stimulant.

ANISE *(Pimpinellaanisum)*

Medicinal Part: Seed.

Actions and Uses: Anise tea promotes digestion, relieves cramps, digestive disorders, and expels gas. Also helps loosen phlegm, and clear congestion. Good for coughs and colds. Also stimulates milk production when sipped by nursing mothers.

Bodily Influence: Anticatarrhal, Carminative, and Nervine.

APPLE *(Pyrusmalus)*

Medicinal Parts: Fruit.

Actions and Uses: A soluble fiber called pectin is found in apples. Pectin has the ability to lower blood cholesterol levels, reducing the risk of heart disease. Used to regulate blood sugar, control normal bowel function, and help prevent constipation and diarrhea.

Bodily Influence: Esculent, Nutritive, and Stomachic.

APPLE MINT *(Menthapiperita)*

Medicinal Part: Leaves, Stems.

Actions and Uses: Apple mint is an agreeable and harmless herb for infants and children as well as adults. Prepared as a herbal tea it is cleansing to the entire system, and will strengthen heart muscles. An excellent remedy for sea sickness, and an effective agent for suppressed menstruation. Useful for cramps and hiccoughs, prevent the gripping effects of cathartics, relieve hysterics, chills colic, influenza, nausea, and vomiting.

External Use: Tincture applied to forehead will relieve most headaches. Also apply oil to burns, neuralgia, rheumatism, and toothaches. Enemas are effective treatments for cholera and colon troubles.

Bodily Influence: Aromatic, Carminative, Stimulant, Stomachic.

APRICOT *(Prunusarmeniaca)*

Medicinal Parts: Kernel.

Actions and Uses: In Chinese traditional medicine, this herb is only used as a nutritive tonic for the lungs. In the west, the apricot kernel is highly regarded as an anti-cancer source of laetrile.

Bodily Influence: Demulcent, Expectorant, and Nutritive.

ARBUTUS, TRAILING *(Epigaearepens)*

Medicinal Part: Leaves.

Actions and Uses: Arbutus is superior to Buchu, and Uva Ursi. An extremely effective treatment in all lithic acid diseases, of the urinary organs associated with irritation. Used for chronic inflammation of the bladder, digestive disorders, gravel, debilitated or relaxed bladder, irritation of the urethra, urine retention, nephritis, cystitis, and catarrh of the bladder.

Warning: Avoid long term use. Do not use if blood or pus is observed in the urine. Arbutus can be irritating to the kidneys.

Bodily Influence: Antiseptic, Diuretic, and Stimulant.

ARNICA *(Arnicamontana)*

Medicinal Part: Flower, Rhizome.

Actions and Uses: Arnica is considered to be natures number one pain killer. Patients recover much more rapidly than under morphine. Used for headaches, pain, and swelling of dental extraction's, mental of physical shock, fractured bones, and sprains of joints.

External Use: Compresses used on any unbroken surface to stop pain, such as bruises, gout, rheumatic joints, etc.

Warning: Care should be taken when given internally, as large amounts are poisonous.

Bodily Influence: Anodyne, and Sedative.

ARTEMISIAS *(Artemisia Compositae)*

Medicinal Parts: Tops and Leaves.

Actions and Uses: Used for aminorrhoes, chronic leukorrhea, diabetes, diarrhea, female complaints, inflammation of tonsils and quinsy. Also small doses are used for dispersing the yellow bile of jaundice from the skin caused by liver conditions.

External Use: Apply Artemisias oil to bruises, local inflammations, sprains, swellings, rheumatism, and lumbago.

Warning: Overdose will irritate the stomach and increase heart action.

Bodily Influence: Anthelmintic, Febrifuge, Narcotic, Stimulant, Stomachic, and Tonic.

ARTICHOKE *(Cynara scolymus)*

Medicinal Parts: Flower, Fruit.

Actions and Uses: The flower of this herb has been used for centuries as an aphrodisiac. Artichoke produces an anti cholesterol drug called cynara that has the ability to lower blood cholesterol levels, reducing the risk of heart disease. Also used to enhance liver function by increasing bile production, and works as a diuretic, relieving excess water weight.

Bodily Influence: Alterative, Cholagogue, Esculent, and Tonic.

ASPARAGUS *(Asparagus officinalis)*

Medicinal Parts: Whole Herb.

Actions and Uses: This herb contains steroidal glycosides that stimulate hormone production and act as an anti inflammatory in the treatment of rheumatism. Also used to promote fertility, increase milk production in nursing mothers, help reduce menstrual cramps, and works as a diuretic, relieving excess water weight.

Bodily Influence: Antirheumatic, Antispasmodic, Diuretic, Galactagogue.

ASTRAGALUS *(Astragalus membranaceous)*

Medicinal Part: Root.

Actions and Uses: An Oriental herb used for a wide variety of ailments such as diabetes, heart disease, high blood pressure, and also improves digestion. Strengthens the immune systems and promotes healing. Astragalus has been used to help restore normal immune function and may prevent the spread of malignant cells in cancer patients.

Bodily Influence: Anhydrotic, Diuretic, and Tonic.

BARBERRY *(Berberisvulgaris)*

Medicinal Parts: Bark, Berries and Root.

Actions and Uses: This herb is an excellent body cleanse, used for consumption, heart burn, rheumatism, sores, and ulcers. A very good cough medicine, and as a blood tonic, it will help convalescent patients recuperate. Antiseptic root tea also used for kidney ailments.

External use — Liquid from the ground root is effective for the treatment of minor injuries, wounds, cuts, and bruises.

Bodily Influence: Alterative, Antiseptic, Aromatic, Laxative, Stimulant, and Tonic.

BARLEY GRASS *(Hordeumdistichum)*

Medicinal Part: Leaves, and Seeds.

Actions and Uses: The leaves are an excellent source of chlorophyll. Barley water steeped from the seed is used to treat rheumatic, and arthritic symptoms, and is effective for relief in fevers, diarrhea, and stomach irritations.

Bodily Influence: Demulcent, and Nutritive.

BASIL *(Ocimumbasilicum)*

Medicinal Part: Leaves, and Seeds.

Actions and Uses: This herb is an effective remedy for digestive disorders. Used to promote normal bowel functions, relieve gas, constipation, nausea, vomiting, stomach cramps, and irritations.

Bodily Influence: Adaptogen, Antiemetic, Carthartic, Stomachic.

BAYBERRY *(Myrica cerifera)*

Medicinal Part: The Root Bark.

Actions and Uses: Bayberry is both a general and special stimulant to the mucous membranes. Effective influence in diseased mucus accumulation of the alimentary canal. Used for bronchopulmonic diseases such as chronic catarrhal diarrhea, dysentery, gastritis, goiter, and leukorrhea. Made into a tea it is excellent as a gargle for sore throats. Valuable for all kinds of hemorrhages.

External Use: Rub liquid mixture on skin ulcers, boils, carbuncles, hemorrhoids, and varicose veins as needed.

Bodily Influence: Astringent, Emetic, Stimulant, and Tonic.

BEARBERRY *(Arctostaphylos uva ursi)*

Medicinal Part: Leaves.

Actions and Uses: Bearberry is a perennial evergreen shrub that grows at very high altitudes (5000 to 9000 Ft.) Extremely effective in the treatment for diseases of the urinary organs, chronic affections of the kidneys, discharges from the bladder, and all derangement's of the water passages. Also useful in the treatment of chronic diarrhea, dysentery, liver, pancreas, piles, spleen, and profuse menstruation.

Bodily Influence: Astringent, Diuretic, Tonic.

BEE POLLEN

Medicinal Part: Fresh pollen from bees.

Actions and Uses: A miracle food from nature rich in vitamins, minerals, and amino acids. Reduces the craving for protein. Used for aging, prostrate gland, fatigue, allergies, and as a sexual rejuvenate. Also contains natural antibodies so is effective against infections.

Warning: Some people may be allergic to bee pollen. Use small amounts at first and discontinue if discomfort or any other symptoms occur.

Bodily Influence: Anti microbial and Antiseptic.

BEECHDROP *(Orobanche Virginiana)*

Medicinal Part: Whole plant.

Actions and Uses: This herb is used by homoepaths to treat cancer. Also good for diarrhoea, asthma, and is valuable in the treatment of obstinate ulcers of the mouth and stomach.

External Use: Apply salve to minor bruises, cuts, and wounds.

Bodily Influence: An eminent astringent.

BEET

Medicinal Part: Root.

Actions and Uses: One of the best-known plant sources of assimil-able iron. Good for toning and rebuilding liver, also gall bladder infections. Also contains Vitamin A, B, C, sodium, potassium, calcium, and chlorine.

Bodily Influence: Adaptogen, Hepatic, and Nutritive.

BETH ROOT *(TrilliumPendulum)*

Medicinal Part: Root.

Actions and Uses: Beth root controls excessive vaginal discharges and excessive menstruation. It is an excellent remedy for coughs, bronchial problems, and hemorrhages from the lungs. Helps restore normal nerve supply to the organs in the thorax and is useful in treating diarrhea and dysentery.

Bodily Influence: Antiseptic, Astringent, Emmenagogue, and Tonic.

BILBERRY *(Vacciniummyrtillus)*

Medicinal Part: Leaves and Berries.

Actions and Uses: Bilberry has a well established reputation as being similar to insulin for sugar diabetes. Helps preserve eyesight and prevent eye damage. Extremely effective for people who suffer from eyestrain or night blindness. Also useful for diarrhea, dropsy, gravel, liver and stomach conditions.

Warning: Leaves can be poisonous if consumed over a long period of time, use only recommended dosage.

Bodily Influence: Astringent, Diuretic, and Refrigerant.

BIRCH *(Betulaalba)*

Medicinal Part: Bark and Leaves.

Actions and Uses: An effective treatment for dropsy, gout, rheumatism, stones in the kidneys and bladder, and is used to expel worms. Also a good remedy for diarrhoea, dysentery, cholera, and all problems of the alimentary tract. Oil of wintergreen is distilled from the inner bark.

External Use: Extract of the buds, bark, and leaves is applied boils, eczema, swelling, and rheumatic pain.

Bodily Influence: Aromatic, Diaphoretic, and Stimulant.

BISTORT *(Polygonumbistorta)*

Medicinal Part: Root.

Actions and Uses: Bistort is a powerful astringent. An excellent herb in the treatment of diarrhea, dysentery, and hemorrhages from the stomach and lungs. Also used as a gargle for throat and mouth infections and as a douche for leukorrhea.

External Use: Used as a poultice for strains, sprains, and sore bruises. Makes an excellent dressing for wounds and cuts when mixed with echinacea, goldenseal, and myrrh.

Bodily Influence: Antiseptic, Astringent, and Styptic.

BITTER MELON *(Momordica charantia)*

Medicinal Part: Fruit.

Actions and Uses: Bitter melon has been used for many years in traditional medicine to treat diabetes, hyperglycemia and other blood sugar abnormalities.

Bodily Influence: Adaptogen, and Depurative.

BITTER ROOT *(Apocynum androsaemifolium)*

Medicinal Part: Root.

Actions and Uses: Bitter root is considered by the American Indians as almost infallible in the treatment of venereal diseases. Recommended to relieve cardial dropsy, rheumatic gout of the joints, and in the treatment of brights disease. Also used for jaundice, chronic liver conditions, emptying the gall ducts, and gall stones.

External Use: Apply two or three times a day to remove warts.

Bodily Influence: Emetic, Expectorant, Diaphoretic, Laxative, and Tonic.

BLACK BERRY *(Rubus villosus)*

Medicinal Part: Leaves and Root bark.

Actions and Uses: A good astringent for watery diarrhea in children. Blackberry syrup is used as a tonic for children with weak stomachs, no appetite and skin pallor. Also an effective treatment for deficient glandular secretions of the stomach and intestines.

External Use: Salve acts as an astringent to haemorrhoids. Gargle the tea of roots or leaves for sore mouth and inflamed throat.

Bodily Influence: Astringent, Diuretic, Hemostatic, Syptic, and Tonic.

BLACK COHOSH *(Cimicifugaracemosa)*

Medicinal Part: Root and Rhizome.

Actions and Uses: A natural precursor to estrogen; helps relieve symptoms such as premenstrual and menstrual cramps. Relieves muscle spasms and swelling and soreness typical of rheumatism. Lowers cholesterol and high blood pressure (equalizes circulation), helpful for poisonous bites, reduces mucus levels, and relieves sinusitis and asthma.

Bodily Influence: Alterative, Anti-spasmodic, Cardiac Stimulant, Diuretic, Diaphoretic, Emmenagogue, Expectorant, and Sedative (arterial and nervous)

Warning: Do not take if you are pregnant or have any type of chronic disease. An overdose will produce nausea and vomiting.

BLACK HAW *(Viburnumpunifolium)*

Medicinal Part: Root bark.

Actions and Uses: Black haw is commonly used to ease contractions and cramps in the pelvic organs. An excellent treatment for painful menstruation, whether due to congested tissue or nerve disability. Used as a sedative to the female reproductive organs and has a tonic effect during pregnancy. Also a valuable remedy in chronic uterine inflammation, congested uterus, and leukorrhea.

Bodily Influence: Antispasmodic, Emmenagogue, and Sedative, and Tonic.

BLACK ROOT *(Leptandravirginica)*

Medicinal Part: Root.

Actions and Uses: Black root acts on the intestines in chronic constipation and is very effective in treating chronic Hepatic diseases. Also used for ascites, bilious fever, dyspepsia, headache, jaundice, pleurisy, and liver disorders.

Bodily Influence: Alterative, Antiseptic, Cholagogue, Emetocathartic, Laxative, and Tonic.

BLACK WALNUT *(Juglansnigra)*

Medicinal Parts: Bark, Husks, Leaves, Rind, Green Nut.

Actions and Uses: Expels internal parasites and tape worms. Helps promote bowel regularity. Aids in treatment of tuberculosis, diarrhea, toxic blood conditions, and promotes healing of sores in mouth and throat. Rich in manganese which is important for nerves, brain, and cartilage, and helps relieve many kinds of skin problems.

External Uses: Should be applied topically to ring worm twice a day until it disappears. Also beneficial for boils, eczema, herpes, psoriasis, and vaginitis.

Bodily Influence: Antiseptic, Astringent, Tonic, and Vermifuge.

BLADDERWRACK *(Blansbindeictus)*

Medicinal Parts: Leaves and Root.

Actions and Uses: A little known American herb with a lot of potential. Eliminates parasites, improves goiter and kidney functions, increases thyroid activity, and absorbs water in the intestines to produce bulk.

Bodily Influence: Adaptogen, and Vermifuge.

BLESSED THISTLE *(Cnicusbenedictus)*

Medicinal Parts: Flower, Leaves, Root, and Seed.

Actions and Uses: Stimulates appetite, helps regulate menstrual cycle, promotes menstrual discharge, regulates hormones, increases milk production while nursing, and used in treating liver problems. Also a stimulant for the brain, circulation, heart, and nerves.

Bodily Influence: Adaptogen, Emmenagogue, Galactagogue, Stomachic, and Stimulant.

Warning: Do not use during pregnancy, and handle carefully to avoid toxic skin effects.

BLOOD ROOT *(Sanguinariacanadensis)*

Medicinal Parts: Root.

Actions and Uses: Small doses stimulate the digestive system. When taken in large doses it is an arterial sedative. This herb is effective in treating asthma, chronic bronchitis, laryngitis, whooping cough, and other complaints of the respiratory organs. The tincture has been used successfully in treating dyspepsia and dropsy of the chest.

External Use: Injections of strong tea is excellent for leucorrhoea and haemorrhoids.

Bodily Influence: Alterative, Diuretic, Febrifuge, Sialagogue, Stimulating expectorant, Systemic emetic, and Tonic.

BLUE COHOSH *(Caulophyllumthalictroides)*

Medicinal Part: Root.

Actions and Uses: Especially valuable in epileptic fits and ulceration's of the mouth and throat. Used for suppressed menstruation and to help regulate menstrual flow. Relieves or prevents spasms, cramps, colic, diabetes, leukorrhea, nervous disorders, rheumatism. Elevates blood pressure, cleanses blood, promotes perspiration, and also increases volume of urine excreted.

Bodily Influence: Antispasmodic, Depurative, Diuretic, Dysmenorrhea, Emmenagogue, Oxytocic, Parturient, Sudorific and Spasmodic.

Warning: Not recommended for pregnant women.

BLUE FLAG *(Iris versicolor)*

Medicinal Parts: Root, Rhizome.

Actions and Uses: A valuable herb for all diseases of the blood, kidney, spleen, and chronic hepatic affections. Has a special influence on the lymphatic glands (pure lymphatic circulation is spontaneous to longevity). Also effective in treating secondary Syphilis.

External Uses: Used in treating infected wounds, ulcers, and fistula.

Bodily Influence: Alterative, Cathartic, Diuretic, Resolvent, Sialagogue, and Vermifuge.

BLUE GUM TREE *(Eucalyptusglobulus,Labill)*

Medicinal Parts: Oil, Bark, Leaves.

Actions and Uses: Oil from this tree is extremely potent. An infusion is effective in treating scarlet, and typhoid fevers. It may be inhaled for asthma, diphtheria, congestion, colds, flu, and sore throat.

External Use: Apply salve as a local antiseptic. Is a stimulant and corrective to boils, carbuncles, growths, sores, ulcers, wounds, and the pain, stiffness and swelling of arthritis and rheumatism.

Warning: Oil may be taken internally only in small doses. Overdose will result in nausea, vomiting, and related effects. Do not use on open wounds.

Bodily Influence: Antiseptic, Antispasmodic, Astringent, and Tonic.

BLUE VERVAIN *(Verbena hastata)*

Medicinal Parts: Leaves, Root, and Stems.

Actions and Uses: Effective treatment for epilepsy, falling sickness, and fits. Also expels worms, increases and restores proper blood circulation, relieves bladder, helps to expel phlegm from the throat and lungs. Good for asthma, colds, epilepsy, female disorders, fever, flu, headaches, and pneumonia.

Bodily Influence: Antiperiodic, Antispasmodic, Diaphoretic, Emetic, Expectorant, Nervine, Sudorific, and Tonic.

BONESET *(Eupatorium perfoliatum)*

Medicinal Parts: Leaves and Tops.

Actions and Uses: Boneset is duel in action: (when warm emetic diaphoretic; when cold a tonic). This duel action herb has a calming effect on the system. Used as a mild laxative, to reduce fevers, good for dropsy, intemperance, and to promote perspiration. Also effective in the treatment of acute and chronic rheumatism.

Bodily Influence: Antispasmodic, Aperient, Diaphoretic, Emetic, Stimulant, and Tonic.

BORAGE *(Borago officinalis)*

Medicinal Parts: Seeds.

Actions and Uses: A good source of essential fatty acids (EFA's). Studies show that Borage lowers blood cholesterol and reduces blood pressure. Early research suggests that this herb could be an effective remedy for heart disease and stroke. Good for female disorders such as PMS, hyperactivity, cramps, hot flashes, and heavy bleeding.

Bodily Influence: Astringent, Nervine, and Sedative

BOWLES MINT *(Mentha rotundifolia)*

Medicinal Part: Leaves, Stems.

Actions and Uses: Bowles Mint is an agreeable and harmless herb for infants and children as well as adults. Prepared as a herbal tea it is cleansing to the entire system, and will strengthen heart muscles. An excellent remedy for sea sickness, and an effective agent for suppressed menstruation. Useful for cramps and hiccoughs, prevent the gripping effects of cathartics, relieve hysterics, chills colic, influenza, nausea, and vomiting.

External Use: Tincture applied to forehead will relieve most headaches. Also apply oil to burns, neuralgia, rheumatism, and toothaches. Enemas are effective treatments for cholera and colon troubles.

Bodily Influence: Aromatic, Carminative, Stimulant, Stomachic.

BRIDEWORT *(Filipendulaulmaria)*

Medicinal Parts: Flower and Buds.

Actions and Uses: Bridewort was the first source of salicylic acid discovered. Used as a mild sedative and painkiller. As a tea it helps rid the body of feverish colds, heartburn, and excess fluids.

Bodily Influence: Nervine, and Sedative

BUCHU *(Barosmabetulina)*

Medicinal Part: Leaves.

Actions and Uses: Buchu and Uva Ursi are slightly milder than Arbutus (Epigaea repens), but still are extremely effective treatments in all lithic acid diseases, of the urinary organs associated with irritation. Used for chronic inflammation of the bladder, digestive disorders, gravel, debilitated or relaxed bladder, irritation of the urethra, urine retention, nephritis, cystitis, and catarrh of the bladder.

Warning: Avoid long term use. Buchu can be irritating to the kidneys.

Bodily Influence: Antiseptic, Diuretic, and Stimulant,

BUCKTHORN *(Rhamnuspurshiana)*

Medicinal Part: Dried Bark.

Actions and Uses: One of the best natural laxatives in the herbal kingdom. Extremely useful in hemorrhoidal conditions and chronic constipation. It is considered suitable for delicate and elderly persons. Also a very good remedy for gallstones; increases secretion of bile.

External Use: Apply locally to skin irritations, burns, and warts.

Bodily Influence: Laxative, and Bitter tonic.

BUGLEWEED *(Lycopus virginicus)*

Medicinal Part: Leaves.

Actions and Uses: An excellent herb for functional or organic heart diseases marked by irregular heartbeat. Used for treating coughs, chronic inflammation of the lungs, and all chest congestive diseases. Bugleweed has also been used successfully in the treatment of hemorrhages from the lungs and bowels.

External Uses: Extremely useful when made into an ointment for bruises and a lotion of Bugle, Alum and Honey is recommended for the treatment of mouth sores.

Bodily Influence: Antibiotic, Astringent, Detergent, and Sedative.

BULLS BLOOD *(Marrubium vulgara)*

Medicinal Parts: Whole Herb.

Actions and Uses: Used for congestion of coughs, colds, and pulmonary affections associated with unwanted phlegm from the chest, and promotes sweating which in turn, cools the body. Good for intestinal gas, when taken in large doses, it is a laxative and will expel worms.

Bodily Influence: Anthelmintic, Diuretic, Diaphoretic, Expectorant, Laxative, Resolvent, Stimulant, Stomachic, and Tonic.

BUPLEURUM *(Bupleurum chinese)*

Medicinal Part: Root.

Actions and Uses: Bupleurum is highly recommended for reducing fever and feverish headache. This herb is regarded as one of the best herbs for detoxifying the liver. Also used to relieve nausea, reduce anxiety, and dizziness.

Bodily Influence: Analgestic, Alterative, Antipyretic.

BURDOCK *(Arctium lappa)*

Medicinal Parts: Leaves, Seed, Stems, Root, (the whole herb).

Actions and Uses: Herbalists from around the world revere this herb, to be the ultimate blood purifier. Burdock effectively cleanses and eliminates impurities from the blood, thus alleviating boils, abscesses, eczema, and other skin disorders. An excellent diuretic, soothing to the kidneys. Excellent for gout, will reduce arthritic swelling and deposits within the joints.

External Use: For relief of pain and to hasten healing. Apply locally to skin irritations and burns.

Warning: Burdock interferes with iron absorption.

Bodily Influence: Alterative, Diaphoretic, Diuretic, and Tonic

BUTCHER'S BROOM *(Ruscusacluteatus)*

Medicinal Parts: Seeds, and Tops.

Actions and Uses: Builds up structure of the veins. Therefore, used for hemorrhoids and other types of varicose veins. Improves poor circulation and reduces swelling caused by arthritis and rheumatism. Also relieves inflammation in the kidney and bladder.

External Use: Apply ointment to hemorrhoids to reduce pain and swelling.

Bodily Influence: Demulcent, Mucilaginous, Rubifacient, and Styptic.

BUTTER NUT *(Juglanscinerea)*

Medicinal Part: Dried Inner Bark and Leaves.

Actions and Uses: A good treatment for diarrhea and dysentery. Also used for acne, angina pectoris, ecthyma, eczema, headache, herpes, and migraines. When combined with bitter root it is a good remedy for consumption.

External Use: Diluted tincture is effective for chronic skin diseases.

Bodily Influence: Cathartic, Tonic, and Vermifuge.

CALENDULA *(Calendulaofficinalis)*

Medicinal Part: Flower, Leaf, and Root.

Actions and Uses: Calindula reduces fevers, relieves menstrual cramps, soothes ulcers, and provides relief from skin virus such as shingles. It is also valued in treating vaginal infections, pruritis, and bleeding.

External Use: Soothes and promotes healing of burns and wounds. When applied directly to the ear the oil will reduce the pain of earache.

Bodily Influence: Anodyne, Antibiotic, Antipyretic, Astringent, Emollient, and Vulnerary.

CANADIAN SNAKE ROOT *(Cimicifugaracemosa)*

Medicinal Part: Root.

Actions and Uses: Accelerates childbirth causing stimulation of the involuntary muscles of the uterus. Effective remedy for the relief of pain during menstrual periods. Relieves gas from stomach and intestines. Promotes perspiration and increases volume of urine excreted.

External Use: The American Indians use the bruised root as an antidote for snake bites.

Bodily Influence: Carminative, Parturient, and Stomachic.

CANCER ROOT *(OrobancheVirginiana)*

Medicinal Part: Whole plant.

Actions and Uses: This herb is used by homoepaths to treat cancer. Also good for diarrhoea, asthma, and is valuable in the treatment of obstinate ulcers of the mouth and stomach.

External Use: Apply salve to minor bruises, cuts, and wounds.

Bodily Influence: An eminent astringent.

CAPSICUM (CAYENNE) *(Capsicumfrutescens)*

Medicinal Part: The fruit.

Actions and Uses: A catalyst for all herbs. Capsicum taken with Burdock, Ginger, Golden Seal, Slippery elm, etc., will soon diffuse itself throughout the whole system. Improves circulation, helps arteries, veins, and capillaries retain their elasticity. It soothes and rebuilds stomach tissue and is therefore, an excellent aid in healing intestinal and stomach ulcers. Combine with Lobelia for nerves. Unlike most stimulants of allopathy, it is not narcotic. Good for the heart, lungs kidneys, pancreas, spleen, and stomach.

External Use: Rub liniment on sprains, bruises, rheumatism, and neuralgia.

Bodily Influence: Carminative, Condiment, Diaphoretic, Rubefacient, Stimulant, and Tonic.

CARAWAY *(Carumcarvi)*

Medicinal Part: Seed.

Actions and Uses: A mild but effective herb for colic in infants. Used for most stomach disorders such as cramps, expulsion of gas, and nausea. Also used for coughs, colds, and stimulates the production of breast milk in nursing mothers.

Warning: Use the extract when administering to infants or young children.

Bodily Influence: Esculent, Galactagogue, Pectoral, Stomachic.

CARROT *(Daucus carota)*

Medicinal Parts: Root.

Actions and Uses: Recent studies sponsored by the National Cancer Institute confirm that people eating diets rich in carotene reduce their risk of developing certain forms of cancer. Carotene strengthens the eyes, helps counteract night blindness, and lowers cholesterol levels, reducing the risk of heart disease. Also soothes indigestion, relieving diarrhea, gas, and heartburn.

Bodily Influence: Adaptogen, Antacid, Carminative, Esculent, Stomachic.

CASCARA SAGRADA *(Rhamnus purshiana)*

Medicinal Part: Dried Bark.

Actions and Uses: One of the best natural laxatives in the herbal kingdom. A stimulant to the whole digestive system. Extremely useful in hemorrhoidal conditions, chronic constipation, and liver and gall bladder complaints. It is considered suitable for delicate and elderly persons. Also a very good remedy for gallstones; increases secretion of bile.

Bodily Influence: Antispasmodic, Hepatic, Laxative, and Bitter tonic.

CATNIP *(Nepata cataria)*

Medicinal Parts: The whole herb.

Actions and Uses: Excellent for small children with colic. Controls fever; catnip enemas reduce fever. Produces perspiration without increasing body temperature. Very good as a sleeping aid, relieves stress, and is soothing to the nerves. Also a digestive aid for gas and diarrhea.

External Use: Rub ointment on piles to ease pain.

Bodily Influence: Antispasmodic, Aphrodisiac (cats), Carminative, Diaphoretic, Emmenagogue, Stimulant, and Tonic.

CELERY *(Apium graveolens)*

Medicinal Parts: Root and Seed.

Actions and Uses: Used in incontinence of dropsical, urine, and liver problems. Good for arthritis, rheumatism, neuralgia, and nervousness. Acts as an antioxidant and a sedative. Enhances appetite, relieves gas, and has a calming effect on the digestive system.

Warning: Celery juice and oil induce menstruation, so should not be used during pregnancy.

Bodily Influence: Aromatic, Carminative, Diuretic, Nerve Sedative, Stimulant, and Tonic.

CHAMOMILE *(Matricaria chamomilla)*

Medicinal Parts: Flowers and Herb.

Actions and Uses: A natural sedative for hysteria, nightmares, delirium, and nervousness. Also used as a digestive aid for weak stomachs and to provide appetite. Effective use in childhood ailments such as colds, colic, earache, infantile convulsions, and stomach pains.

External Use: Oil from the Chamomile flower will comfort the side pain of liver and spleen. Also effective when rubbed on skin irritations and hemorrhoids.

Warning: Do not use for long periods of time. Do not use if allergic to ragweed.

Bodily Influence: Antispasmodic, Anodyne, Carminative, Diaphoretic, Emmenagogue, Nervine, Sedative, and Tonic.

CHAPARRAL *(Larrea divaricata)*

Medicinal Parts: Leaves and Stem.

Actions and Uses: Chaparral is an extremely effective blood purifier. One of natures best antibiotics, very useful in cases of acne, arthritis, chronic backache, tumor warts, and skin blotches. Protects from harmful effects of radiation and sun exposure. May help slow down the aging process by preventing the formation of free radicals. Also used for liver problems, lymphatic troubles, and digestive disorders.

External Use: Apply extract on injuries, skin diseases, herpes, scabies, arthritic pains and rheumatism.

Bodily Influence: Alterative, Antiseptic, Diuretic, Expectorant, Parasiticide, and Tonic.

CHASTE TREE *(Vitex verbenaceae)*

Medicinal Parts: Leaves, Flowers.

Actions and Uses: A hormone balancer and natural alternative to estrogen. European herbalists use Chaste tree for the treatment of female complaints. Useful for side effects associated with menopause, fibroid tumors, and PMS.

Bodily Influence: Adaptogen, Discutient, and Nervine.

CHERRY BIRCH *(Betulaalba)*

Medicinal Part: Bark and Leaves.

Actions and Uses: An effective treatment for dropsy, gout, rheumatism, stones in the kidneys and bladder, and is used to expel worms. Also a good remedy for diarrhoea, dysentery, cholera, and all problems of the alimentary tract. Oil of wintergreen is distilled from the inner bark.

External Use: Extract of the buds, bark, and leaves is applied boils, eczema, swelling, and rheumatic pain.

Bodily Influence: Aromatic, Diaphoretic, and Stimulant.

CHERVIL *(Anthruscus cerefolium)*

Medicinal Parts: Leaves.

Actions and Uses: A good source of vitamins and minerals. Stimulates digestion and alleviates circulation disorders and chronic catarrh.

Bodily Influence: Adaptogen, Condiment, and Esculent.

CHICKWEED *(Stellaria Media)*

Medicinal Parts: Whole Herb.

Actions and Uses: Used extensively to help lose weight. Excellent herb for the digestive system, kidney trouble, and inflammation or weakness of the bowels. Excellent bronchial cleanser. Good for bronchitis, colds, coughs, fevers, hoarseness, pleurisy, and inflammation of the lungs.

External Use: One of the best remedies for boils, tumors, hemorrhoids, and swollen testes.

Bodily Influences: Alterative, Antipyretic, Demulcent, Emollient, Pectoral, and Refrigerant.

CHICORY *(Cichoriumintybus)*

Medicinal Part: Root.

Actions and Uses: The root is ground to make a tonic, diuretic, and a mild laxative. Chicory is also useful in the treatment of gallstones, kidney stones, and inflammation of the urinary tract and liver.

Bodily Influence: Adaptogen, Laxative, and Tonic.

CHIVES *(Allium schoenoprasum)*

Medicinal Part: Leaves.

Actions and Uses: Used to stimulate the appetite, aid digestion, and good for most stomach disorders such as cramps, expulsion of gas, and nausea.

Bodily Influence: Esculent, Stomachic.

CHLORELLA

Medicinal Parts: Fresh spear leaves. (barley or wheat)

Actions and Uses: Highest known source of natural chlorophyll stimulates the natural immune system. Also very effective in detoxifying the liver, bloodstream and in cleansing the bowel. Chlorella helps clear heavy metals and harmful chemicals from the body.

Bodily Influences: Alterative, Depurative, Hepatic, Nutritive, and Stimulant.

CHRYSANTHEMUM *(Chrysanthemum morrifolium)*

Medicinal Parts: Flowers.

Actions and Uses: In China the dried chrysanthemum flowers are a symbol of longevity. Effective in detoxifying the liver, as a blood cleanser, and in lowering blood pressure. Also used in the treatment of conjunctivitis, dizziness, fevers, headaches, and pneumonia.

External Use: Tincture is used to reduce abscesses, boils, and inflammation of the skin.

Bodily Influences: Alterative, Antipyretic, and Carminative.

CLEAVERS *(Galium aparine)*

Medicinal Part: Whole Herb.

Actions and Uses: Cleavers is excellent when used to help break fevers and is one of our most effective herbs for obstructions of the urinary organs; acts as a solvent of stones in the bladder. Helps with urinary secretion. Also used for treatment of scurvy and treating children for bed wetting (it should be drunk three times a day).

External Use: Rub salve on burns, scalds, eczema, psoriasis, sunburn, skin diseases and eruption generally.

Bodily Influences: Alterative, Aperient, Diuretic, Refrigerant, and Tonic.

CITRUS PEEL *(Citrusreticulata)*

Medicinal Parts: Orange or tangerine peel.

Actions and Uses: The strength of citrus peel improves with drying and age. Peel is added to herbal formulas to stimulate and promote the circulation of energy. Effective treatment for abdominal swelling, diarrhea, indigestion, and vomiting.

Bodily Influences: Antiemetic, Antitussive, Digestant, Expectorant, Stimulant, and Stomachic.

CLOVES *(Caryophyllumaromaticus)*

Medicinal Part: Dried Buds and Fruit.

Actions and Uses: Cloves have been used in the Orient for over two thousand years as an aphrodisiac. Used to help control vomiting. Cloves are stimulating and warming to the system promoting sweating in colds, flu, and fevers. As a carminative it is good for gas and intestinal spasms.

External Use: Clove oil is highly antiseptic, and a highly praised remedy for toothache.

Bodily Influences: Antiemetic, Antiseptic, Aphrodisiac, Aromatic, Carminative, Stimulant, and Stomachic.

CODONOPSIS *(Panaxcodonopsis)*

Medicinal Part: Root.

Actions and Uses: Called "poor mans ginseng" in China. Has very similar qualities as ginseng, and can be used by both sexes in any climate.

Bodily Influences: Adaptogen and Tonic.

COLTSFOOT *(Tussilagofarfara)*

Medicinal Parts: Berries and Leaves.

Actions and Uses: For congestion of the pulmonary system, especially if inclined to consumption. Also used for asthma, bronchitis, coughs, catarrh, diarrhea, fever, inflammation, and ulcers.

External Use: Tincture used on open wounds to draw out injurious matter, salve is used for piles, and as a poultice in scrofulous tumors.

Warning: Carcinogenic properties have been discovered.

Bodily Influence: Demulcent, Emollient, Expectorant, Pectoral, and Tonic.

COMFREY *(Symphytum officinale)*

Medicinal Parts: Leaves and Root.

Actions and Uses: Comfrey contains allantoin, a substance that stimulates the growth of new cells. An effective blood cleanser and tissue builder, helps to heal broken bones, sprains and slow healing sores. Recommended for healing ulcers and kidney problems. Best remedy for blood in urine. Also a powerful remedy for coughs and catarrh.

External Use: Rub Comfrey salve or tincture on burns, bruises, ruptures, and fresh wounds.

Warning: Do not use for longer than 3 months at a time. May cause liver damage.

Bodily Influence: Astringent, Demulcent, Expectorate, Mucilage, and Vulnerary.

CORNSILK *(Tigmata maydis)*

Medicinal Part: The green pistils.

Actions and Uses: Corn Silk will assist all inflammatory conditions of the bladder, kidney, and urethra. Controls general malfunction of the body due to uric acid retention. Good for hypertension, edema, urinary tract dysfunction, and stones, bedwetting, and enlarged prostrate gland.

External Use: Rub ointment on wounds and ulcer-like skin disturbances.

Bodily Influence: Alterative, Demulcent, Diuretic, and Lithotriptic.

CORSICAN MINT *(Mentha piperita)*

Medicinal Part: Leaves, Stems.

Actions and Uses: An agreeable and harmless herb for infants and children as well as adults. Prepared as a herbal tea it is cleansing to the entire system, and will strengthen heart muscles.

An excellent remedy for sea sickness, and an effective agent for suppressed menstruation. Useful for cramps and hiccoughs, prevent the gripping effects of cathartics, relieve hysterics, chills colic, influenza, nausea, and vomiting.

External Use: Tincture applied to forehead will relieve most headaches. Also apply oil to burns, neuralgia, rheumatism, and toothaches. Enemas are effective treatments for cholera and colon troubles.

Bodily Influence: Aromatic, Carminative, Stimulant, Stomachic.

COWSLIP *(Primula officinalis)*

Medicinal Part: Flowers, Leaves.

Actions and Uses: Cowslip strengthens the brain and nervous systems. Highly recommended for convulsions, cramps, frenzy, false apprehension, palsy, and trembling. Also used to ease pain in the back and bladder.

External Use: Rub ointment on scalds and burns.

Bodily Influence: Antispasmodic, Sedative.

CRAMPBARK *(Viburnum opulis)*

Medicinal Part: Bark.

Actions and Uses: Crampbark is used for asthma, hysteria, spasms of involuntary muscles, and menstural cramps. This herb is also used for heart palpitation, nervous conditions and cramps during pregnancy.

Bodily Influence: Antispasmodic, Astringent, and Nervine.

CRANBERRY *(Vaccinium macrocarpon)*

Medicinal Part: Fruit.

Actions and Uses: Good for chronic kidney infections, prevents the spread of bacterial infection in the urinary tract. Also used as a treatment for relief of cramps and spasms of involuntary muscular contractions, such as in asthma and hysteria.

Bodily Influence: Diuretic, Mucilaginous, and Nervine.

CRANESBILL *(Geranium maculatum)*

Medicinal Part: Dried Root and Leaves.

Actions and Uses: Cranesbill is a powerful, non-irritating astringent. This herb controls diarrhea, secondary dysentery, and infantile cholera. Also used for diabetes, brights disease, and excessive chronic mucus discharges.

External Use: Rub ointment on hemorrhages, indolent ulcers, and piles. Apply powder to check bleeding from nose, wounds, and tooth extractions.

Bodily Influence: Astringent, Diuretic, Styptic, Tonic.

CREEPING PENNYROYAL *(Mentha pulegium)*

Medicinal Part: Leaves, Stems.

Actions and Uses: Creeping Pennyroyal is an agreeable and harmless herb for infants and children as well as adults. Prepared as a herbal tea it is cleansing to the entire system, and will strengthen heart muscles. An excellent remedy for sea sickness, and an effective agent for suppressed menstruation. Useful for cramps and hiccoughs, prevent the gripping effects of cathartics, relieve hysterics, chills colic, influenza, nausea, and vomiting.

External Use: Tincture applied to forehead will relieve most headaches. Also apply oil to burns, neuralgia, rheumatism, and toothaches. Enemas are effective treatments for cholera and colon troubles.

Bodily Influence: Aromatic, Carminative, Stimulant, Stomachic.

CULVER'S PHYSIC *(Leptandra virginica)*

Medicinal Part: Root.

Actions and Uses: Black root acts on the intestines in chronic constipation and is very effective in treating chronic Hepatic diseases. Also used for ascites, bilious fever, dyspepsia, headache, jaundice, pleurisy, and liver disorders.

Bodily Influence: Alterative, Antiseptic, Cholagogue, Emetocathartic, Laxative, and Tonic.

DAMIANA *(Turnera aphrodisiaca)*

Medicinal Part: Leaves.

Actions and Uses: A great sexual rejuvenator and stimulant to the central nervous system. Gives energy; helps to balance female hormones. Controls bed wetting, expels excess water from the body. Stimulates muscular contractions of the intestinal tract (relieves constipation) and increases blood circulation. Helps relieve anxiety and promotes a feeling of well-being.

Warning: Damiana interferes with iron absorption when taken internally. This herb has a tendency to overstimulate if used excessively.

Bodily Influence: Aphrodisiac, Cholagogue, Emmenagogue, Laxative, Stimulant, and Tonic.

DANDELION *(Leontodon taraxacum)*

Medicinal Part: Leaf and Root.

Actions and Uses: Strengthens kidneys and bladder, and removes excess fluids. Protects against liver and gallbladder disorders. Effective for the obstructions of the liver, gall, and spleen. A highly praised agent for skin diseases, scrofula, and scurvy. Excellent for anemia because it is high in iron, calcium and other vitamins and minerals. A very good diuretic.

Bodily Influence: Aperient, Deobstruent, Diuretic, Hepatic, Lithotriptic, Stomachic, and Tonic.

DEAD NETTLE *(Lamium maculatum)*

Medicinal Parts: Roots and Leaves.

Actions and Uses: Traditionally thought to have astringent properties. Dead Nettle is also prescribed as a blood purifier and used to encourage perspiration.

External Use: bruised leaves are used to stop bleeding and to cleanse wounds and ulcers.

Bodily Influence: Astringent, Alterative, and Tonic.

DEVILS CLAW *(Harpagophytum procumbens)*

Medicinal Part: Leaves and Root.

Actions and Uses: Recent studies compare the anti inflammatory action of Devil's Claw to the drugs cortisone and phenylbutazone. A blood cleanser which will remove deposits in the joints and aid in the elimination of uric acid from the body. A very effective painkiller for arthritis, gout, and rheumatism, and a recommended treatment for liver and kidney disorders.

Warning: Do not use during pregnancy.

Bodily Influence: Adaptogen, Alterative, Antirheumatic, and Depurative.

DEW BERRY *(Rubus villosus)*

Medicinal Part: Leaves and Root bark.

Actions and Uses: A good astringent for watery diarrhea in children. Blackberry syrup is used as a tonic for children with weak stomachs, no appetite and skin pallor. Also an effective treatment for deficient glandular secretions of the stomach and intestines.

External Use: Salve acts as an astringent to haemorrhoids. Gargle the tea of roots or leaves for sore mouth and inflamed throat.

Bodily Influence: Astringent, Diuretic, Hemostatic, Syptic, and Tonic.

DEWCUP *(Alchemilla vulgaris)*

Medicinal Part: Leaves, Rhizome.

Actions and Uses: Anciently known as a female hormone, used for beauty, youth, and longevity. Acts as a tonic, stimulates the appetite, and gives one a general feeling of well-being. Used for problems arising in menopause, such as hot flashes and helps to correct irregular menstruation. Also makes a soothing douche for vaginal irritations.

External Use: Apply tincture to open sores and wounds. Promotes healing and coagulation of blood.

Bodily Influence: Adaptogen, Emollient, Styptic, Vulnerary, Tonic.

DILL *(Aniethumgraveolens)*

Medicinal Part: Leaves, Stem, Seed.

Actions and Uses: A mild but effective herb for colic in infants. Used for most stomach disorders such as cramps, expulsion of gas, and nausea. Also stimulates the production of breast milk in nursing mothers.

Warning: Use the extract when administering to infants or young children.

Bodily Influence: Esculent, Galactagogue, Stomachic.

DOG'S BANE *(Apocynumandrosaemifolium)*

Medicinal Part: Root.

Actions and Uses: Bitter root is considered by the American Indians as almost infallible in the treatment of venereal diseases. Recommended to relieve cardial dropsy, rheumatic gout of the joints, and in the treatment of brights disease. Also used for jaundice, chronic liver conditions, emptying the gall ducts, and gall stones.

External Use: Apply two or three times a day to remove warts.

Bodily Influence: Emetic, Expectorant, Diaphoretic, Laxative, and Tonic.

DROP BERRY *(Polygonatumcommutatum)*

Medicinal Part: Rhizome.

Actions and Uses: Helps to mend broken bones. Also pulmonary consumption and bleeding of the lungs, female complaints, bruises, hemorrhoids, inflammations of the stomach, and tumors.

External Use: Tincture is used to close fresh and bleeding wounds. and the root extract is effective in diminishing freckles and discoloration of the skin.

Bodily Influence: Astringent, Demulcent, and Tonic.

ECHINACEA *(Echinaceaangustifolia)*

Medicinal Parts: Leaves, Dried Rhizome, and Root.

Actions and Uses: Glandular balancer, especially lymphatic and liver areas. Also blood purifier, antiseptic, and anti-infection herb. Good for boils, blood poisoning, carbuncles, all pus diseases, snake and spider bites. Helps boost immune response. Echinacea is also used to restore normal immune function in patients receiving chemotherapy.

External Use: Apply tincture to all infected wounds and insect bites.

Warning: Alcohol tincture may destroy polysaccharides in echinacea that stimulate the immune system.

Bodily Influence: Alterative, Antiseptic, Diaphoretic, Lymphatic, and Sialagogue.

ELDERBERRY *(Sambucuscanadensis)*

Medicinal Parts: Berries, Leaves, Flowers, Inner bark, and Root.

Actions and Uses: Elderberry is effective in the treatment of children's diseases, such as erysipelas, and liver derangement's. Also recommended for colds, epilepsy, headache due to colds, jaundice, palsy, rheumatism, scofula, and syphilis.

External Use: Apply ointment to skin to remove spots, and freckles. Useful for burns, rashes, and minor skin problems. Helps to soften and preserve skin.

Warning: Raw Elderberries are toxic. Do not eat the berries unless they are cooked.

Bodily Influence: Alterative, Cathartic, Diaphoretic, Discutient, Diuretic, Emetic, Emollient, Hydragogue, and Mild Stimulant.

ELECAMPANE *(Inulahelenium)*

Medicinal Part: Root.

Actions and Uses: This herb strengthens, cleanses, and tones the pulmonary and gastric membranes. A treatment for pulmonary affections that have symptoms of cough, wheezing, and shortness of breath. Also effective for malignant fevers, dyspepsia, and heptic torpor. Assists the pancreas with a large amount of natural insulin contained in the root.

External Use: Used for itching skin, rash, and wounds.

Warning: Bodily Influence: Diuretic, Diaphoretic, Expectorant, Emmenagogue, Stimulant, and Tonic.

EPHEDRA *(Ephedrasinica)*

Medicinal Parts: Leaves and Berries.

Actions and Uses: A long acting stimulant that can last up to one full day. In China this herb is known as ma huang and has been used for four thousand years to treat respiratory infections and asthma. An effective decongestant used to relieve headaches, hay fever, fevers, watery eyes, stuffy nose, and other allergy and cold symptoms.

Warning: Do not use this herb if you have diabetes, thyroid disease, heart disease, or high blood pressure.

Bodily Influence: Demulcent, Emollient, Expectorant, Pectoral, and Tonic.

EUCALYPTUS *(Eucalyptusglobulus)*

Medicinal Parts: Oil, Bark, Leaves.

Actions and Uses: Oil from this tree is extremely potent. An infusion is effective in treating scarlet, and typhoid fevers. It may be inhaled for asthma, diphtheria, congestion, colds, flu, and sore throat.

External Use: Apply salve as a local antiseptic. Is a stimulant and corrective to boils, carbuncles, growths, sores, ulcers, wounds, and the pain, stiffness and swelling of arthritis and rheumatism.

Warning: Oil may be taken internally only in small doses. Overdose will result in nausea, vomiting, and related effects. Do not use on open wounds.

Bodily Influence: Antiseptic, Antispasmodic, Astringent, and Tonic.

EVENING PRIMROSE *(Oenothera biennis)*

Medicinal Parts: Bark, Leaves, and Seeds.

Actions and Uses: An excellent source of essential fatty acids (EFA's). Studies show that Evening Primrose Oil lowers blood cholesterol and reduces blood pressure. Effective remedy for heart disease and stroke. Good for female disorders such as PMS, hyperactivity, cramps, hot flashes, and heavy bleeding. Helps maintain healthy skin and controls topic diseases such as eczema.

Bodily Influence: Astringent, Nervine, and Sedative

EYEBRIGHT *(Euphrasia officinalis)*

Medicinal Part: Leaves.

Actions and Uses: It is the main herb for protecting and maintaining the health of the eye. Acts as an internal medicine for the constitutional tendency to eye weakness. Relieves itchy or sore eyes due to allergies and colds. Will remove cysts that have been caused by chronic conjunctivitis.

External Use: Commercial eyewash preparations made of Eyebright and compatible herbs can be soothing to irritated and inflamed eyes.

Bodily Influence: Adaptogen, Alterative, Astringent, Nutritive, and Tonic.

FALSE UNICORN *(Chamailirium luteum)*

Medicinal Part: Root.

Actions and Uses: Most commonly used for female infertility and impotence. Also used for treating intestinal weakness, female hormone imbalances, irregular menstruation, leukorrhea, uterine problems, and as a urinary tract tonic.

Bodily Influence: Diuretic, Emetic, Parasiticide, Stimulant, and Tonic.

FENNEL *(Foeniculum vulgare)*

Medicinal Part: Whole Herb.

Actions and Uses: Helps suppress the appetite. Aids digestion when uric acid is the problem. Effective for gas, acid stomach, kidneys, liver, spleen, and gout. In larger doses, Jethro Kloss used it to remove obstructions of the liver, spleen and gall bladder. Use mixed with catnip in tincture form, as an aid to colic in infants. Also helps to relieve pain for cancer patients, after chemotherapy and radiation.

External Use: Fennel oil can be rubbed on arthritis and rheumatism to alleviate pain. It can also be used as an eyewash.

Bodily Influence: Antispasmodic, Aromatic, Carminative, Diuretic, Expectorant, and Galactagogue.

FENUGREEK *(Trigonella graecum)*

Medicinal Part: Seeds.

Actions and Uses: Fenugreek lowers blood sugar and is useful for all mucous conditions of the lungs. An effective remedy for bronchitis, coughs, colds, fevers, gout, and inflammation of stomach and intestines. As a gargle it can relieve sore throats. This herb also acts as a bulk laxative.

External Use: Pulverized seeds can be made into a poultice and applied against tumors, abscesses, boils, carbuncles, neuralgia, and swollen glands for pain relief.

Bodily Influence: Aphrodisiac, Demulcent, Emollient, Expectorant, Galactagogue, Laxative, and Tonic.

FEVERFEW *(Chrysanthemum parthenium)*

Medicinal Parts: Whole Herb.

Actions and Uses: This highly praised herb is most helpful in the prevention of migraines. Research shows that Feverfew reduces the severity of migraine symptoms, (relieves dizziness, nausea, vomiting, brain and nerve pressure). Feverfew also stimulates uterine contractions, promotes menses, increases fluidity of lung and bronchial tube mucus. Also an effective remedy used in alleviating inflammation and discomfort of arthritis. A recommended corrective for female disorders such as scanty or delayed monthly periods.

External Use: Salve applied to chest area for pain of congestion, or inflammation of the lungs.

Bodily Influence: Aperient, Carminative, Emmenagogue, Stimulant, Tonic, and Vermifuge.

FLAG LILY *(Iris versicolor)*

Medicinal Parts: Root, Rhizome.

Actions and Uses: A valuable herb for all diseases of the blood, kidney, spleen, and chronic hepatic affections. Has a special influence on the lymphatic glands (pure lymphatic circulation is spontaneous to longevity). Also effective in treating secondary Syphilis.

External Uses: Used in treating infected wounds, ulcers, and fistula.

Bodily Influence: Alterative, Cathartic, Diuretic, Resolvent, Sialagogue, and Vermifuge.

FLAX *(Linumvsitatissimum)*

Medicinal Parts: Seed.

Actions and Uses: Flax is an excellent treatment for all intestinal inflamations. Relieves coughs, asthma, and pleurisy. Also used to strengthen teeth and bones. As a tea it is a good laxative, people with bleeding, painful hemorrhoids have experienced easy bowel movments without pain.

External Use: Combine with slippery elm bark for a very effective poultice for boils, burns, oozing sores and pimples.

Bodily Influence: Demulcent, Emollient, Laxative, and Mucilage.

FOLGATE *(Folgateangustifolia)*

Medicinal Part: Flower.

Actions and Uses: When taken as a tea it calms nerves, soothes headaches, eases flatulence, dizziness, fainting and halitosis. Herbalists use the neat essential oil as a mild sedative, antiseptic, and painkiller on insect bites and burns

External Uses: Used as a massage oil for skin sores, insomnia, infections, and rheumatic aches.

Note: May be poisonous. Do not take more than two drops of undiluted oil internally.

Bodily Influence: Antiseptic, Nervine, and Tonic.

FORGET- ME-NOT *(Myosotis sylvatica)*

Medicinal Parts: Leaves and Flowers.

Actions and Uses: This herb is most helpful in the treatment of respiratory problems and is sometimes made into a syrup for pulmonary disorders

Bodily Influence: Adaptogen, Anticatarrhal, and Tonic.

FRENCH LAVENDER *(Dentataangustifolia)*

Medicinal Part: Flower.

Actions and Uses: When taken as a tea it calms nerves, soothes headaches, eases flatulence, dizziness, fainting and halitosis. Herbalists use the neat essential oil as a mild sedative, antiseptic, and painkiller on insect bites and burns

External Uses: Used as a massage oil for skin sores, insomnia, infections, and rheumatic aches.

Note: May be poisonous. Do not take more than two drops of undiluted oil internally.

Bodily Influence: Antiseptic, Nervine, and Tonic.

GARLIC *(Alliumsativum)*

Medicinal Part: Bulb.

Actions and Uses: Natural antibiotic, stimulates activity of the digestive organs, therefore relieves problems associated with poor digestion. This herb is excellent for both high and low blood pressure and it is used to emulsify the cholesterol and loosen it from the arterial walls. Proven useful in the treatment of asthma, whooping cough, lung and respiratory ailments. Its anti fungal properties make it a good adjunct in treating vaginal yeast infections *(candida albicans)*. Valuable in intestinal infections and effective in reducing high blood pressure. Recent studies show that Garlic has cancer-inhibiting properties (Garlic is toxic to some tumor cells).

External Use: Apply directly on affected parts for aches, sprains and skin disorders. Drops in ear relieves earache. Garlic tea is used as an enema for the expulsion of parasites.

Bodily Influence: Alterative, Antibiotic, Antispasmodic, Diaphoretic, Esculent, Expectorant, and Stimulant.

GELSEMIUM *(Gelsemiumsempervirens)*

Medicinal Part: Root.

Actions and Uses: Gelsemium is an unrivaled febrifuge, possessing antispasmodic and relaxing properties. Effective for colds, nervous and bilious headache, fevers, pneumonia, promoting perspiration, and quieting of nervous irritability. A useful treatment for inflammation of the bowels, dysentery, and diarrhea. Also used in pelvic disorders of women, spermatorrhoea, various cardiac diseases, and genital diseases.

Bodily Influence: Antiperiodic, Antispasmodic, Mydriatic, Nervine, and Sedative.

GENTAIN *(Gentaina lutea)*

Medicinal Parts: Leaves and Root.

Actions and Uses: Gentain is most useful in states of exhaustion from chronic disease, and all cases of general debility, weakness of digestive organs and want of appetite. Also effectively controls colds, fever, gout, and spleen and liver function. Kills plasmodia (organisms that cause malaria) and worms. Many dyspeptic complaints are effectively relieved with gentain.

Bodily Influence: Adaptogen, Cholagogue, Fubrifuge, Nutritive, Stimulant, Stomachic, Tonic, and Vermifuge.

GINGER *(Zangiber officinale)*

Medicinal Part: Root and rhizomes.

Actions and Uses: Hot (as tea), promotes cleansing of the body through perspiration and is useful for suppressed menstruation. Relieves indigestion, gas, morning sickness, and nausea. In a recent university study, ginger root capsules proved to be far more effective at controlling motion-induced nausea than either a drug or placebo. It helps absorb toxins, restore gastric activities to normal, and helps control diarrhea and vomiting that often accompanies gastro-intestinal flu.

External Use: Apply tincture to soothe, and promote the healing of skin infections and minor burns.

Bodily Influence: Aromatic, Carminative, Diaphoretic, Diuretic, Stimulant, and Tonic.

GINKGO *(gingko biloba)*

Medicinal Part: Leaves.

Actions and Uses: A cerebal/vascular conditioner. Widens blood vessels, increases circulation and speeds blood flow in the capillaries. Expands mental perception and provides increased clarity during intense study sessions or examinations. Useful for depression, hearing, vision, memory loss, senile dementia, dizziness, tinnitus (ringing in the ears), and heart and kidney disorders. Studies show that ginkgo is an antioxidant (slows formation of free radicals) which are considered responsible for cancer, and premature aging.

Bodily Influence: Cardiac, Rubifacient, and Vasodilator.

GINSENG - AMERICAN *(Panax quinquefolius)*

Medicinal Part: Root.

Actions and Uses: It is very similar to panax ginseng. Works as a mild stimulant, normalizes body functions, and helps the body adapt to stress. The American Indians used it in their love potions.

Warning: Do not use large amounts of ginseng on elderly or weak persons when there there is inflammation or during high fevers.

Bodily Influence: Alterative, Aphrodisiac, Demulcent, Nervine, Stimulant, Stomachic, and Tonic.

GINSENG - KOREAN *(Panaxginseng)*

Medicinal Part: Root.

Actions and Uses: A physical restorative. Helps the entire body adapt to stress; regenerates and rebuilds sexual centers. Impotency and low sperm count have been corrected by using Korean Ginseng. Stimulates the appetite, and normalizes blood pressure. Anciently known as a male hormone, and used for longevity.

Warning: Do not use large amounts of ginseng on elderly or weak persons when there there is inflammation or during high fevers.

Bodily Influence: Alterative, Aphrodisiac, Demulcent, Nervine, Stimulant, Stomachic, and Tonic.

GINSENG-SIBERIAN *(Eleutherococcus senticosus)*

Medicinal Part: Root.

Actions and Uses: Strengthens the entire endocrine glandular system, a tonic and toner of the body, promotes mental and physical vigor, stamina, endurance, metabolism, appetite and digestion. Mildly stimulates the central nervous system, also helpful in problems arising in menopause such as hot flashes and irregular periods. Also good for cocaine withdrawal, radiation protection, and enhances lung and immune functions.

Warning: Avoid if hyperactive or under high nervous tension.

Bodily Influence: Aphrodisiac, Demulcent, Nervine, Stimulant, and Stomachic.

GOLDEN SEAL HERB *(Hydrastiscanadensis)*

Medicinal Part: Rhizomes.

Actions and Uses: For all problems of the mucous membranes. Contains many of the same properties as the root but, in milder form. Relieves nausea, colds, and flu.

External Use: The infusion makes a good vaginal douche. Salve is effective in treating skin inflammations such as eczema.

Warning: Do not use large amounts during pregnancy. When used over a long period, will reduce vitamin B absorption.

Bodily Influence: Alterative, Antibiotic, Antiseptic, Emmenagogue, Stomachic, Tonic.

GOLDEN SEAL ROOT *(Hydrastis conadensis)*

Medicinal Part: Root.

Actions and Uses: One of the best substitutes for quinine. A natural antibiotic herb used with all infections. A powerful agent used in treating ulcers, diphtheria, tonsillitis, spinal meningitis, and aids indigestion and constipation. Combined with Gota Kola, Goldenseal acts as a brain tonic.

External Use: Mouthwash can help prevent gum disease. Rub tincture on irritated gums and canker sores.

Warning: Long-term use may weaken bacterial flora of the colon.

Bodily Influence: Alterative, Antibiotic, Antiseptic, Laxative, and Tonic.

GOTU KOLA *(Centella Asiatica)*

Medicinal Parts: Nuts, Root, and Seeds.

Actions and Uses: Known in India as the longevity herb. Contains remarkable rejuvenating properties. May promote hair growth when combined with eclipta. It strengthens the heart, and liver functions. Good for mental disorders, blood diseases, high blood pressure, sore throat, tonsillitis, hepatitis, measles, rheumatism, and venereal diseases. Promotes healing after childbirth and reduces swelling and pain due to phlebitis. Used by students as a brain cell activator to help memory.

Warning: Gota Kola should not be used if you have an overactive thyroid, and do not use this herb during pregnancy.

Bodily Influence: Alterative, Antipyretic, Antibiotic, Diuretic, Nervine, Rubifacient, and Tonic.

GOUT BERRY *(Rubus villosus)*

Medicinal Part: Leaves and Root bark.

Actions and Uses: A good astringent for watery diarrhea in children. Blackberry syrup is used as a tonic for children with weak stomachs, no appetite and skin pallor. Also an effective treatment for deficient glandular secretions of the stomach and intestines.

External Use: Salve acts as an astringent to haemorrhoids. Gargle the tea of roots or leaves for sore mouth and inflamed throat.

Bodily Influence: Astringent, Diuretic, Hemostatic, Syptic, and Tonic.

GRAVEL ROOT *(Eupatoriompurpureum)*

Medicinal Part: Root, and Flower.

Actions and Uses: This herb is almost infallible when used for the expulsion of gravel. One of the best known herbs for kidney, bladder, and urinary infections. An effective treatment for dropsy, gout, lumbago, neuralgia, rheumatism, and joint stiffness caused by uric acid deposits. Used for many female problems such as endrometritis, chronic uterine disease, labor pains, threatened abortions and dysmenorrhea. Also valuable in diarrhea, especially for children. Imparts to the bowels some nourishment as well as an astringency.

Bodily Influences: Astringent, Diuretic, Nervine, Relaxant, Stimulant, and Tonic.

GUAR GUM *(Grindelia squarrosa)*

Medicinal Part: Leaves and Seed.

Actions and Uses: Used as a diet aid because it absorbs liquids and swells; also reduces serum cholesterol levels and has a mild bulk-forming laxative effect.

Bodily Influence: Esculent, and Laxative.

HAWTHORN *(Crataegusoxyacantha)*

Medicinal Part: Berries and Leaves.

Actions and Uses: High in magnesium chloride. A dietary herb that aids in burning off excess calories. As a diuretic it helps rid the body of excess salt and water. Relieves abdominal distention and diarrhea. A herbal aid for circulation and specific nutritional resources for building heart tone (increases the flow of oxygen and blood to the heart). It helps prevent hardening of the arteries, and facilitates cardiac healing and restoration. Valuable in angina pectoris or inflammation of the heart muscle. The tea is also good for nervous conditions and insomnia.

Bodily Influences: Adaptogen, Antispasmodic, Astringent, Cardiac, Circulatory Diuretic, Sedative, and Tonic.

HIDCOTE *(Lavandulaangustifolia)*

Medicinal Part: Flower.

Actions and Uses: When taken as a tea it calms nerves, soothes headaches, eases flatulence, dizziness, fainting and halitosis. Herbalists use the neat essential oil as a mild sedative, antiseptic, and painkiller on insect bites and burns

External Uses: Used as a massage oil for skin sores, insomnia, infections, and rheumatic aches.

Note: May be poisonous. Do not take more than two drops of undiluted oil internally.

Bodily Influence: Antiseptic, Nervine, and Tonic.

HONEYSUCKLE *(Lonicerajaponica)*

Medicinal Parts: Flowers.

Actions and Uses: Honeysuckle is mostly used for acute infectious and inflammatory conditions. A valuable herb for the treatment of colds, acute flu, and fevers.

External Use: Tincture may also be applied externally for skin infections.

Bodily Influence: Alterative, and Antipyretic.

HOPS *(Humuluslupulus)*

Medicinal Parts: Strobiles or Cones.

Actions and Uses: A powerful sedative, strong yet safe to use. Decreases the desire for alcohol, improves appetite, and induces sleep. Good for the heart, relieves indigestion, liver problems, nervousness, restlessness, pain, toothaches, earaches, and stress. Extremely high in B vitamins.

External Use: As a poultice this herb is effective for boils, tumors, and skin inflammations.

Bodily Influence: Anodyne, Anthelmintic, Diuretic, Febrifuge, Hypnotic, Nervine, Sedative and Tonic.

HOREHOUND *(Marrubiumvulgara)*

Medicinal Parts: Whole Herb.

Actions and Uses: Used for congestion of coughs, colds, and pulmonary affections associated with unwanted phlegm from the chest, and promotes sweating which in turn, cools the body. It is very useful in chronic sore throats; use as a syrup for children.

Good for intestinal gas, when taken in large doses, it is a laxative and will expel worms.

Bodily Influence: Anthelmintic, Diuretic, Diaphoretic, Expectorant, Laxative, Resolvent, Stimulant, Stomachic, and Tonic.

HORSE CHESTNUT *(Aesculus hippocastum)*

Medicinal Part: Leaves, Rhizomes.

Actions and Uses: Horse Chestnut is an effective remedy for colds and flu. Promotes sweating which helps to break fevers. Used to treat coughs, feverish headaches, nausea, and sore throat. A useful remedy to strengthen and tone veins and arteries.

External Use: Apply tincture gently on hemorrhoids, and varicose veins.

Bodily Influence: Adaptogen, Antiseptic, Emollient, and Tonic.

HORSE RADISH *(Cochlearia armoracia)*

Medicinal Part: Root.

Actions and Uses: Horse radish is used as a digestive agent. Promotes sweating which helps to break fevers and is especially good for the treatment of dropsy occurring after fevers. Used to treat weak digestive organs, pancreas disorders, neuralgia, and rheumatism.

External Use: Use poultice mixed with powdered mustard seed and slippery elm for swellings of liver and spleen.

Warning: Avoid contact with the eyes. Fresh horseradish left in contact with the skin will cause blistering.

Bodily Influence: Diaphoretic, Digestive, Diuretic, Expectorant, Stimulant, and Stomachic.

HORSE TAIL *(Equisetum arvense)*

Medicinal Parts: Leaves and Stems.

Actions and Uses: Contains a great deal of silica, so herbalists use it for skin and eye conditions. Increases calcium absorption, promotes healthy skin, strengthens bones, hair, nails, teeth, and helps eliminate excess oil from hair and skin. Horsetail helps coagulate the blood and is useful during excessive bleeding and menstruation. Also a diuretic. Helps with kidney disorders, especially kidney stones, glandular swellings and pus discharges. This herb works best in small frequent doses.

External Use: Used as poultice to depress bleeding and accelerate healing of wounds and ulcers.

Warning: Horsetail can be irritating to the kidneys when used for prolonged periods.

Bodily Influence: Astringent, Diuretic, Emmenagogue, Galactagogue, Lithotriptic, Nutritive, and Tonic.

HUCKLEBERRY *(Vacciniom myrtillus)*

Medicinal Parts: Whole Plant.

Actions and Uses: Used to lower insulin, blood sugar levels, and to ease inflammation. Proven beneficial to cool feverish liver, and stomach conditions. Effective remedy for diabetes, kidney and bladder infections, sinusitis, and ulcers. Also a useful agent for dropsy and gravel.

External Use: Apply tincture to sores, ulcers, and wounds.

Warning: Interferes with iron absorption when taken internally.

Bodily Influences: Alterative, Depurative, Nutritive, and Stomachic.

HYSSOP *(Hyssopus officinalis)*

Medicinal Parts: Tops and Leaves.

Actions and Uses: Highly Praised as a blood regulator, both increasing the circulation of the blood and reducing blood pressure. An effective tonic for mucous tissue of both gastro-intestinal and respiratory tract in weakened conditions. Recommended for dropsy, gravel, jaundice, scrofula, various stomach complaints, and spleen malfunction.

External Use: Apply salve to heal wounds and ulcers. A formentation made from the leaves is used to relieve muscular rheumatism.

Warning: Do not take internally for more than two weeks with out seeking medical advise.

Bodily Influences: Aromatic, Carminative, Cholagogue, Expectorant, Stimulant, Tonic, and Vulnerary.

INDIAN PLANT *(Sanguinaria canadensis)*

Medicinal Parts: Root.

Actions and Uses: Small doses stimulate the digestive system. When taken in large doses it is an arterial sedative. This herb is effective in treating asthma, chronic bronchitis, laryngitis, whooping cough, and other complaints of the respiratory organs.

The tincture has been used successfully in treating dyspepsia and dropsy of the chest.

External Use: Injections of strong tea is excellent for leucorrhoea and haemorrhoids.

Bodily Influence: Alterative, Diuretic, Febrifuge, Sialagogue, Stimulating expectorant, Systemic emetic, and Tonic.

INDIAN TOBACCO *(Lobelia inflata)*

Medicinal Parts: Leaves, Flower, Seeds and Stem.

Actions and Uses: A powerful relaxant used extensively for persons wishing to stop smoking or drinking. Aids in hormone production. Reduces palpitation of the heart and strengthens muscle action. An effective remedy for fevers, pneumonia, meningitis, pleurisy, hepatitis and peritonitis. The Indians used this herb for syphilis and for expelling or destroying intestinal worms. Emetic in large amounts.

External Use: Apply salve or tincture to swellings and inflammations.

Bodily Influence: Antispasmodic, Diaphoretic, Emetic, Expectorant, Nauseant, Relaxant, Sedative, and Stimulant.

IRISH MOSS *(Cypripedium pubescens)*

Medicinal Parts: Whole Plant.

Actions and Uses: Used in cosmetics to soften and promote elasticity of the skin. Also effective in the treatment of thyroid problems (goiter), colon disorders, kidney and bladder irritations, ulcers of the throat and stomach, and obesity.

External Use: Used in hair rinses for dry hair and as a fomentation for dry and burning skin diseases.

Bodily Influences: Adaptogen, Demulcent, Emollient, and Nutritive.

JERUSALEM COWSLIP *(Pulmonaria officinalis)*

Medicinal Parts: Leaves.

Actions and Uses: Lungwort is an effective and reliable herb for all weakened and chronic lung conditions. Extremely effective when there is bleeding from the lung structure. Used for the treatment of asthma, bronchial and catarrhal infections, colds, coughs, throat irritation, and helps cure diarrhea.

External Use: Lungwort is an antiseptic. Used for washing and dressing wounds.

Bodily Influence: Demulcent, Mucilaginous, Pectoral.

JUJUBE DATE *(Ziziphus jujuba)*

Medicinal Parts: Whole date.

Actions and Uses: Jujube date is grown in the Orient and warmer climates of America. This date is sold in dried form in most Chinese herb shops. This herb has a calming effect on the body, and is recommended for the treatment of apprehension, dizziness, forgetfulness, insomnia, and to relieve nervous exhaustion.

Bodily Influences: Digestive, Nervine, Nutritive, Tonic.

JUNIPER BERRY *(Juniperus communis)*

Medicinal Part: Ripe dry berries.

Actions and Uses: Useful in digestive problems, gastrointestinal infections, inflammations, cramps, dropsy kidney, and bladder diseases. It is a good douche for vaginal infections. Also effective for gout, and other arthritic conditions associated with uric acid waste.

External Use: The salve is used for skin parasites, eczema, psoriasis, and wounds.

Warning: Not intended for use during pregnancy. Avoid prolonged use during urinary tract or inflammatory problems.

Bodily Influence: Antispasmodic, Anodyne, Aromatic, Astringent, Carminative, Diuretic, Lithotriptic, and Stimulant.

KAVA KAVA *(Piper methysticum)*

Medicinal Part: Root.

Actions and Uses: A mild diuretic and an excellent herb for insomnia and nervousness. Invokes sleep and relaxes the nervous system. Taken as a tea it will relieve stress after injury. This herb is an antiseptic which makes it useful as a douche and valuable for urinary tract infections.

Warning: Long term usage of high dosages can interfere with elimination of toxins from the liver.

Bodily Influence: Anodyne, Antiseptic, Antispasmodic, Diuretic, Sedative, and Tonic.

KELP *(Fucus visiculosis)*

Medicinal Part: Whole plant.

Actions and Uses: Source of olkaki, calcium, sulfur, iodine, silicon, and vitamin k. Beneficial to reproductive organs and tones the walls of the blood vessels. Kelp absorbs wastes from the body f;uids and is excellent for the thyroid gland and goiters. Has a remedial and normalizing action on the sensory nerves. Also good for nails, hair, and radiation poisoning.

Warning: Excessive use of kelp can produce goiter-like symptoms due to the high content of iodine.

Bodily Influence: Alterative, Demulcent, Diuretic, Thyroid restorative, and Nutritive.

KUDZU VINE *(Pueraria lobata)*

Medicinal Parts: Root.

Actions and Uses: This herb is used to treat bronchial congestion and respiratory problems. Effective for asthma, bronchitis, coughs, sore throat, pneumonia, and related lung ailments. Kudzu root also relieves acidity in the body and thus relieves minor aches and pains

Bodily Influence: Antipyretic, Demulcent, Diaphoretic, Refrigerant, and Spasmolytic.

LADY'S MANTLE *(Alchemilla vulgaris)*

Medicinal Part: Leaves, Rhizome.

Actions and Uses: Anciently known as a female hormone, used for beauty, youth, and longevity. Acts as a tonic, stimulates the appetite, and gives one a general feeling of well-being. Used for problems arising in menopause, such as hot flashes and helps to correct irregular menstruation. Also makes a soothing douche for vaginal irritations.

External Use: Apply tincture to open sores and wounds. Promotes healing and coagulation of blood.

Bodily Influence: Adaptogen, Emollient, Styptic, Vulnerary, Tonic.

LADY'S SLIPPER *(Cypripedium pugescins)*

Medicinal Part: Root.

Actions and Uses: Acts as a tonic to the exhausted nervous system, improving circulation and nutrition of the nerve centers. This in turn calms nerves, mental irritation and quiets spasms of voluntary muscles with no harmful or narcotic effects. Effective in treating reflex functional disorders, chorea, low fevers, hysteria, insomnia, nervous unrest, and nervous depression. Combined with chamomile and dandelion, it is excellent for digestive and liver problems.

Bodily Influence: Antiperiodic, Antispasmodic, Nervine, Sedative, and Tonic.

LAVENDER *(Lavandula angustifolia)*

Medicinal Part: Flower.

Actions and Uses: When taken as a tea it calms nerves, soothes headaches, eases flatulence, dizziness, fainting and halitosis. Herbalists use the neat essential oil as a mild sedative, antiseptic, and painkiller on insect bites and burns

External Uses: Used as a massage oil for skin sores, insomnia, infections, and rheumatic aches.

Note: May be poisonous. Do not take more than two drops of undiluted oil internally.

Bodily Influence: Antiseptic, Nervine, and Tonic.

LEMON BALM *(Melissa officinalis)*

Medicinal Part: Tops.

Actions and Uses: Lemon balm is specific for infants and children with colds, fever, and flu complaints. Also useful when combined with catnip tea for nervous fevers, or hyperactive children with digestive disturbances.

Bodily Influence: Antitryptic, Antispasmodic, Diaphoretic, and Sedative.

LEMON VERBENA *(Aloysia triphylla)*

Medicinal Part: Leaf.

Actions and Uses: Lemon verbena is used to soothe bronchial and nasal congestion, to relieve flatulence, indigestion, stomach cramps, palpitations, and nausea. When taken as a tea it has a mild sedative effect.

Warning: Long term use or large amounts of the leaf may cause stomach irritations.

Bodily Influence: Sedative, Stomachic.

LEMON WALNUT *(Juglanscinerea)*

Medicinal Part: Dried Inner Bark and Leaves.

Actions and Uses: A good treatment for diarrhea and dysentery. Also used for acne, angina pectoris, ecthyma, eczema, headache, herpes, and migraines. When combined with bitter root it is a good remedy for consumption.

External Use: Diluted tincture is effective for chronic skin diseases.

Bodily Influence: Cathartic, Tonic, and Vermifuge.

LEPTANDRA *(Leptandravirginica)*

Medicinal Part: Root.

Actions and Uses: Black root acts on the intestines in chronic constipation and is very effective in treating chronic Hepatic diseases. Also used for ascites, bilious fever, dyspepsia, headache, jaundice, pleurisy, and liver disorders.

Bodily Influence: Alterative, Antiseptic, Cholagogue, Emetocathartic, Laxative, and Tonic.

LICORICE ROOT *(Glycyrrhiza globra)*

Medicinal Part: The dried root.

Actions and Uses: Hormone balancer. Natural cortisone. Used for hypoglycemia, adrenal glands, stress, and female problems (menstrual and menopause). Decreases muscle or skeletal spasms, and reduces pain from ulcers. Also used to increase fluidity of mucus from the lungs and bronchial tubes. Also used for coughs and chest complaints, gastric ulcers, and throat conditions. Licorice root is added to bitter tonics to make them more palatable and to combinations of herbs to balance the formula. New studies in the United States and Japan have found that licorice root may help retard growth of certain cancerous tumors.

Warning: Licorice increases production of aldosterone causing an increase in blood pressure. Large doses of licorice root should be avoided by people with high blood pressure.

Bodily Influence: Alterative, Demulcent, Expectorant, Laxative, and Pectoral.

LILY OF THE VALLEY *(Convallaria majalis)*

Medicinal Parts: Bark, Leaves, and Seeds.

Actions and Uses: An excellent source of essential fatty acids (EFA's). Studies show that this herb lowers blood cholesterol and reduces blood pressure. Effective remedy for heart disease and stroke. Good for female disorders such as PMS, hyperactivity, cramps, hot flashes, and heavy bleeding. Helps maintain healthy skin and controls topic diseases such as eczema.

Note: This highly toxic plant should never be used without strict medical supervision.

Bodily Influence: Astringent, Nervine, and Sedative

LIPPIA *(Lippia dulcis)*

Medicinal Parts: Whole Herb.

Actions and Uses: Used to enhance the healing powers of other herbs. Stimulates the mind, and nervous system, retards aging, and stimulates the production of cortisone. Also good for allergies, coughs, colds, hay fever, arthritis, fluid retention, and constipation.

Bodily Influences: Adaptogen, Alterative, Anodyne, Antirheumatic, Nervine, Nutritive, and Sedative.

LIVER LILY *(Iris versicolor)*

Medicinal Parts: Root, Rhizome.

Actions and Uses: A valuable herb for all diseases of the blood, kidney, spleen, and chronic hepatic affections. Has a special influence on the lymphatic glands (pure lymphatic circulation is spontaneous to longevity). Also effective in treating secondary Syphilis.

External Uses: Used in treating infected wounds, ulcers, and fistula.

Bodily Influence: Alterative, Cathartic, Diuretic, Resolvent, Sialagogue, and Vermifuge.

LOBELIA *(Lobelia inflata)*

Medicinal Parts: Leaves, Flower, Seeds and Stem.

Actions and Uses: A powerful relaxant used extensively for persons wishing to stop smoking or drinking. Aids in hormone production. Used for spasmodic lung and respiratory conditions. Reduces palpitation of the heart and strengthens muscle action.

An effective remedy for fevers associated with pneumonia, meningitis, pleurisy, hepatitis, and peritonitis. The Indians used Red Lobelia for syphilis and for expelling or destroying intestinal worms. Emetic in large amounts.

External Use: Apply salve or tincture to arthritis, bites, poison ivy, ringworm, tumors, swellings, and inflammations.

Bodily Influence: Antispasmodic, Diaphoretic, Emetic, Expectorant, Nauseant, Relaxant, Sedative, and Stimulant.

LODDON PINK *(Lavandula angustifolia)*

Medicinal Part: Flower.

Actions and Uses: When taken as a tea it calms nerves, soothes headaches, eases flatulence, dizziness, fainting and halitosis. Herbalists use the neat essential oil as a mild sedative, antiseptic, and painkiller on insect bites and burns.

External Uses: Used as a massage oil for skin sores, insomnia, infections, and rheumatic aches.

Note: May be poisonous. Do not take more than two drops of undiluted oil internally.

Bodily Influence: Antiseptic, Nervine, and Tonic.

LONGAN BERRY *(Euphoria longana)*

Medicinal Parts: Berries.

Actions and Uses: A powerful tonic used to strengthen the reproductive organs in women, stimulate the mind, nervous system, and counteract forgetfulness, and hyperactive mental activity. Also an effective remedy for hypoglycemia.

Bodily Influences: Nutritive, Tonic.

LOVAGE *(Ligusticum chuanxiong)*

Medicinal Part: Root.

Actions and Uses: A great sexual rejuvenator. Gives energy, helps to balance female hormones. Controls bed wetting, expels excess water from the body. Increases blood circulation, relieves abdominal pains, helps relieve anxiety, and promotes a feeling of well-being.

Bodily Influence: Antispasmodic, Emmenagogue, Stimulant, and Tonic.

LUNGWORT *(Pulmonariaofficinalis)*

Medicinal Parts: Leaves.

Actions and Uses: Lungwort is an effective and reliable herb for all weakened and chronic lung conditions. Extremely effective when there is bleeding from the lung structure. Used for the treatment of asthma, bronchial and catarrhal infections, colds, coughs, throat irritation, and helps cure diarrhea.

External Use: Lungwort is an antiseptic. Used for washing and dressing wounds.

Bodily Influence: Astringent, Demulcent, Emollient, Expectorant, Mucilaginous, Pectoral, Tonic, and Vulnerary.

LYCII *(Lyciumchinensis)*

Medicinal Parts: Berries.

Actions and Uses: Lycii is effective for the treatment of bronchial inflammation and an aid in the removal of toxins from the blood. Lycii clears the eyes and is good for those that suffer from cloudy vision. Also used to nourish liver and kidneys, and lower high blood pressure.

Bodily Influence: Alterative, Antipyretic, Nutrient, and Tonic.

MANDRAKE (AMERICAN) *(Podophyllumpeltatum)*

Medicinal Part: Root.

Actions and Uses: This herb is a powerful glandular stimulant in small doses. Used to treat constipation, obstructions of the liver and gall bladder, digestive problems, lymphatic problems, skin diseases, and mercurial poisoning.

External Use: Tincture is used for skin diseases and warts.

Warning: Do not use during pregnancy or in large doses. Discontinue its use if any uncomfortable symptoms are noticed.

Bodily Influence: Alterative, Cholagogue, Emetic, Hepatic, Laxative, and Stimulant.

MARIGOLD *(Marigold officinalis)*

Medicinal Part: Leaf, Root.

Actions and Uses: Marigold reduces fevers, relieves menstrual cramps, soothes ulcers, and provides relief from skin virus such as shingles.

External Use: Soothes and promotes healing of burns and wounds. When applied directly to the ear the oil will reduce the pain of earache.

Bodily Influence: Anodyne, Antibiotic, Antipyretic, Emollient.

MARSHMALLOW *(Althea officinalis)*

Medicinal Parts: Whole Herb.

Actions and Uses: This herb is high in mucilage. Useful in inflammation and irritation of the alimentary canal, urinary and respiratory organs. Relieves pain caused by colitis, enteritis, and ulcers. Also used in combination with other diuretic herbs during kidney treatment to assist in release of stones.

External Use: Douche for vaginal irritations and a poultice for bee stings, burns, open wounds, and skin inflammations.

Bodily Influence: Alterative, Demulcent, Diuretic, Emollient, Lithotriptic, Nutritive, and Vulnery.

MEADOWSWEET *(Filipendula ulmaria)*

Medicinal Parts: Flower and Buds.

Actions and Uses: Meadowsweet was one of the first sources of salicylic acid discovered. Used as a mild sedative and painkiller. As a tea it helps rid the body of feverish colds, heartburn, and excess fluids.

Bodily Influence: Nervine, and Sedative

MILFOIL *(Achillea millefolium)*

Medicinal Parts: Whole Herb.

Actions and Uses: Very high in tannic acid thus helps to stop bleeding wounds, hemorrhaging stomach, bowels, and lungs. Yarrow is an effective treatment for acute catarrhs of the respiratory tract, colds, chickenpox, fevers, influenza, measles, and smallpox. Also useful in menstrual irregularities and has a soothing effect on nervous conditions of the heart.

External Use: Salve has a soothing effect on hemorrhoids, skin ulcers and wounds.

Warning: Interferes with the absorption of iron.

Bodily Influence: Alterative, Astringent, Diuretic, and Tonic.

MILK THISTLE *(cardusmarianus)*

Medicinal Parts: Fruit, Leaves and Seeds.

Actions and Uses: Milk Thistle enhances overall liver function. Regenerates liver cells and protects them against the action of liver poisons (leukotrienes). Increases the production of bile, used for the breakdown of fats. Beneficial to those with psoriasis. Aids rehabilitation process after acute hepatitis, gall bladder disease or exposure to alcohol, drug, or chemical pollution abuse.

Bodily Influence: Cholagogue, Liver Tonic.

MILKWEED *(Asclepias syriaca)*

Medicinal Part: Root.

Actions and Uses: An effective treatment for inflammatory rheumatism, dyspepsia and scrofulous conditions of the blood. A helpful remedy for bowel, kidney, and stomach complaints. Good for female complaints, asthma, arthritis, and bronchitis. Effective remedy for gallstones and is used for dropsy as it increases the flow of urine.

External Use: Milkweed tincture will cause warts to disappear if applied often to the elevated part.

Warning: May be harmful to children and people over 55.

Bodily Influence: Diaphoretic, and Expectorant.

MINT *(Menthapiperita)*

Medicinal Part: Leaves, Stems.

Actions and Uses: Mint is an agreeable and harmless herb for infants and children as well as adults. Prepared as a herbal tea it is cleansing to the entire system, and will strengthen heart muscles. An excellent remedy for sea sickness, and an effective agent for suppressed menstruation. Useful for cramps and hiccoughs, prevent the gripping effects of cathartics, relieve hysterics, chills colic, influenza, nausea, and vomiting.

External Use: Tincture applied to forehead will relieve most headaches. Also apply oil to burns, neuralgia, rheumatism, and toothaches. Mint enemas are effective treatments for cholera and colon troubles.

Bodily Influence: Aromatic, Carminative, Stimulant, Stomachic.

MISTLETOE *(Viscum album)*

Medicinal Part: Leaves.

Actions and Uses: Specific Mistletoe extracts have anti-tumor properties and are being used to treat certain types of cancer. European mistletoe is used as a cardiac tonic and to stimulate circulation. Extracts dilate blood vessels, decrease blood pressure, and heart rate.

External Use: Fomentation on chilblains(frostbite) and leg ulcers.

Warning: Mistletoe may be fatal in high doses and should be used only under strict medical consultation.

Bodily Influence: Cardiac, Discutient, Diuretic, Stimulant, and Tonic.

MOTHERWORT *(Leonurus cardiaca)*

Medicinal Parts: Leaves, Tops.

Actions and Uses: Motherwort is a nervine and is excellent for female problems, such as suppressed menstruation. Effective treatment for albumen in the urine, chest colds, convulsion, delirium, hysteria, neuritis, rheumatism, sciatica, sleeplessness, and urinary cramps. Also good for the expulsion of worms.

External Use: Hot, strong tea fomentation's will relieve pain in painful menstruation and cramps.

Bodily Influence: Antispasmodic, Diaphoretic, Emmenagogue, Laxative, Nervine, and Tonic.

MOUNTAIN MAHOGANY *(Betula alba)*

Medicinal Part: Bark and Leaves.

Actions and Uses: An effective treatment for dropsy, gout, rheumatism, stones in the kidneys and bladder, and is used to expel worms. Also a good remedy for diarrhoea, dysentery, cholera, and all problems of the alimentary tract. Oil of wintergreen is distilled from the inner bark.

External Use: Extract of the buds, bark, and leaves is applied boils, eczema, swelling, and rheumatic pain.

Bodily Influence: Aromatic, Diaphoretic, and Stimulant.

MUGWORT *(Artemisia vulgaris)*

Medicinal Parts: Tops.

Actions and Uses: This herb is excellent for female complaints such as menstrual cramps and suppressed menstruation. Drink tea for pains in the stomach and bowels. Mugwort is also good in combinations when there are stones or gravel.

External Use: Apply as a poutice to abscesses, boils, and carbuncles.

Bodily Influence: Diaphoretic, Diuretic, Emmenagogue, Nervine, and Stomachic.

MULLEIN *(Verbascum thapsus)*

Medicinal Parts: Leaves and Flowers.

Actions and Uses: Pain reliever, glandular rebuilder. The only herb known that is a narcotic without being harmful or poisonous. Good for coughs, colds, hay fever, shortness of breath, and hemorrhages in the lungs. Also effective for gastrointestinal stress, helps control diarrhea, and relieves stomach cramps.

External Use: Salve is used to treat diaper rash, hemorrhoids, sciatica, spinal tenderness, tumors, and ulcers. The oil is considered one of the best remedies for ear infection.

Bodily Influence: Anodyne, Antispasmodic, Astringent, Demulcent, Diuretic, Pectoral, and Vulnerary.

MUNSTEAD *(Lavandula munstead angustifolia)*

Medicinal Part: Flower.

Actions and Uses: When taken as a tea it calms nerves, soothes headaches, eases flatulence, dizziness, fainting and halitosis. Herbalists use the neat essential oil as a mild sedative, antiseptic, and painkiller on insect bites and burns

External Uses: Used as a massage oil for skin sores, insomnia, infections, and rheumatic aches.

Note: May be poisonous. Do not take more than two drops of undiluted oil internally.

Bodily Influence: Antiseptic, Nervine, and Tonic.

MUSK MALLOW *(Malva moschata)*

Medicinal Parts: Whole Herb.

Actions and Uses: Useful in treating inflammation and irritation of the throat. Leaves and roots are used as a syrups and ointments for coughs.

Bodily Influence: Emollient, and Pectoral.

MYRRH *(Commiphora nyrrha)*

Medicinal Part: Gum.

Actions and Uses: Stimulator, appetite and flow of gastric juices. Myrrh destroys putrification in the intestines and prevents blood absorption of toxins. A powerful antiseptic which is generally used in equal parts with golden seal for intestinal ulcer, catarrh of the intestines and other mucous membrane conditions. Also used for bronchial and lung diseases. Tightening the gums and preventing pyorrhea is one of its most outstanding qualities.

External Use: Apply tincture to cuts, skin disease, and wounds. Gargle for bad breath, cankers, bleeding gums, and mouth sores.

Warning: Do not use if you are pregnant or have kidney disease. Myrrh gum taken in large amounts or over a long period of time can be toxic.

Bodily Influence: Antiseptic, Carminative, Emmenagogue, Expectorant, Digestive Aid, and Stimulant.

NETTLE *(Urtica dioica)*

Medicinal Parts: Roots and Leaves.

Actions and Uses: Tradition use, asthma relief. Also used for kidney diseases, colon and urinary disorders, checking hemorrhage of uterus, nose, lungs and other internal organs. Nettle is valuable in diarrhea, dysentery, piles, neuralgia, gravel, and tea made from the young or dried root is of great help in dropsy of the first stages.

External Use: Cleansing wounds and ulcers. Used as a hair rinse to restore natural color.

Bodily Influence: Alterative, Antiseptic, Astringent, Diuretic, Expectorant, Hemostatic, Pectoral, and Tonic.

OAT FIBER *(Avena sativa)*

Medicinal Part: Seed.

Actions and Uses: Oat seed contains soluble and insoluble fiber, which have cholesterol-lowering benefits. Reducing cholesterol helps prevent heart disease. Good for gas, upset stomach, kidney and chest ailments, and is useful in maintaining a healthy colon. Will help overcome most diseases caused by nervous disorders and is especially effective for ovarian and uterine disorders. Oat seed is an excellent source of vitamin B.

External Use: Apply oatmeal boiled in vinegar for the removal of freckles and face and body spots.

Bodily Influence: Adaptogen, Antispasmodic, Esculent, Nervine, Stimulant, and Tonic.

OIL NUT BARK *(Juglanscinerea)*

Medicinal Part: Dried Inner Bark and Leaves.

Actions and Uses: A good treatment for diarrhea and dysentery. Also used for acne, angina pectoris, ecthyma, eczema, headache, herpes, and migraines. When combined with bitter root it is a good remedy for consumption.

External Use: Diluted tincture is effective for chronic skin diseases.

Bodily Influence: Cathartic, Tonic, and Vermifuge.

OLIVE *(Olea europaea)*

Medicinal Part: Leaves, Fruit.

Actions and Uses: Olive oil is high in monosaturated fats, so it has the ability reduce LDLs (bad cholesterol) without reducing HDLs (good cholesterol). Helps prevent heart disease. Also used to promote contraction of the bowels, relieving constipation.

Warning: Do not use as a laxative if you are pregnant.

External Use: Olive oil is soothing to skin irritations and insect bites. The warm oil is used as conditioner for dry hair and scalp.

Bodily Influence: Adaptogen, Emollient, Esculent, Laxative.

ONION *(Allium cepa)*

Medicinal Part: Bulb.

Actions and Uses: Natural source of energy and a good antiseptic, stimulates activity of the digestive organs, therefore relieves problems associated with poor digestion. Valuable in intestinal infections, relieves gas, helps prevent blood clots, lowers cholesterol and effective in reducing high blood pressure. Recent studies show that allium vegetables such as onion and garlic help prevent stomach cancer.

External Use: Apply juice directly on raised portion of warts, and rub between toes to fight athletes foot.

Bodily Influence: Carminative, Condiment, Diuretic, Expectorant, Nutritive, Stimulant.

OREGON GRAPE ROOT *(Berberisaquifolium)*

Medicinal Part: Root.

Actions and Uses: Blood purifier and liver activator. Recommended in all chronic skin disease such as acne, eczema, herpes, and psoriasis. Builder of the reproductive organs.

Increases the power of digestion and aids assimilation. Recommended as an alterative for treatment of psoriasis, syphilis, and unpure blood conditions. Combine with Cascara Sagrada for constipation. It is rich in iron and other natural vitamins and minerals.

External Use: Douche for leukorrhea.

Bodily Influence: Alterative, Antiseptic, Cholagogue, Laxative, and Tonic.

PAPAYA *(Carica Papaya)*

Medicinal Part: Fruit.

Actions and Uses: Papaya in an excellent antacid, contains papain which has similar chemical characteristics to pepsin, an enzyme that helps to breakdown protein in the body. Good for the metabolism of protein, increased energy, gastrointestinal problems, and helps relieve indigestion.

Bodily Influence: Antacid, Esculent, and Stimulant.

PAPPOOSE ROOT *(Caulophyllumthalictroides)*

Medicinal Part: Root.

Actions and Uses: Especially valuable in epileptic fits and ulceration's of the mouth and throat. Used for suppressed menstruation and to help regulate menstrual flow. Relieves or prevents spasms, cramps, colic, diabetes, leukorrhea, nervous disorders, rheumatism. Elevates blood pressure, cleanses blood, promotes perspiration, and also increases volume of urine excreted.

Bodily Influence: Antispasmodic, Depurative, Diuretic, Dysmenorrhea, Emmenagogue, Oxytocic, Parturient, Sudorific and Spasmodic.

Warning: Not recommended for pregnant women.

PARSLEY *(Petroselinumsativum)*

Medicinal Parts: Leaves, Seeds, and Root.

Actions and Uses: Rich in vitamin B and potassium. An excellent diuretic, and one of the most excellent herbs for gall bladder problems, expels gallstones. Soothing for asthma, and an effective treatment for bed wetting, edema, fluid retention, goiter, gas, indigestion, menstrual disorders, and worms. This herb is an excellent treatment for cancer due to the high chlorophyll content of the leaves. Also useful as a preventative in treating epilepsy.

External Use: Tincture will relieve insect bites and stings.

Warning: Parsley can be warming and should not be used if the kidney is inflamed. Avoid heavy consumption during pregnancy.

Bodily Influence: Anthelmintic, Aperient, Carminative, Diuretic, Esculent, Expectorant, Stimulant, and Tonic.

PASSION FLOWER *(Passifloraincarnata)*

Medicinal Parts: Plant and Flower.

Actions and Uses: Passion Flower is one of the best herbal tranquilizers. An effective treatment when in need of help for nervousness, unrest, agitation and exhaustion without pain, such as unrest, agitation, and exhaustion. Also used to control convulsions, particularly in the young, as indicated by muscular twitching, and also for asthenic insomnia in childhood and the elderly.

External Use: Poultice for rheumatic pains.

Warning: Do not take during pregnancy. This herb is a strong tranquilizer and should not be used before driving or operating machinery.

Bodily Influence: Anodyne, Antispasmodic, Diuretic, and Nerve Sedative.

PAU D'ARCO *(Tabecuiaimpetiginosa)*

Medicinal Parts: Inner Bark.

Actions and Uses: Undoubtedly the greatest treasure the Incas left us. Medical literature confirms that this South American herb possesses antibiotic, tumor inhibiting, virus killing, anti fungal, and anti-malarial properties. Consumer publications report success for the symptoms of anemia, asthma, candida, psoriasis, colitis, and resistance to various infections by building the immune system. This herb also lowers blood sugar levels so is helpful in the prevention of diabetes.

Bodily influence: Adaptogen, Antibiotic, Nutritive, and Resolvent.

PEACH TREE *(Amygdaluspersica)*

Medicinal Parts: Bark, Flowers, and Leaves

Actions and Uses: Peach tree leaves have a sedative effect on the the nervous system. Tea from the leaves is good for dyspepsia, jaundice, stomach problems, and can be used to expel worms.

Decoction of bark is used for coughs, bronchitis, and bladder congestion. Leaves are also added to lung remedies to help expectorate mucus. Syrup made from the leaves or flowers are laxative.

Warning: Large doses cause a purging of the bowels so should be avoided in pregnant women.

Bodily influence: Demulcent, Mucilage, Sedative, and Stomachic.

PENNYROYAL *(Hedeoma pulegioides)*

Medicinal Parts: Whole Plant:

Actions and Uses: Diuretic, corrective nervine used to induce perspiration and promote menstruation. Purifies the blood, stimulates uterine contractions, relieves gas and intestinal pains. Also for nervousness and hysteria, cramps, gout, colic, jaundice, nausea, griping, colds, and skin disorders.

External Use: A few drops of pennyroyal oil on your pet makes an excellent bug repellent.

Warning: Do not use during pregnancy. Overdose may cause kidney and liver damage.

Bodily Influence: Corrective, Diaphoretic, Diuretic, and Nervine.

PEONY *(Paeonia lactiflora)*

Medicinal Parts: Root:

Actions and Uses: Peony is effective in treating menstrual irregularity and abdominal pains associated with the menstrual cycle. This herb is a liver tonic. Purifies the blood, and is used for all diseases stemming from an unbalanced liver function.

Warning: Do not use during pregnancy.

Bodily Influence: Alterative, Antispasmodic, and Hepatic tonic.

PEPPERMINT *(Mentha piperita)*

Medicinal Part: Leaves, Stems.

Actions and Uses: Mint is an agreeable and harmless herb for infants and children as well as adults. Prepared as a herbal tea it is cleansing to the entire system, and will strengthen heart muscles. An excellent remedy for sea sickness, and an effective agent for suppressed menstruation. Useful for cramps and hiccoughs, prevent the gripping effects of cathartics, relieve hysterics, chills colic, influenza, nausea, and vomiting.

External Use: Tincture applied to forehead will relieve most headaches. Also apply oil to burns, neuralgia, rheumatism, and toothaches. Mint enemas are effective treatments for cholera and colon troubles.

Bodily Influence: Aromatic, Carminative, Stimulant, Stomachic.

PERSIAN ROOT *(Rhamnuspurshiana)*

Medicinal Part: Dried Bark.

Actions and Uses: One of the best natural laxatives in the herbal kingdom. A stimulant to the whole digestive system. Extremely useful in hemorrhoidal conditions, chronic constipation, and liver and gall bladder complaints. It is considered suitable for delicate and elderly persons. Also a very good remedy for gallstones; increases secretion of bile.

Bodily Influence: Antispasmodic, Hepatic, Laxative, and Bitter tonic.

PIPSISSEWA *(Chimaphilaumbellata)*

Medicinal Part: Tops.

Actions and Uses: A good remedy for bladder and kidney problems such as cattarrh of the bladder, relaxed bladder, burning urine, and urethral and prostrate irritation. Also used for all blood troubles and diseases of the urinary organs when combined with dandelion, golden seal, and yellow dock

External Use: Apply oil to Painful joints and skin disease..

Bodily Influence: Alterative, Astringent, Diuretic, and Tonic.

PLANTAIN *(Plantago major)*

Medicinal Parts: Whole Plant:

Actions and Uses: Influences lymphatic system and builds tissue. Good for inflammation of the intestines, excessive menstrual flow and pain of ulcers. Excellent remedy for kidney and bladder problems including bed-wetting, diarrhea, and infections. Seeds are used for dropsy, epilepsy, and yellow jaundice.

External Use: Apply tincture to inflamed skin, eczema, erysipelas, scalds, external hemorrhaging, insect bites, burns, scalds and ulcers.

Bodily Influence: Alterative, Antiseptic, Astringent, Deobstruent, Diuretic, Emollient, Expectorant, and Vulnerary.

PLATYCODON *(Platycodon grandiflorum)*

Medicinal Parts: Root.

Actions and Uses: This herb is used to treat lung and bronchial congestion and respiratory problems. Effective for asthma, bronchitis, coughs, sore throat, pneumonia, and related lung ailments.

Bodily Influence: Expectorant, and Tonic.

PLEURSY ROOT *(Asclepias tuberosa)*

Medicinal Part: Root.

Actions and Uses: Pleursy root is used for ailments involving the lungs and upper respiratory system. This herb relieves the pain and difficulty of breathing without being a stimulant. Also good for indigestion, dysentery, all bronchial congestion's, inflammation of the lungs, fevers, diseases of the respiratory system, consumption, and catarrhal affections.

Warning: Use commercial preparations, the fresh root can be toxic.

Bodily Influence: Adaptogen, Carminative, Diaphoretic, Expectorant, Febrifuge, Stomachic, and Tonic.

POKE *(Phytolacca americana)*

Medicinal Part: Root and Fruit.

Actions and Uses: Poke root is an excellent treatment for enlargement of the liver, spleen, and thyroid glands. Also good for breast tumors, lymphatic swelling, mumps, tonsillitis, and rheumatism.

External Use: Salve applied to goiter and swollen breasts.

Warning: Poke root contains toxic substances and should be limited to one gram per day.

Bodily Influence: Alterative, Emetic, Laxative, and Lymphatic.

PRICKLY ASH *(Xanthoxylum americanum)*

Medicinal Part: Bark.

Actions and Uses: Prickly ash bark is a good blood purifier for deposits in the joints. Also used for arthritis, colds, poor digestion, and is excellent when used to increase circulation and to produce warmth during chills.

External Use: Salve applied to wounds to bring down swelling and speed healing.

Bodily Influence: Alterative, Antispasmodic, Astringent, Emmenagogue, Rubefacient, and Stimulant.

PROPOLIS

Bees manufacture propolis to prevent disease from entering the hive. As it is a natural antibiotic it wards off all kinds of infections such as colds, flu, fevers, digestive disorders, etc.

PSYLLIUM *(Plantagopsyllium)*

Medicinal Part: Seed.

Actions and Uses: Psyllium assists in easy evacuation by increasing water in the colon, cleans out compacted pockets thereby making bowel movements easier for people with colitis and hemorrhoids. Creates bulk. Relieves auto-intoxication. Also used for treating ulcers, gastro- intestinal irritations, and colitis. Recent studies show that Psyllium helps reduce cholesterol, so this herb could be used as a preventative against heart disease.

Warning: Because Psyllium forms an indigestible mass, it should be taken at different times than other supplements.

Bodily Influence: Demulcent, and Laxative.

PUMPKIN

Medicinal Part: Seed and Husks.

Actions and Uses: Used for worms, stomach problems, morning sickness, nausea, and toning the prostate gland.

Bodily Influence: Adaptogen, Anthelmintic, Nervine, and Vermifuge.

PURPLE CONEFLOWER *(Echinaceaangustifolia)*

Medicinal Parts: Leaves, Dried Rhizome, and Root.

Actions and Uses: Glandular balancer, especially lymphatic and liver areas. Also blood purifier, antiseptic, and anti-infection herb. Good for boils, blood poisoning, carbuncles, all pus diseases, snake and spider bites. Helps boost immune response. This herb is also used to restore normal immune function in patients receiving chemotherapy.

External Use: Apply tincture to all infected wounds and insect bites.

Warning: Alcohol tincture may destroy polysaccharides in echinacea that stimulate the immune system.

Bodily Influence: Alterative, Diaphoretic, Sialagogue.

QUEEN OF THE MEADOW

(Eupatoriompurpureum)

Medicinal Part: Root, Flower.

Actions and Uses: This herb is almost infallible when used for the expulsion of gravel. One of the best known herbs for kidney, bladder, and urinary infections. An effective treatment for dropsy, gout, lumbago, neuralgia, rheumatism and joint stiffness caused by uric acid deposits. Also valuable in diarrhea, especially for children. Imparts to the bowels some nourishment as well as an astringency.

Bodily Influences: Astringent, Diuretic, Relaxant, Stimulant, and Tonic.

RED CLOVER *(Trifolium pratense)*

Medicinal Part: Blossoms, and Leaves..

Actions and Uses: An excellent blood purifier, glandular restorer and mineralizer. Contains silica and other earthy salts. Good for tuberculoses and to fight other bacteria, inflamed lungs, arthritis, gout, malignant ulcers, whooping coughs, and renal problems. Relaxing to nerves and entire system. Also used for many years as an antidote to cancer.

External Use: Apply salve for the removal of external cancer and indolent ulcers.

Bodily Influence: Alterative, Antibiotic, Deobstruent, Nutritive, Sedative, and Tonic.

RED PUCCOON *(Sanguinaria canadensis)*

Medicinal Parts: Root.

Actions and Uses: Small doses stimulate the digestive system. When taken in large doses it is an arterial sedative. This herb is effective in treating asthma, chronic bronchitis, laryngitis, whooping cough, and other complaints of the respiratory organs. The tincture has been used successfully in treating dyspepsia and dropsy of the chest.

External Use: Injections of strong tea is excellent for leucorrhoea and haemorrhoids.

Bodily Influence: Alterative, Diuretic, Febrifuge, Sialagogue, Stimulating expectorant, Systemic emetic, and Tonic.

RED RASPBERRY *(Rubus idaeus)*

Medicinal Parts: Whole plant.

Actions and Uses: Effective in menstrual problems, decreasing the blood flow without stopping it abruptly. Promotes healthy nails, bones, teeth, and skin. Remedy for dysentery and diarrhea in infants. As a tea, excellent for morning sickness in pregnancy. Helps prevent miscarriage, strengthens uterine walls prior to giving birth, and may help shorten delivery. Long-term usage may be required to achieve optimal results.

External Use: Poultic of leaves mixed with slippery elm is used for wounds and burns.

Warning: Use only under doctors supervision during pregnancy. May interfere with iron absorption.

Bodily Influence: Alterative, Antispasmodic, Astringent, Stimulant, and Tonic.

RED SPEARMINT *(Mentha smithiana)*

Medicinal Part: Leaves, Stems.

Actions and Uses: An agreeable and harmless herb for infants and children as well as adults. Prepared as a herbal tea it is cleansing to the entire system, and will strengthen heart muscles. An excellent remedy for sea sickness, and an effective agent for suppressed menstruation. Useful for cramps and hiccoughs, prevent the gripping effects of cathartics, relieve hysterics, chills colic, influenza, nausea, and vomiting.

External Use: Tincture applied to forehead will relieve most headaches. Also apply oil to burns, neuralgia, rheumatism, and toothaches. Enemas are effective treatments for cholera and colon troubles.

Bodily Influence: Aromatic, Carminative, Stimulant, Stomachic.

RESHI MUSHROOM *(ganoderma lucidum)*

Medicinal Part: Top.

Actions and Uses: Reshi has been used for over two thousand years. It has the long and distinguished reputation as the ultimate longevity herb in Oriental history. Reshi has a positive effect on the immune system. Good for allergies and auto-immune diseases. Acts as an immune modulator. Reshi has also been used to help eradicate the side effects of radiation and chemotherapy in cancer patients, and has a reported anti-tumor activity. Aids the liver and is helpful for digestion. Has antibacterial and anti viral properties. It has been used for bronchitis, coronary disease, senility and general debility. In recent years, it has been used to treat patients suffering with AIDS.

Bodily Influence: Adaptogen, Alterative, Demulcent, Discutient, Esculent, Nutritive, and Tonic.

RHUBARB ROOT *(Rheum palmatum)*

Medicinal Part: Root.

Actions and Uses: Rhubarb root is used to treat chronic blood diseases and is useful for colon, spleen, and liver disorders. Enhances gallbladder functions and has a positive effect on duodenal ulcers. Also good for headaches, constipation, diarrhea, and hemorrhoids.

Warning: Do not use during pregnancy. Prolonged use tends to aggravate any tendency toward chronic constipation

Bodily Influence: Adaptogen, Antibiotic, Hepatic, and Stomachic

ROMAN WORMWOOD *(Artemisia pontica)*

Medicinal Parts: Tops and Leaves.

Actions and Uses: Used for aminorrhoes, chronic leukorrhea, diabetes, diarrhea, female complaints, inflammation of tonsils and quinsy. Also small doses are used for dispersing the yellow bile of jaundice from the skin caused by liver conditions.

External Use: Apply Worm Wood oil to bruises, local inflammations, sprains, swellings, rheumatism, and lumbago.

Warning: Overdose will irritate the stomach and increase heart action.

Bodily Influence: Anthelmintic, Febrifuge, Narcotic, Stimulant, Stomachic, and Tonic.

ROSEHIPS *(Sabbatia angularis)*

Medicinal Part: Seed and Pod.

Actions and Uses: An extremely high source of Vitamin C. Relieves bladder problems and is recommended for all infections. Effective for colds, diarrhea, coughs, consumption, dysentery and scurvy. Also helps to combat stress.

Bodily Influence: Adaptogen, Antiseptic, and Nervine.

ROSEMARY *(Rosarinus officinalis)*

Medicinal Part: Flowers and Leaves.

Actions and Uses: An effective treatment for colic, indigestion, nausea, and fevers. This herb will raise the blood pressure and promotes liver function, the production of bile, and improves circulation.

External Use: Salve is used to treat eczema, arthritis, and rheumatism.

Bodily Influence: Aromatic, Astringent, Carminative, Diaphoretic, and Stimulant.

RUE *(Ruta graveolens)*

Medicinal Part: Leaves.

Actions and Uses: An excellent treatment for cramps in the bowel, gas, poor digestion, hysteria, nervousness, spasms, dizziness, and congestion in the female organs. Rue is also a good herb to add to cough medicines.

External Use: Oil applied for headache and sciatica.

Bodily Influence: Antispasmodic, Emmenagogue, Rubefacient, and Stimulant.

SACRED ROOT *(Rhamnus purshiana)*

Medicinal Part: Dried Bark.

Actions and Uses: One of the best natural laxatives in the herbal kingdom. A stimulant to the whole digestive system. Extremely useful in hemorrhoidal conditions, chronic constipation, and liver and gall bladder complaints. It is considered suitable for delicate and elderly persons. Also a very good remedy for gallstones; increases secretion of bile.

Bodily Influence: Antispasmodic, Hepatic, Laxative, and Bitter tonic.

SAFFLOWER *(Carthamus tinctorious)*

Medicinal Part: Flowers.

Actions and Uses: This herb is recommended to sooth the nerves in cases of hysteria. Safflower tea taken hot will produce perspiration and is used during colds, flu, and fevers.

Bodily Influence: Diaphoretic, Emmenagogue, and Laxative.

SAFFRON *(Nepeta safiria)*

Medicinal Part: Leaves and Root.

Actions and Uses: A natural hydrochloric acid (utilizes sugar of fruits and oils), thus helping arthritics get rid of the uric acid which holds the calcium deposited in joints. Also reduces lactic acid build up.

Bodily Influence: Antacid, and Antirheumatic.

SAGE *(Salvia officinalis)*

Medicinal Part: Leaves.

Actions and Uses: Best known effect is the reduction of perspiration and stopping the flow of milk in a nursing mother. Also used for nervous conditions, trembling, depression, vertigo, and to decrease secretions of the lungs, sinuses, throat, and mucus membranes.

External Use: Used to cleanse old ulcers and wounds.

Bodily Influence: Anthelmintic, Antispasmodic, Aromatic, Astringent, Diaphoretic, Expectorant, Tonic, and Vulnerary.

SALVIA *(Salvia miltiorrhiza)*

Medicinal part: Root.

Actions and Uses: An all purpose herb used To treat various female gynecological problems. Relieves symptoms of menopause, and PMS. Restores menstrual regularity and controls hot flashes. Also an effective treatment for boils, distention, erysipelas, and spasmodic rheumatism.

Warning: Should not be used during pregnancy.

Bodily Influence: Alterative, Blood stimulant, and Emmenagogue.

SANGUINARIA *(Sanguinaria canadensis)*

Medicinal Parts: Root.

Actions and Uses: Small doses stimulate the digestive system. When taken in large doses it is an arterial sedative. This herb is effective in treating asthma, chronic bronchitis, laryngitis, whooping cough, and other complaints of the respiratory organs. The tincture has been used successfully in treating dyspepsia and dropsy of the chest.

External Use: Injections of strong tea is excellent for leucorrhoea and haemorrhoids.

Bodily Influence: Alterative, Diuretic, Febrifuge, Sialagogue, Stimulating expectorant, Systemic emetic, and Tonic.

SANICLE *(Saniculamarilandica)*

Medicinal Parts: Root and Leaves.

Actions and Uses: Possesses powerful cleansing and healing properties both internally and externally. Good for asthma, bee stings, boils, debility diabetes, diarrhea, gastritis, dysentery, intermittent fevers, lungs, intestines, ozaena, reproductive organs, renal tract, and throat discomfort.

External Use: Rub salve on chapped hands and bleeding skin ulcerations.

Bodily Influence: Alterative, Anodyne, Astringent, Discutient, Depurative. Nervine, and Vulnerary.

SARSAPARILLA *(Aralia nudicaulis) (Smilax ornata)*

Medicinal Part: Root.

Actions and Uses: Widely used by athletes as a natural steroid and as a source of precursors of muscle building hormones. Contains the male hormone testosterone which tends to restore sexual power and mental alertness. Clears skin disorders such as eczema, and psoriasis. Increases energy, and protects against harmful radiation. Eliminates poisons from the blood and helps cleanse the system of infections. Useful for rheumatism, gout, skin eruptions, ringworm, scrofula, internal inflammation, colds, and catarrh.

External Use: Rub tincture on skin infections. The tea may be used as an eyewash for sore or irritated eyes.

Bodily Influence: Alterative, Antiscorbutic, Demulcent, Diuretic, and Stimulant.

SASSAFRAS *(Sassafras officonale)*

Medicinal Part: Root bark.

Actions and Uses: This herb is given for painful menstruation. Relieves suffering and is effective in afterpains from childbirth. When combined with alterative herbs sassafas is effective to purify the blood.

External Use: Oil is effective as a disinfectant. Alao used as a liniment for rheumatic pains.

Bodily Influence: Alterative, Aromatic, Carminative, Diaphoretic, Diuretic, and Stimulant.

SAW PALMETTO *(Serenoa serrulata)*

Medicinal Part: Berries.

Actions and Uses: A tissue builder. It is recommended in all wasting diseases as it has a marked effect upon all the glandular tissue. A valuable herb when recovering from diseases of the reproductive organs, ovaries, prostate, and testes. Capable of increasing nutrition of the testicles and mamma in functional atony of these organs. Builds stamina and endurance and rids respiratory membranes of mucus. Also of use in renal conditions, internal inflammations, diabetes, rheumatism, and gout.

Warning: Saw palmetto may suppress cancer symptoms. Men having difficulty with urination or experiencing pain or swelling of the prostate should see a health professional for diagnosis before using this herb.

Bodily Influence: Anticatarrhal, Anyiseptic, Diuretic, Expectorant, Nutritive, Sedative, and Tonic

SCHIZANDRA FRUIT *(South american)*

Medicinal Part: Root.

Actions and Uses: Used to enhance the immune system. Has an a positive effect on the lungs. Used in some cases for forgetfulness. Also used for insomnia.

Bodily Influence: Adaptogen, Anti-catarrhal, Nervine, and Sedative.

SCULLCAP *(Scutellaria lateriflora)*

Medicinal Part: Whole Herb.

Actions and Uses: A natural anti-depressant. Used for most nervous system malfunctions. More effective than quinine, and not harmful. Good for neuralgia, aches and pains, rheumatism, convulsions, nervous tension, and relieves severe hiccups. Helps reduce high blood pressure, helps heart conditions and disorders of the central nervous systems such as palsy, hydrophobia and epilepsy.

Bodily Influence: Antispasmodic, Antipyretic, Nervine, Relaxant, and Restorative.

SEED OF HORUS *(Marrubium vulgara)*

Medicinal Parts: Whole Herb.

Actions and Uses: Used for congestion of coughs, colds, and pulmonary affections associated with unwanted phlegm from the chest, and promotes sweating which in turn, cools the body. Good for intestinal gas, when taken in large doses, it is a laxative and will expel worms.

Bodily Influence: Anthelmintic, Diuretic, Diaphoretic, Expectorant, Laxative, Resolvent, Stimulant, Stomachic, and Tonic.

SENNA *(Cassia marilandica)*

Medicinal Part: Leaves and Pods.

Actions and Uses: A stimulant laxative, extremely powerful, should be combined with ginger or fennel to prevent cramping. Will help eliminate most types of worms from the colon if used following wormwood.

External Use: Apply salve to skin diseases and pimples.

Warning: Do not use during pregnancy or if there is inflammation in intestinal tract.

Bodily Influence: Cathartic, Diuretic, Laxative, and Vermifuge.

SHAVE GRASS *(Equisetum arvense)*

Medicinal Parts: Leaves and Stems.

Actions and Uses: Contains a great deal of silica. Increases calcium absorption, promotes healthy skin, strengthens bone, hair, nails, teeth, and helps eliminate excess oil from hair and skin. Also a diuretic. Helps with kidney disorders, especially kidney stones. Works best in small frequent doses.

External Use: Used as poultice to depress bleeding and accelerate healing of wounds.

Bodily Influence: Astringent, Diuretic, Lithotriptic, and Tonic.

SHEEP'S SORREL *(Rumex acetosella)*

Medicinal Part: Leaves.

Actions and Uses: Sheep's Sorrel is highly praised as a vermifuge. Intestinal worms have no resistance to the properties of this herb. A good remedy for stomach hemorrhage, and profuse menstruation. Also extremely effective for kidney, bladder, and liver problems, such as gravel, stones, and jaundice.

External Use: Extract is used for boils, cancerous tumors, tetters, and ringworm.

Bodily Influence: Antiscorbutic, Diuretic, Refrigerant, Vermifuge.

SHEPHERD PURSE *(Capsella bursa pastoris)*

Medicinal Part: Whole Herb.

Actions and Uses: Controls hemorrhaging of stomach, lungs, uterus, and kidneys. Successfully used in cases of hemorrhaging after childbirth and excessive menstruation. Also valuable when used for dysentery, vulnerary, rheumatism, catarrh, dropsy, scrofula, skin diseases, and chronic menorrhagia.

External Use: Fresh juice stops external bleeding and heals bruises.

Bodily Influence: Antiscorbutic, Astringent, Diuretic, and Stimulant.

SHITAKI MUSHROOM *(Lentinus edodes)*

Medicinal Part: Top.

Actions and Uses: Used as both food and healing agent in the Orient. Taken to enhance the immune system. Has an anti-tumor activity, and helps to enhance the natural protective defenses of the body. Shitaki is used as a cancer fighting agent in China and Japan. Also used to lower blood cholesterol levels and help to pull fat from the system. May be helpful for those diagnosed with clinical depression.

Bodily Influence: Adaptogen, Discutient, Esculent, and Stimulant.

SILERIS *(Ledebouriella divaricata)*

Medicinal part: Root.

Actions and Uses: Sileris relieves muscle spasms and pain of the joints. Taken on a daily basis as a tonic it will bolster the immune system. Effective treatment for chills, flu, headache, and rheumatoid numbness.

Bodily Influence: Antispasmodic, and Tonic.

SLIPPERY ELM *(Ulmus fulva)*

Medicinal Part: Inner Bark (fresh or dried).

Actions and Uses: Considered one of the most valuable remedies in herbal practice, having wonderful strengthening and healing qualities. Used extensively for inflammation of the lungs, bowels, stomach, heart, diseases of female organs, kidney and bladder. Slippery Elm will soothe an ulcerated or a cancerous stomach when nothing else will.

External Use: Apply salve to swollen glands of the neck, enlarged prostate, and groin.

Bodily Influence: Astringent, Demulcent, Emollient, and Nutritive.

SNAKE LILY *(Iris versicolor)*

Medicinal Parts: Root, Rhizome.

Actions and Uses: A valuable herb for all diseases of the blood, kidney, spleen, and chronic hepatic affections. Has a special influence on the lymphatic glands (pure lymphatic circulation is spontaneous to longevity). Also effective in treating secondary Syphilis.

External Uses: Used in treating infected wounds, ulcers, and fistula.

Bodily Influence: Alterative, Cathartic, Diuretic, Resolvent, Sialagogue, and Vermifuge.

SNAKEROOT *(Saniculamarilandica)*

Medicinal Parts: Root and Leaves.

Actions and Uses: Possesses powerful cleansing and healing properties both internally and externally. Good for asthma, bee stings, boils, debility diabetes, diarrhea, gastritis, dysentery, intermittent fevers, lungs, intestines, ozaena, reproductive organs, renal tract, and throat discomfort.

External Use: Rub salve on chapped hands and bleeding skin ulcerations.

Bodily Influence: Alterative, Anodyne, Astringent, Discutient, Depurative. Nervine, and Vulnerary.

SOLOMON'S SEAL *(Polygonatumcommutatum)*

Medicinal Part: Rhizome.

Actions and Uses: Helps to mend broken bones. Also pulmonary consumption and bleeding of the lungs, female complaints, bruises, hemorrhoids, inflammations of the stomach, and tumors.

External Use: Tincture is used to close fresh and bleeding wounds, and the root extract is effective in diminishing freckles and discoloration of the skin.

Bodily Influence: Astringent, Demulcent, and Tonic.

SORREL *(Rumex acetosa)*

Medicinal Part: Leaves.

Actions and Uses: Sorrel is highly praised as a vermifuge. Intestinal worms have no resistance to the properties of this herb. A good remedy for stomach hemorrhage, and profuse menstruation. Also extremely effective for kidney, bladder, and liver problems, such as gravel, stones, and jaundice.

External Use: Extract is used for boils, cutaneous tumors, tetters, and ringworm.

Bodily Influence: Antiscorbutic, Diuretic, Refrigerant, and Vermifuge.

SPANISH SAGE *(Salvia lavandulifolia)*

Medicinal Part: leaves.

Actions and Uses: Best known effect is the reduction of perspiration and stopping the flow of milk in a nursing mother. Also used for nervous conditions, trembling, depression, and vertigo.

External Use: Used to cleanse old ulcers and wounds.

Bodily Influence: Astringent, Diaphoretic, Expectorant, and Tonic.

SPEARMINT *(Mentha viridas)*

Medicinal Part: Leaves.

Actions and Uses: Spearmints main uses are during colds, flu, gas, indigestion, cramps, and spasms. This herb is non-toxic and is soothing to the stomach with mild diaphoretic and diuretic properties. Also used for enemia and to stop vomiting.

Bodily Influence: Aromatic, Antispasmodic, Carminative, Diaphortic, Diuretic, and Stimulant.

SPICE BIRCH *(Betula alba)*

Medicinal Part: Bark and Leaves.

Actions and Uses: An effective treatment for dropsy, gout, rheumatism, stones in the kidneys and bladder, and is used to expel worms. Also a good remedy for diarrhoea, dysentery, cholera, and all problems of the alimentary tract. Oil of wintergreen is distilled from the inner bark.

External Use: Extract of the buds, bark, and leaves is applied boils, eczema, swelling, and rheumatic pain.

Bodily Influence: Aromatic, Diaphoretic, and Stimulant.

STAGBUSH *(Viburnumpunifolium)*

Medicinal Part: Root bark.

Actions and Uses: Black haw is commonly used to ease contractions and cramps in the pelvic organs. An excellent treatment for painful menstruation, whether due to congested tissue or nerve disability. Used as a sedative to the female reproductive organs and has a tonic effect during pregnancy. Also a valuable remedy in chronic uterine inflammation, congested uterus, and leukorrhea.

Bodily Influence: Antispasmodic, Emmenagogue, and Sedative, and Tonic.

ST. JOHN'S WART *(Hypericum perforatum)*

Medicinal Parts: Tops and Flowers.

Actions and Uses: This is one of the most useful herbs. It can be used by young or elderly. Useful in stopping bed wetting. Also for treatment of dysentery, diarrhea, bleeding of the lungs, hysteria and nervous irritability, worms, jaundice, and suppressed urine. Will also correct irregular menstruation and is an excellent remedy for painful menstruation.

External Use: Salve promotes healing of bruises, eruptive skin, skin wounds, and ulcers.

Bodily Influence: Astringent, Alterative, Aromatic, Diuretic, Expectorant, Nervine, and Sedative.

STRAWBERRY *(Fragaria vesca)*

Medicinal Part: Leaves, Root and Berries.

Actions and Uses: A good blood purifier, clears eczema and other skin conditions. Very effective in treating intestinal malfunctions (diarrhea, dysentery and weakness of intestines and urinary organs).

External Use: Tincture used to cleanse and heal eczema and other skin conditions.

Bodily Influence: Mild Astringent, Diuretic, and Tonic.

SQUAW VINE *(Mitchella repens)*

Medicinal Part: Root.

Actions and Uses: Particularly good for women in building of female organs. It has been used for years by expectant mothers six weeks prior to delivery to aid parturition. Alleviates painful menstruation and is a diuretic. Used for insomnia and also used successfully for gravel and urinary ailments.

Bodily Influence: Adaptogen, Astringent, Diuretic, Emmenagogue, Nutritive, and Tonic.

STONE ROOT *(Collinsoniacanadensis)*

Medicinal Part: Root.

Actions and Uses: A good remedy for varicose veins in the legs and rectum. Relaxes the walls on veins and arterioles. Especially good for piles and hemorrhoids. Also improves general circulation and strengthens the heart.

Bodily Influence: Astringent, Diuretic, and Hepatic.

SUCORY *(Cichoriumintybus)*

Medicinal Part: Root.

Actions and Uses: The root is ground to make a tonic, diuretic, and a mild laxative. Sucory is also useful in the treatment of gallstones, kidney stones, and inflammation of the urinary tract and liver.

Bodily Influence: Adaptogen, Laxative, and Tonic.

SUMA *(Pfaffiapaniculata)*

Medicinal Parts: Bark, Berries, Leaves, and Roots.

Actions and Uses: Also called Brazilian Ginseng. It is the richest source of naturally-occurring germanium and an immune system booster. It has a positive tonic effect on the endocrine system and helps the body to regulate hormone levels. As a female hormone balancer, Suma will act as a precursor to the production of estrogen if the body needs it. It will not cause the production of more estrogen then the body can handle. Also useful for anemia, diabetes, fatigue, and stress.

Bodily Influences: Adaptogen, and Tonic.

SWEET CICLY *(myrrhis odorata)*

Medicinal Part: Leaves.

Actions and Uses: Stimulator, appetite and flow of gastric juices. A powerful antiseptic which is generally used in equal parts with golden seal for intestinal ulcer, catarrh of the intestines and other mucous membrane conditions. Also used for bronchial and lung diseases. Tightening the gums and preventing pyorrhea is one of its most outstanding qualities.

Warning: Do not use if you are pregnant or have kidney disease.

Bodily Influence: Antiseptic, Digestive Aid, and Stimulant.

TALL SPEEDWELL *(Leptandravirginica)*

Medicinal Part: Root.

Actions and Uses: Black root acts on the intestines in chronic constipation and is very effective in treating chronic Hepatic diseases. Also used for ascites, bilious fever, dyspepsia, headache, jaundice, pleurisy, and liver disorders.

Bodily Influence: Alterative, Antiseptic, Cholagogue, Emetocathartic, Laxative, and Tonic.

TANSY *(Tanacetumvulgare)*

Medicinal Parts: Whole Herb.

Actions and Uses: An effective treatment for hysteria, and other nervous disorders of women. Used for colds, fevers, dyspepsia, jaundice. and kidney disorders. Tansy is also used for expelling worms in both children and adults.

External Use: Salve is excellent for bruises, freckles, inflammations, sunburn, swellings, and tumors.

Warning: Do not exceed the manufactures recommended dosage. Overdose can cause vomiting, feeble respiration and pulse, convulsions, and coma.

Bodily Influences: Anthelmintic, Diaphoretic, Emmenagogue, Stimulant, and Tonic.

TEA TREE *(Meleleucaalternifolia)*

Medicinal Part: Leaves.

Actions and Uses: Tea tree is grown primarily in the Pacific Rim. Extremely effective as a germicide and fungicide, the antiseptic power of the Tea Tree Oil is 12 times that of carbolic acid. Good for athletes foot, cold sores, cystitis, dermatitis, wounds, and yeast infections.

Warning: Oral consumption of the oil is not recommended. Internal use of the oil may cause increased heart rate and sever indigestion.

Bodily Influence: Antiseptic and Antifungal.

TETTERWORT *(Sanguinariacanadensis)*

Medicinal Parts: Root.

Actions and Uses: Small doses stimulate the digestive system. When taken in large doses it is an arterial sedative. This herb is effective in treating asthma, chronic bronchitis, laryngitis, whooping cough, and other complaints of the respiratory organs. The tincture has been used successfully in treating dyspepsia and dropsy of the chest.

External Use: Injections of strong tea is excellent for leucorrhoea and haemorrhoids.

Bodily Influence: Alterative, Diuretic, Febrifuge, Sialagogue, Stimulating expectorant, Systemic emetic, and Tonic.

THYME *(Thymusvulgaris)*

Medicinal Parts: Whole Plant.

Actions and Uses: An effective remedy for hysteria, and nervous disorders. Also good for sinusitis, asthma, and chronic respiratory problems such as bronchial irritation, colic, colds, fever, headaches, irritable stomach, mucus, and spasms of whooping cough. Recent research indicates Thyme lowers cholesterol levels, so it may also be helpful in the prevention of heart disease.

External Use: Oil is used for painful swellings, Neuralgia, and toothaches.A salve made from thyme, myrrh, and goldenseal is a very effective remedy for herpies.

Bodily Influence: Antiseptic, Antispasmodic, Carminative, Diuretic, Emmenagogue, Expectorant, Parasiticide, and Tonic.

TORMENTIL ROOT *(Potentillatormentilla)*

Medicinal Parts: Root.

Actions and Uses: This herb is used for diarrhea, enteritis, and stomach inflamation. Also used for prostrate enlargement, prolapsed anus, and hemorrhoids. Effective as a gargle for tonsilitis, canker sores, and laryngitis. Also some homeopathic practicioners use it as a douche for leukorrhea.

External Use: Salve is used for varicose veins and wounds.

Bodily Influence: Anticatarrhal, Astringent, Styptic, and Styptic.

TRICOLOR *(Salviaofficinalis)*

Medicinal Part: leaves.

Actions and Uses: Best known effect is the reduction of perspiration and stopping the flow of milk in a nursing mother. Also used for nervous conditions, trembling, depression, and vertigo.

External Use: Used to cleanse old ulcers and wounds.

Bodily Influence: Astringent, Diaphoretic, Expectorant, and Tonic.

TURKEY RHUBARB ROOT *(Rheum palmatum)*

Medicinal Part: Root.

Actions and Uses: Useful for colon, spleen, and liver disorders. Enhances gallbladder functions and has a positive effect on duodenal ulcers. Good for headaches, constipation, diarrhea, and hemorrhoids. Low doses increase gastric secretion, increase the secretion of bile, and acts as an appetite stimulant.

Bodily Influence: Adaptogen, Antibiotic, anti-inflammatory, Antiseptic, Aperient, Hepatic, Stomachic, and Tonic.

TURMERIC *(Circuma longa)*

Medicinal Part: Leaves, Seeds, Root.

Actions and Uses: Turmeric is a potent anti-inflammatory used for the relief of pain and arthritic symptoms. Also an effective blood cleanser, good for liver related ailments such as jaundice, helps prevent blood clots, and is an excellent remedy for gallbladder diseases.

Note: Some individuals may be allergic to this herb.

Bodily Influence: Antibiotic, Antirheumatic, Hepatic, Mucilaginous.

TWICKLE PURPLE *(Lavandula angustifolia)*

Medicinal Part: Flower.

Actions and Uses: When taken as a tea it calms nerves, soothes headaches, eases flatulence, dizziness, fainting and halitosis. Herbalists use the neat essential oil as a mild sedative, antiseptic, and painkiller on insect bites and burns.

External Uses: Used as a massage oil for skin sores, insomnia, infections, and rheumatic aches.

Note: May be poisonous. Do not take more than two drops of undiluted oil internally.

Bodily Influence: Antiseptic, Nervine, and Tonic.

UVA URSI *(Arctostaphylos uva ursi)*

Medicinal Parts: Leaves.

Actions and Uses: Very useful in diabetes and all kinds of kidney and bladder infections. Helps disorders of the small intestines, spleen, liver, pancreas, and eliminates excessive bloating due to water retention. Strengthens heart muscle, and imparts tone to the urinary passages. Excellent remedy for piles, hemorrhoids, kidney stones, and helpful in the treatment of gonorrhea. Also good where there are mucus discharges from the bladder with pus and blood.

External Use: Salve used for hemorrhoids and piles. Douche for dysentery and leukorrhea.

Bodily Influence: Adaptogen, Alterative, Antisyphilitic, Astringent, Cardiac, Diuretic, Hemostatic, Stimulant, and Tonic.

VALERIAN ROOT *(Valeriana officinalis)*

Medicinal Parts: Root and Rhizomes.

Actions and Uses: A strong nervine without a narcotic effect. Soothes and quiets the nervous system, beneficial in cardiac palpitation. Used for epileptic fits, nervous tension or irritations. Also relieves gas pains, stomach cramps, and promotes sleep. Excellent for children with measles and scarlet fever.

External Use: Vapor baths given to children will quieten and encourage restful sleep.

Warning: Do not exceed recommended dose. Extremely high dosages of valerian may cause weakening of the heartbeat and paralysis.

Bodily Influence: Antispasmodic, Calmative, Nervine, Stimulant, and Tonic.

VARIEGATA *(Mentha variegata)*

Medicinal Part: Leaves, Stems.

Actions and Uses: Variegata is an agreeable and harmless herb for infants and children as well as adults. Prepared as a herbal tea it is cleansing to the entire system, and will strengthen heart muscles. An excellent remedy for sea sickness, and an effective agent for suppressed menstruation. Useful for cramps and hiccoughs, prevent the gripping effects of cathartics, relieve hysterics, chills colic, influenza, nausea, and vomiting.

External Use: Tincture applied to forehead will relieve most headaches. Also apply oil to burns, neuralgia, rheumatism, and toothaches. Enemas are effective treatments for cholera and colon troubles.

Bodily Influence: Aromatic, Carminative, Stimulant, Stomachic.

VERVAIN *(Verbena officinalis)*

Medicinal Part: Top.

Actions and Uses: An effective herb for colds, coughs, fevers, and pleurisy. Also used for pain in the bowels, convulsions, nerve weakness, and headaches. Vervain tea will also settle a nervous stomach and is good for insomnia.

External Use: Salve used to treat neuralgia, rheumatism, and sciatica.

Bodily Influence: Antispasmodic, Astringent, Diaphoretic, Emetic, Expectorant, Galactagogue, and Vulnerary.

VIOLET *(Viola odorata)*

Medicinal Parts: Leaves, Flowers.

Actions and Uses: Useful for pain in cancerous growths. Soothing and healing effect on inflamed mucal surfaces. Good for colds, hoarseness, inflammation of the lungs, and whooping cough.

Externally: Apply tincture to inflamed tumors, sore throat, and swollen breasts.

Bodily Influence: Antiseptic, and Expectorant.

VITEX *(Vitex verbenaceae)*

Medicinal Parts: Leaves, Flowers.

Actions and Uses: A hormone balancer and natural alternative to estrogen. European herbalists use vitex for the treatment of female complaints. Useful for side effects associated with menopause, fibroid tumors, and PMS.

Bodily Influence: Adaptogen, Discutient, and Nervine.

WALNUT *(Juglans cinerea)*

Medicinal Part: Dried Inner Bark and Leaves.

Actions and Uses: A good treatment for diarrhea and dysentery. Also used for acne, angina pectoris, ecthyma, eczema, headache, herpes, and migraines. When combined with bitter root it is a good remedy for consumption.

External Use: Diluted tincture is effective for chronic skin diseases.

Bodily Influence: Cathartic, Tonic, and Vermifuge.

WATER CRESS *(Nasturtium officinale)*

Medicinal Parts: Leaves, Root.

Actions and Uses: Helps the body to use oxygen, stimulates rate of metabolism, increasing physical endurance and stamina and improves heart response. Also used for bladder, kidney, and liver problems, and to dissolve kidney stones.

Bodily Influence: Alterative, Nutritive, Stimulant, and Tonic.

WATER FLAG *(Iris versicolor)*

Medicinal Parts: Root, Rhizome.

Actions and Uses: A valuable herb for all diseases of the blood, kidney, spleen, and chronic hepatic affections. Has a special influence on the lymphatic glands (pure lymphatic circulation is spontaneous to longevity). Also effective in treating secondary Syphilis.

External Uses: Used in treating infected wounds, ulcers, and fistula.

Bodily Influence: Alterative, Cathartic, Diuretic, Resolvent, Sialagogue, and Vermifuge.

WESTERNWALL *(Apocynum androsaemifolium)*

Medicinal Part: Root.

Actions and Uses: Bitter root is considered by the American Indians as almost infallible in the treatment of venereal diseases. Recommended to relieve cardial dropsy, rheumatic gout of the joints, and in the treatment of brights disease. Also used for jaundice, chronic liver conditions, emptying the gall ducts, and gall stones.

External Use: Apply two or three times a day to remove warts.

Bodily Influence: Emetic, Expectorant, Diaphoretic, Laxative, and Tonic.

WHITE OAK BARK *(Quercus robur)*

Medicinal Parts: Bark and Acorn.

Actions and Uses: Good for varicose veins. Used in douches and enemas, for internal tumors, vaginal infections, and swellings. One of the best remedies for hemorrhoids, hemorrhages, varicose veins, tumors, womb troubles, goiter or any trouble of the rectum. Normalizes the liver, kidneys, spleen, and dissolves kidney stones and gallstones. Tea is taken for bleeding of the stomach, lungs, and rectum.

External Use: Salve applied for relief of painful bleeding and itching hemorrhoids. As it is an antiseptic it is also a good salve for wounds.

Bodily Influence: Antiseptic, Astringent , Diuretic, Hemostatic, and Tonic.

WHITE WILLOW BARK *(Salix alba)*

Medicinal Part: Bark.

Actions and Uses: It is one of nature's greatest gifts to mankind as a pain-relieving, fever-lowering, anti-inflammatory agent without any side effects. Helps relieve symptoms of headache, fever, arthritis, rheumatism, bursitis, dandruff, eye problems (eyewash), influenza, chills, eczema, and nosebleed. Most effective in concentrated extract form.

External Use: Use as a gargle for mouth sores and tonsillitis.

Bodily Influence: Anodyne, Antispasmodic, Astringent, Diaphoretic, Diuretic, Febrifuge, and Tonic.

WILD CHERRY BARK *(Prunus serotina)*

Medicinal Part: Inner bark.

Actions and Uses: This herb soothes nerve irritations of the lungs and stomach and loosens mucus in the throat and chest. Wild cherry is a common remedy for heart palpitations when this condition is caused by a stomach disorder. Also used to improve digestion by stimulating the gastric glands.

Bodily Influence: Astringent, Sedative, Stimulant, Stomachic, and Tonic.

WILD YAM *(Dioscorea villosa)*

Medicinal Part: Root.

Actions and Uses: Yam is a source of the male sex hormone testosterone and is used for rejuvenating effects. Relieves nauseous symptoms of pregnancy, and will help to prevent miscarriage when combined with ginger. Also good for acne, angina, biliousness, diarrhea, dysentery, gallbladder, and liver disorders.

Bodily Influence: Antispasmodic, Antibilious, Cholagogue, and Diaphoretic.

WINTERGREEN *(Gaultheriaprocumbens)*

Medicinal Part: Whole Plant.

Actions and Uses: Used for centuries for its ability to relieve pains of rheumatism. Also good for headaches, colic, flatulence, gastritis, neuralgia, pleurodynia, and urinary ailments.

External Use: Tincture effective for joint pains and swelling.

Bodily Influence: Anodyne, Astringent, and Stimulant.

WITCH HAZEL *(Hamamelisvirginica)*

Medicinal Parts: Bark and Leaves.

Actions and Uses: One of the best known herbs to check internal bleeding, especially for excessive menstruation, hemorrhages from the lungs, stomach, uterus, and bowels. Also useful in reducing pain associated to diarrhea, dysentery, and hemorrhoids.

External Use: Apply salve or tincture to varicose veins, also used for skin irritations and wounds.

Bodily Influence: Astringent, Hemostatic, Sedative, and Tonic.

WOOD BETONY *(Betonicaofficinalis)*

Medicinal Part: Leaves.

Actions and Uses: Strengthens and stimulates the heart muscle. Expels worms. Good for headache, colic, colds, gout, indigestion, and stomach cramps. Also used for jaundice, Parkinson's disease, and tuberculosis.

External Use: Salve is used for sores, ulcers, and wounds.

Bodily Influence: Alterative, Anodyne, Antacid, Aromatic, Hepatic, Nutritive, Parasiticide, Stomachic, and Vermifuge.

WORM WOOD *(Artemisiaabsinthium)*

Medicinal Parts: Tops and Leaves.

Actions and Uses: Used for aminorrhoes, chronic leukorrhea, diabetes, diarrhea, female complaints, inflammation of tonsils and quinsy. Also small doses are used for dispersing the yellow bile of jaundice from the skin caused by liver conditions.

External Use: Apply Worm Wood oil to bruises, local inflammations, sprains, swellings, rheumatism, and lumbago.

Warning: Overdose will irritate the stomach and increase heart action.

Bodily Influence: Anthelmintic, Antiseptic, Aromatic, Diaphoretic, Febrifuge, Narcotic, Stimulant, Stomachic, and Tonic.

YARROW *(Achillea millefolium)*

Medicinal Parts: Whole Herb.

Actions and Uses: Very high in tannic acid thus helps to stop bleeding wounds, hemorrhaging stomach, bowels, and lungs. Yarrow is an effective treatment for acute catarrhs of the respiratory tract, colds, chickenpox, fevers, influenza, measles, and smallpox. Also useful in menstrual irregularities and has a soothing effect on nervous conditions of the heart.

External Use: Salve has a soothing effect on hemorrhoids, skin ulcers and wounds.

Warning: Interferes with the absorption of iron.

Bodily Influence: Alterative, Astringent, Diaphoretic, Diuretic, Hemostatic, Stimulant, and Tonic.

YELLOW DOCK *(Rumex crispus)*

Medicinal Parts: Leaves, and Roots.

Actions and Uses: Mineral rich plant, especially in iron. It is a powerful restorer of the lymphatic system. Also a blood purifier, laxative, astringent, and effective in skin problems such as psoriasis, eczema, and urticarea. Combine with Sarsaparilla as a tea for chronic skin disorders.

External Use: When made into an ointment it is valuable to use for swelling, open sores, and itching eruptions.

Bodily Influence: Alterative, Antiscorbutic, Astringent, Cholagogue, Laxative, Nutritive, and Tonic.

YERBAMATE *(Lippia dulcis)*

Medicinal Parts: Whole Herb.

Actions and Uses: Used to enhance the healing powers of other herbs. Stimulates the mind, and nervous system, retards aging, and stimulates the production of cortisone. Also good for allergies, coughs, colds, hay fever, arthritis, fluid retention, and constipation.

Bodily Influences: Adaptogen, Alterative, Anodyne, Anti-rheumatic, Nervine, Nutritive, and Sedative.

YERBA SANTA *(Eriodictyon californicum)*

Medicinal Parts: Leaves.

Actions and Uses: Yerba Santa is a leading herb for all respiratory conditions. An effective treatment for allergies, asthma, catarrh, coughs, colds, hay fever, vomiting, and diarrhea. Also used for rheumatic pain and kidney conditions.

External Use: Tincture used to relieve pain of rheumatism, swellings, sores, etc.

Bodily Influences: Aromatic, Expectorant, Stimulant, Tonic.

YUCCA *(Yucca liliaceae)*

Medicinal Part: Root.

Actions and Uses: New hope for arthritics. Contains special steroid saponins which are effective in treating acute forms of arthritis and rheumatism. Also a good blood purifier, relieves stress, migraine headaches, shingles, gout, colitis, diarrhea, and an effective remedy for urethritis and prostatitis. Tests at the University of Wyoming show that Yucca may also have an anti-cancer potential.

Bodily Influence: Alterative, Antirheumatic, and Discutient.

COMMON ORIENTAL HERBS

Chinese herbs have a very long history of use. The first tabloids on traditional Chinese herbal medicine titled "Shen Nong Ben Cao Jing" were written around 2700 BC by a tribal chief named Shen Nong that lived on the great Yellow River Plateau of China. These tabloids described 252 healing plants and laid the foundation for the development of Chinese herbal medicine. China's first bonified book on herbal medicine is called the Materia Medica (Xin Xiu Ben Cao), and held 1,746 entries. This book was written by the government of the Tang Dynasty in 618 AD. The latest revision to the Materia Medica was written by the Jiangsu College of New Medicine in 1977. It now holds over 4,000 entries on medicinal plants. The Chinese approach to medicine is an interesting blend of philosophy and healing. Their emphasis is not to eradicate disease, but to promote health.

Many of the Chinese herbs are available in western herb shops or health food stores. Some of the herbs listed require special preparation. You should first consult your local Chinese herbal practitioner, if you want to try some of the more exotic herbs. The following list describes the most popular Chinese herbs that are available to the west.

BA DAN XING REN *(Prunusamygdalus)*

Medicinal Part: Seed.

Actions and Uses: The Chinese have used Ba Dan Xing Ren (almond oil) for over two thousand years as a muscle relaxer and a local anesthetic. According to a study at the Health Research and Studies Center in Los Altos, California, almond oil was a more effective cholesterol-reducing agent than olive oil, so may also help prevent heart disease.

External Use: Ba Dan Xing Ren can moisturize and soften the skin.

Bodily Influence: Antibiotic, Emollient, and Nervine.

CH' AI HU *(Bupleurumchinese)*

Medicinal Part: Root.

Actions and Uses: Ch' ai hu is recommended for reducing fevers and feverish headache. This herb is regarded as one of the best herbs for detoxifying the liver. Also used to relieve nausea, reduce anxiety, and dizziness.

Bodily Influence: Analgestic, Alterative, and Antipyretic.

CHEN PI *(Citrusreticulata)*

Medicinal Parts: Orange or tangerine peel.

Actions and Uses: The strength of citrus peel improves with drying and age. Peel is added to herbal formulas to stimulate and promote the circulation of energy. Effective treatment for abdominal swelling, diarrhea, indigestion, and vomiting.

Bodily Influences: Antiemetic, Antitussive, Digestant, Expectorant, Stimulant, and Stomachic.

CHUANXIONG *(Ligusticumchuanxiong)*

Medicinal Part: Root.

Actions and Uses: A great sexual rejuvenator. Gives energy, helps to balance female hormones. Controls bed wetting, expels excess water from the body. Increases blood circulation, relieves abdominal pains, helps relieve anxiety, and promotes a feeling of well-being.

Bodily Influence: Antispasmodic, Emmenagogue, Stimulant, and Tonic.

CHU HUA *(Chrysanthemummorrifolium)*

Medicinal Parts: Flowers.

Actions and Uses: In China the dried Chu hua flowers are a symbol of longevity. Effective in detoxifying the liver, as a blood cleanser and to lower blood pressure. Also used in the treatment of conjunctivitis, dizziness, fevers, headaches, and pneumonia.

External Use: Tincture is used to reduce abscesses, boils, and inflammation of the skin.

Bodily Influences: Alterative, Antipyretic, and Carminative.

DANG SHEN *(Salvia miltiorrhiza)*

Medicinal part: Root.

Actions and Uses: An all purpose herb used To treat various female gynecological problems. Relieves symptoms of menopause and PMS. Restores menstrual regularity and controls hot flashes. Also an effective treatment for boils, distention, erysipelas, and spasmodic rheumatism.

Warning: Should not be used during pregnancy.

Bodily Influence: Alterative, Blood stimulant, and Emmenagogue.

DA T'SAO *(Ziziphus jujuba)*

Medicinal Parts: Whole date.

Actions and Uses: Da T'sao is sold in dried form in most Chinese herb shops. This herb has a calming effect on the body, and is recommended for the treatment of apprehension, dizziness, forgetfulness, insomnia, and to relieve nervous exhaustion.

Bodily Influences: Digestive, Nervine, Nutritive, and Tonic.

DON SEN *(Codonopsis pilosula)*

Medicinal Part: Root.

Actions and Uses: Don Sen is very similar but a milder version of panax ginseng. Works as a mild stimulant, normalizes body functions, and helps the body adapt to stress. The Orientals used it in their love potions.

Bodily Influence: Aphrodisiac, Demulcent, Nervine, Stimulant, and Stomachic

DONG QUAI *(Angelica sinensis)*

Medicinal part: Root.

Actions and Uses: An all purpose herb used to treat various female gynecological problems. Restores menstrual regularity and relieves symptoms of menopause and PMS. Controls hot flashes and reduces high blood pressure. It is the female equivalent of Korean ginseng. Also relieves constipation by moistening the intestinal tract.

Warning: Should not be used during pregnancy.

Bodily Influence: Adaptogen, Laxative, and Nutritive.

ELEUTHERO *(Eleutherococcus sentocosus)*

Medicinal Part: Leaves and Root.

Actions and Uses: A relative of ginseng but considerably weaker. Used for its tonic properties and calming effects. Relieves anxiety and promotes a feeling of well-being. A good sexual rejuvenator, gives energy, used to treat low blood pressure, impotence and stress.

Bodily Influence: Antispasmodic, and Cardiac tonic.

FANG-FENG *(Ledebouriella divaricata)*

Medicinal part: Root.

Actions and Uses: Fang-Feng relieves muscle spasms and pain of the joints. Taken on a daily basis as a tonic, it will bolster the immune system. Effective treatment for chills, flu, headache, and rheumatoid numbness.

Bodily Influence: Antispasmodic, and Tonic.

FAN MU GUA *(Carica Papaya)*

Medicinal Part: Fruit.

Actions and Uses: Fan mu gua in an excellent antacid, contains papain which has similar chemical characteristics to pepsin, an enzyme that helps to breakdown protein in the body. Good for the metabolism of protein, increased energy, gastrointestinal problems, and helps relieve indigestion.

Bodily Influence: Antacid, Esculent, and Stimulant.

FO-TI *(Polygonum multiforum)*

Medicinal Part: Root.

Actions and Uses: The Chinese claim that fo-ti prevents premature aging. This herb is excellent for mental depression and has been used to enhance the memory. Recent scientific studies verify cholesterol-lowering effects of this herb. Also helps to rejuvenate the endocrine glands which in turn, strengthen the body. This herb may have potential in the prevention of cancer, as recent animal tests using fu-ti extract, show an anti tumor activity.

Bodily Influence: Stimulant and Tonic.

FU LING *(Poria cocos)*

Medicinal Part: Whole fungus.

Actions and Uses: The Chinese claim that Fu ling is one of the best diuretics in the world today. This herb is excellent for hyperactivity in children. Also nervous conditions, restlessness, and mental depression in adults. Fu ling is also an effective treatment for lung congestion, and helps tone the pancreas, spleen, and stomach.

Bodily Influence: Diuretic, Expectorant, and Nervine.

FU TZU *(Aconitum carmichaeli)*

Medicinal Parts: The prepared root.

Actions and Uses: Because of this herbs powerful Yang properties, it should be used with extreme caution. This herb is always used in combination with other herbs to balance the Yin. An effective remedy for sciatica, arthritis, and other severely painful conditions. Also used to stimulate sexual potency and relieve flatulence.

External Use: Apply liniment locally for the relief of rheumatism and neuralgia

Bodily Influence: Analgestic, Antispasmodic, Diaphoretic, Diuretic, Stimulant, and Tonic.

GAY GEE *(Lycium chinensis)*

Medicinal Parts: Berries.

Actions and Uses: Gay gee is effective for the treatment of bronchial inflammation and an aid in the removal of toxins from the blood. Gay gee clears the eyes and is good for those that suffer from cloudy vision. Also used to nourish liver and kidneys, and lower high blood pressure.

Bodily Influence: Alterative, Antipyretic, Nutrient, and Tonic.

GAN CAO or GAN T'SAO *(Glycyrrhiza globra)*

Medicinal Part: The dried root.

Actions and Uses: Used by the Chinese for over five thousand years. A hormone balancer and natural cortisone. Used for hypoglycemia, adrenal glands, stress, and female problems (menstrual and menopause). Decreases muscle or skeletal spasms, and reduces pain from ulcers. Also used to increase fluidity of mucus from the lungs and bronchial tubes. Also used for coughs and chest complaints, gastric ulcers, and throat conditions. New studies in the United States and Japan have found that Gan Cao may help retard growth of certain cancerous tumors.

Warning: Gan Cao increases production of aldosterone causing an increase in blood pressure. Large doses of licorice root should be avoided by people with high blood pressure.

Bodily Influence: Demulcent, Expectorant, Laxative, and Pectoral.

GAN JIANG *(Zangiber officinale)*

Medicinal Part: Root and rhizomes.

Actions and Uses: Hot tea promotes cleansing of the body through perspiration and is useful for suppressed menstruation. Relieves indigestion, gas, morning sickness, and nausea. In a recent university study, gan jiang capsules proved to be far more effective at controlling motion-induced nausea than either a drug or placebo. It helps absorb toxins, restore gastric activities to normal, and helps control diarrhea and vomiting that often accompanies gastro-intestinal flu.

External Use: Apply tincture to soothe, and promote the healing of skin infections and minor burns.

Bodily Influence: Carminative, Diaphoretic, Diuretic, Stimulant, and Tonic.

HO SHOU WO *(Polygonummultiforum)*

Medicinal Part: Root.

Actions and Uses: The Chinese claim that Ho shou wo prevents premature aging. This herb is excellent for mental depression and has been used to enhance the memory. Recent scientific studies verify cholesterol-lowering effects of this herb. Also helps to rejuvenate the endocrine glands which in turn, strengthen the body. This herb may have potential in the prevention of cancer, as recent animal tests using ho shou wo extract, show anti-tumor activity.

Bodily Influence: Stimulant and Tonic.

HUANG CHI *(Astragalus membranaceous)*

Medicinal Part: Root.

Actions and Uses: An Oriental herb used for a wide variety of ailments such as diabetes, heart disease, high blood pressure, and also improves digestion. Strengthens the immune systems and promotes healing. Huang Chi has been used to help restore normal immune function and may prevent the spread of malignant cells in cancer patients.

Bodily Influence: Anhydrotic, Diuretic, and Tonic.

HU SUAN *(Alliumsativum)*

Medicinal Part: Bulb.

Actions and Uses: Natural antibiotic, stimulates activity of the digestive organs, therefore relieves problems associated with poor digestion. It is used to emulsify the cholesterol and loosen it from the arterial walls. Proven useful in asthma and whooping cough. Its anti fungal properties make it a good adjunct in treating vaginal yeast infections *(candida albicans)*. Valuable in intestinal infections and effective in reducing high blood pressure. Recent studies show that Hu Suan has cancer-inhibiting properties (Garlic is toxic to some tumor cells).

External Use: Apply directly on affected parts for aches, sprains and skin disorders. Drops in ear relieves earache.

Bodily Influence: Alterative, Antibiotic, and Esculent.

JEN SHENG *(Panax ginseng)*

Medicinal Part: Root.

Actions and Uses: A physical restorative. Helps the entire body adapt to stress, regenerates and rebuilds sexual centers. Impotency and low sperm count have been corrected by using Panax Ginseng. Stimulates the appetite, and normalizes blood pressure. Anciently known as a male hormone, and used for longevity.

Bodily Influence: Aphrodisiac, Demulcent, Nervine, Stimulant, and Stomachic.

JIE ENG or JIE GENG *(Platycodon grandiflorum)*

Medicinal Parts: Root.

Actions and Uses: This herb is used to treat lung and bronchial congestion and respiratory problems. Effective for asthma, bronchitis, coughs, sore throat, pneumonia, and related lung ailments.

Bodily Influence: Expectorant, and Tonic.

KO KEN *(Pueraria lobata)*

Medicinal Parts: Root.

Actions and Uses: This herb is used to treat bronchial congestion and respiratory problems. Effective for asthma, bronchitis, coughs, sore throat, pneumonia, and related lung ailments. Ko Ken also relieves acidity in the body and thus relieves minor aches and pains

Bodily Influence: Antipyretic, Demulcent, Diaphoretic, Refrigerant, and Spasmolytic.

KU XING REN *(Prunus armeniaca)*

Medicinal Parts: Kernel.

Actions and Uses: In Chinese traditional medicine this herb is only used as a nutritive tonic for the lungs. In the west Ku xing ren is highly regarded as an anti-cancer source of laetrile.

Bodily Influence: Demulcent, Expectorant, and Nutritive.

LONG YEN ROU *(Euphoria longana)*

Medicinal Parts: Berries.

Actions and Uses: A powerful tonic used to strengthen the reproductive organs in women, stimulate the mind, nervous system, and counteract forgetfulness, and hyperactive mental activity. Also an effective remedy for hypoglycemia.

Bodily Influences: Nutritive, and Tonic.

LU HUI *(Aloe barbadenis)*

Medicinal Part: Leaves.

Actions and Uses: Lu Hui is a potent medicine and healer, used by the Chinese for over two thousand years. An excellent colon cleanser. Healing and soothing to the stomach as well as liver, kidneys, spleen, and bladder. Works with your immune system to keep you healthy, strong and vibrant.

External use: An excellent remedy for piles and hemorrhoids. Keeps skin soft and supple, useful for minor burns, mild skin irritations, and bug bites.

Warning: Lu Hui is an effective laxative, and should not be taken internally during pregnancy.

Bodily Influence: Anthelmintic, Emmenagogue, Purgative, and Tonic.

LU RONG *(Deer antler)*

Medicinal Part: Powdered antler.

Actions and Uses: Oriental herbalists believe that Lu Rong contains male hormones. Used in various forms as tonics, and as an aphrodisiac in many Chinese herbal preparations.

Bodily Influence: Tonic.

MA HUANG *(Ephedra sinica)*

Medicinal Parts: Leaves Berries.

Actions and Uses: A long acting stimulant that can last up to one full day. In China this herb has been used for four thousand years to treat respiratory infections and asthma. An effective decongestant used to relieve headaches, hay fever, fevers, watery eyes, stuffy nose, and other allergy and cold symptoms.

Warning: Do not use this herb if you have diabetes, thyroid disease, heart disease, or high blood pressure.

Bodily Influence: Demulcent, Emollient, Expectorant, Pectoral, and Tonic.

MUXU *(Medicago sativia)*

Medicinal Parts: Flowers, Leaves, Petals, and Sprouts.

Actions and Uses: The Chinese have used this herb since the sixth century. Very high in vitamins and minerals, thus nourishes the entire system. Excellent for pregnant women and nursing mothers. Good for the pituitary gland. It alkalizes the body rapidly and helps detoxify the liver. Helps rebuild decayed teeth, relieves fluid retention, dissolves kidney stones, and relieves arthritic and rheumatic pain. Also aids in the assimilation of protein, fats and carbohydrates. Contains an anti fungus agent.

Bodily Influence: Nutrient and Tonic.

PAI SHU *(Atractylodes macrocephala)*

Medicinal Parts: Root.

Actions and Uses: Pai shu increases energy by eliminating excess moisture through a process that first eliminates sodium and other electrolytes, so does not exhaust the kidneys as some other diuretics do. The Chinese also use this herb as a tonic for the spleen and pancreas.

Bodily Influence: Diuretic and Tonic.

PU GONG YING *(Leontodon taraxacum)*

Medicinal Part: Root.

Actions and Uses: This herb is a popular treatment for upper respiratory infections. Strengthens kidneys and bladder, and removes excess fluids. Protects against liver and gallbladder disorders. Effective for the obstructions of the liver, gall, and spleen. A highly praised agent for skin diseases, scrofula, and scurvy. Excellent for anemia because it is high in iron, calcium, and other vitamins and minerals. A very good diuretic.

Bodily Influence: Aperient, Deobstruent, Diuretic, Stomachic, and Tonic.

REN SHEN *(Eleutherococcussenticosus)*

Medicinal Part: Root.

Actions and Uses: Strengthens the entire endocrine glandular system, a tonic and toner of the body, promotes mental and physical vigor, stamina, endurance, metabolism, appetite, and digestion. Mildly stimulates the central nervous system, also helpful in problems arising in menopause such as hot flashes and irregular periods. Also good for cocaine withdrawal, radiation protection, and enhances lung and immune functions.

Warning: Avoid if hyperactive or under high nervous tension.

Bodily Influence: Aphrodisiac, Demulcent, Nervine, Stimulant, and Stomachic.

SHAO YAO *(Paeonialactiflora)*

Medicinal Parts: Root:

Actions and Uses: Shao yao is effective in treating menstrual irregularity and abdominal pains associated with menstrual cycle. This herb is a liver tonic. Purifies the blood, and is used for all diseases stemming from an imbalanced liver function.

Warning: Do not use during pregnancy.

Bodily Influence: Alterative, Antispasmodic, and Hepatic tonic.

SOK DAY- SANG DAY *(Rehmanniaglutinosa)*

Medicinal Parts: Root:

Actions and Uses: An effective herb in treating infertility, menstrual irregularities, and taken as a tonic during pregnancy and to stop postpartum hemorrhage. Promotes the healing of injured bones. Used to eliminate excess acids from the body, and for treating weakened kidneys. This herb is also a liver tonic. Purifies the blood, and is used for all diseases stemming from an imbalanced liver function.

Bodily Influence: Hemostatic, and Uterine tonic.

TANG KUEI *(Angelicasinensis)*

Medicinal part: Root.

Actions and Uses: An all purpose herb used to treat various female gynecological problems. Restores menstrual regularity and relieves symptoms of menopause and PMS. Controls hot flashes and reduces high blood pressure. It is the female equivalent of Korean ginseng. Also relieves constipation by moistening the intestinal tract.

Warning: Should not be used during pregnancy.

Bodily Influence: Adaptogen, Laxative, and Nutritive.

TANG SHEN *(Codonopsis pilosula)*

Medicinal Part: Root.

Actions and Uses: Tang Shen is very similar, but a milder version of panax ginseng. Works as a mild stimulant, normalizes body functions, and helps the body adapt to stress. The Orientals used it in their love potions.

Bodily Influence: Aphrodisiac, Demulcent, Nervine, Stimulant, and Stomachic.

TIENCHI *(Panax notoginseng)*

Medicinal Part: Root.

Actions and Uses: Tienchi is effective in maintaining normal body weight, helps one withstand stress, and prevents fatigue. This herb controls heart rate, normalizes blood pressure, and improves circulation.

Bodily Influence: Cardiac tonic and Hemostatic.

XI XIN *(Asarum heterotropoides)*

Medicinal Part: Root and rhizomes.

Actions and Uses: Hot tea promotes cleansing of the body through perspiration and is useful for suppressed menstruation. Relieves indigestion, gas, morning sickness, nausea. It helps absorb toxins, restore gastric activities to normal, and helps control diarrhea and vomiting that often accompanies gastro-intestinal flu.

External Use: Apply tincture to soothe, and promote the healing of skin infections and minor burns.

Bodily Influence: Antispasmodic, Carminative, Diuretic, Diaphoretic, Stimulant, and Tonic.

YE JU *(Chrysanthemum morrifolium)*

Medicinal Parts: Flowers.

Actions and Uses: In China the dried Ye ju flowers are a symbol of longevity. Effective in detoxifying the liver, as a blood cleanser, and to lower blood pressure. Also used in the treatment of conjunctivitis, dizziness, fevers, headaches, and pneumonia.

External Use: Tincture is used to reduce abscesses, boils, and inflammation of the skin.

Bodily Influences: Alterative, Antipyretic, and Carminative.

YIN HUA *(Lonicera japonica)*

Medicinal Parts: Flowers.

Actions and Uses: Yin hua is mostly used for acute infectious and inflammatory conditions. A valuable herb for the treatment of colds, acute flu, and fevers.

External Use: Tincture may also be applied externally for skin infections.

Bodily Influence: Alterative and Antipyretic.

ZIMU *(Medicago sativia)*

Medicinal Parts: Flowers, Leaves, Petals, and Sprouts.

Actions and Uses: The Chinese have used this herb since the sixth century. Very high in vitamins and minerals thus nourishes the entire system. Excellent for pregnant women and nursing mothers. Good for the pituitary gland. It alkalizes the body rapidly and helps detoxify the liver. Helps rebuild decayed teeth, relieves fluid retention, dissolves kidney stones, and relieves arthritic and rheumatic pain. Also aids in the assimilation of protein, fats, and carbohydrates. Contains an anti fungus agent.

Bodily Influence: Nutrient, and Tonic.

.HERBAL GLOSSARY

Term

Definition

Adaptogen -- Balances and restores tone to a particular area.

Alterative -- Blood purifier, promotes cleansing and detoxification of blood.

Amara -- Term used to designate bitter-constituent drugs.

Analgestic -- Taken to relieve pain without causing loss of consciousness.

Anodyne -- Herb used to ease or relieve pain.

Antacid -- Helps regulate acid conditions in the stomach.

Anthelmintic -- Used to expel intestinal worms.

Antiabortive -- Help to inhibit abortive tendencies.

Antiarthritics -- Relieves problems of gout and other arthritic problems.

Antiasthmatic -- Relieves the symptoms of asthma.

Antibilious -- Acts on the bile, relieving biliousness.

Antibiotic -- Inhibits the growth of, or eradicates viruses and bacteria.

Anticatarrhal -- Eliminate or counteract the formation of mucus.

Antiemetic -- Stops vomiting.

Antihydropics -- Aids in voiding or evacuating urine.

Antileptic -- Relieves fits.

Antilithics -- To relieve calculus problems.

Antioxidant -- Stops oxidation.

Antiperiodic -- Arrests morbid periodic movements.

Antipyretic -- Cools system reducing fevers.

Antirheumatic -- Relieves or cures rheumatism.

Antiscorbutic -- Cures or prevents scurvy.

Antiseptic -- Helps prevent putrefaction.

Antispasmodic -- Relieves or prevents spasms.

The Complete Natural Health Encyclopedia

Term		Definition
Antisyphilitic	--	Having effect or curing venereal diseases.
Aperitive	--	Medication that has a gentle, laxitive effect.
Aphrodisiacs	--	Improve sexual potency and power.
Aromatics	--	Fragrant or spicy tasting herbs that stimulate the gastro-intestinal mucous membranes.
Astringent	--	Constricting or binding effect, checks hemorrhages and secretions.
Calmative	--	Reduces nervousness or excitment.
Cardiac	—	Pertaining to, or affecting the heart.
Carminative	--	Expels gas from the bowels.
Carthartic	--	Cause evacuating from the bowels.
Cephalic	--	Remedies used in diseases of the head.
Cholagogue	--	Increases the flow of bile.
Condiment	--	Improves the flavor of food.
Convulsants	--	Herbs that cause convulsions. Stimulants should be used before convulsants
Cordial	--	Dilates the pupil of the eye.
Demulcent	--	Soothing, relieves internal inflammation.
Deobstruent	--	Removes obstructions in the alimentary canal.
Depressants	--	Sedatives.
Depurative	--	Purifies the blood.
Detergent	--	Cleansing boils, ulcers, wounds, etc.
Diaphoretic	--	Produces and increases perspiration.
Digestive	--	Aids digestion.
Discutient	--	Dissolves and heals tumors and abnormal growths.
Disinfectants	--	Destroy noxious properties of decaying organic matter.
Diuretic	--	Increases the secretion and flow of urine
Ecbolics	--	Induce abortions.
Electuary	--	Medication that has been sweetened.

Term   ## Definition

Term	Definition
Embrocation	-- Liquid medication that is applied to the skin to relieve pain or inflammation.
Emetic	-- Induces vomiting.
Emmenagogue	-- Promotes and stimulates menstrual flow.
Emollient	-- Softens and soothes inflamed tissue.
Esculent	-- Edible as a food.
Essential Oil	-- Highly volatile oils found in most plants.
Evacuants	-- Purgatives
Exanthematous	-- Remedy for skin eruptions and diseases.
Expectorant	-- Expulsion of phlegm from mucus membrane.
Febrifuge	-- Abates and reduces fevers.
Flavonoids	-- Collective term for substances found in plants.
Galactagogue	-- Promotes secretion of breast milk.
Hemostatic	-- Agent that arrests internal bleeding.
Hepatic	-- For liver diseases, stimulates secretive functions.
Herpatic	-- A remedy for skin diseases of all types.
Hydragogues	-- Promotes a water evacuation of the bowel.
Hypnotics	-- Relax and promote sleep.
Hypoglycemics	-- Lowers blood sugar.
Laxative	-- Promotes bowel action.
Lithontryptic	-- Dissolves and discharges calculi in urinary organs.
Lymphatic	-- Used to stimulate and cleanse lymphatic system.
Maturating	-- Ripens or brings boils to a head.
Mucilaginous	-- Soothing to all inflammation.
Mucolytic	-- Causing mucus to break down into a more watery liquid.
Narcotic	-- Powerful anodynes and/or hypnotics.
Nauseant	-- Produces vomiting.

Term		Definition
Nephritics	--	Influence nephritia tubes of kidneys.
Nervine	--	Acts on nervous system, stops nervous excitement.
Nutritive	--	Supplies nutrients, aids building and toning body.
Opthalmicum	--	A remedy for the healing of eye diseases.
Palliative	--	To relieve or alleviate symptoms without curing.
Parasiticide	--	Kills and expels parasites from the skin or digestive tract.
Parturient	--	Induces and promotes labor at childbirth.
Pectoral	--	A remedy for chest affections.
Peristaltics	--	Muscular contraction in the bowels.
Phytotherapy	--	Therapeutic use of medicinal plants.
Precursor	--	Starts a chain reaction which accelerates growth.
Prophylactics	--	Prevent disease.
Purgative	--	Causes copious excretions from the bowels.
Refrigerant	--	Cooling, reduces body temperature.
Resolvent	--	Dissolves boils and tumors.
Rubifacient	--	Increases circulation and produces red skin.
Sedative	--	Nerve tonic, relieves excitement, promotes sleep.
Sialogogue	--	Increases the secretion of saliva.
Soperifics	--	Cause sleep, Also known as somnifacients.
Sorbefacients	--	Cause absorption.
Spasmolytic	--	Relieves muscular cramps or spasms.
Specifics	--	Direct curing powers to certain tissues.
Stimulant	--	Increases energy, assists functional activity.
Stomachic	--	Strengthens and tones stomach. Relieves indigestion.

Term   Definition

Term   ## Definition

Term		Definition
Styptic	--	Contracts tissues, blood vessels, arrests bleeding.
Sudorific	--	Produces profuse perspiration.
Taenicides	--	Kill tapeworms.
Tonic	--	A remedy which is invigorating and strengthening.
Vermicides	--	Kill intestinal worms.
Vermifuge	--	Destroys and expels worms from the system.
Vulnerary	--	Promotes healing by stimulating cell growth.

THE SPICE RACK

The kitchen spice rack is often used as a safe and natural alternative to the synthetic drugs that we normally have in the medicine cabinet. The majority of the common culinary spices that enhance the flavor of our foods, also have a genuine medicinal value. The following natural spices are used to treat and control ailments ranging from headaches and nausea to acute infections and heart attacks.

ANISE (Pimpinella anisum)

Therapeutic Uses: Good for coughs, breaks up mucus.
Bodily Influence: Carminative and stimulant.

BASIL (Ocimum Basilicum)

Therapeutic Uses: Recommended for the treatment of constipation, indigestion, kidney and bladder troubles, cramps, nervous conditions, nausea, and vomiting.
Bodily Influence: Alterative, antipyretic, carminative, diuretic, stimulant, and nervine.

BAY LEAVES (Laurus nobilis)

Therapeutic Uses: Helps to prevent indigestion and gas. When used as a poultice it will relieve rheumatic and arthritic pains.
Bodily Influence: Antirheumatic, carminative, and rubifacient.

BLACK PEPPER (Piper nigrum)

Therapeutic Uses: A preventive and cure for colds and sore throats.
Bodily Influence: Anticatarrhal and demulcent.

CALAMUS (Acorus calamus)

Therapeutic Uses: A versatile herbal stimulant that is of great benefit to circulation and stomach problems. When used externally it will relieve pain, stiff joints, and inflammations.
Bodily Influence: Carminative, diaphoretic, diuretic, stimulant, and tonic.

CARAWAY (Carum carvi)

Therapeutic Uses: Taken for colic, griping, indigestion, gas, and nervous conditions.
Bodily Influence: Carminative and nervine.

CARDAMOM (Elettaria cardamomum)

Therapeutic Uses: A treatment for colic, diarrhea, and headaches.
Bodily Influence: Carminative and stimulant.

CAYENNE (Capsicum anuum)

Therapeutic Uses: A remedy for colds, flu, headaches, and indigestion. Also improves circulation; helps prevent heart attacks and strokes.
Bodily Influence: Antispasmodic, astringent, carminative, and stimulant.

CINNAMON (Cinnomomum zeylanicum)

Therapeutic Uses: Used for abdominal, heart, and lower back pains. Also an effective treatment for chronic diarrhea, cramps, dysentery, indigestion, and gas.
Bodily Influence: Astringent, carminative, and demulcent.

CLOVES (Syzygium aromaticum)

Therapeutic Uses: Treats flatulence, increases circulation, and improves digestion.
Bodily Influence: Stimulant.

CORIANDER (Coriandrum sativum)

Therapeutic Uses: Helps prevent griping.
Bodily Influence: Alterative, carminative, and diuretic.

CUMIN (Cuminum cyminum)

Therapeutic Uses: Increases breast milk production and when used externally as a liniment, it will stimulate circulation.
Bodily Influence: Antispasmodic, carminative, and stimulant.

FENNEL (Foeniculum vulgare)

Therapeutic Uses: When made into a tea it will expel mucus and treat colic and gas.

Bodily Influence: Antispasmodic, carminative, diuretic, expectorant, and stimulant.

FENUGREEK (Trigonella foenumgraecum)

Therapeutic Uses: Used for stomach disorders, mucus conditions, and lung congestion.

Bodily Influence: Astringent, demulcent, emollient, expectorant, and tonic.

GARLIC (Allium sativum)

Therapeutic Uses: Garlic is known as the cure all. It regulates blood-pressure, treats lung ailments, bronchial congestion, and infectious diseases, such as colds and flu, and kills parasites.

Bodily Influence: Alterative, antibiotic, antispasmodic, carminative, diaphoretic, expectorant, nervine, and vulnerary.

GINGER (Zingiber officinale)

Therapeutic Uses: A versatile herbal stimulant that is of great benefit to circulation and stomach problems. When used externally it will relieve pain, stiff joints, and inflammations.

Bodily Influence: Carminative, diaphoretic, diuretic, stimulant, and tonic.

MACE (Myristica fragans)

Therapeutic Uses: Relieves heart problems, chronic nervous disorders, relieves nausea, and helps digestion.

Bodily Influence: Cardiac, carminative, and nervine.

MARJORAME (Origanum majorana)

Therapeutic Uses: When used as a tea it is a good remedy for problems associated with menstruation, such as abdominal cramps and nausea. It is also a good treatment for colic, upset stomach, and nervous complaints.

Bodily Influence: Antispasmodic, carminative, diaphoretic, emmenagoge, expectorant, stimulant, and tonic.

MUSTARD SEED (Brassica nigra)

Therapeutic Uses: Taken internally, it acts as a blood purifier and a mild laxative. Externally, the oil is used to stimulate local circulation.

Bodily Influence: Alterative, diuretic, emetic, rubefacient, and stimulant.

NUTMEG (Myristica fragans)

Therapeutic Uses: Relieves heart problems, chronic nervous disorders, relieves nausea, and helps digestion.

Bodily Influence: Cardiac, carminative, and nervine.

ROSEMARY (Rosmarinus officinalis)

Therapeutic Uses: May be used as a substitute for aspirin in treating headaches. Also a good remedy for colic, fevers, and nausea due to indigestion and gas. Coltsfoot is smoked with rosemary to treat mucous congestion of the lungs and asthma.

Bodily Influence: Astringent, diaphoretic, and stimulant.

SAGE (Salvia officinalis)

Therapeutic Uses: A good remedy for bladder infections, diarrhea, dysentery, and inflammatory conditions. Also used to stop the flow of milk and to clear vaginal discharge.

Bodily Influence: Antispasmodic and astringent.

STAR ANISE (Illicium anisum)

Therapeutic Uses: Good for coughs, breaks up mucus.

Bodily Influence: Carminative and stimulant.

TABASCO PEPPER (Capsicum frutescens)

Therapeutic Uses: A remedy for colds, flu, headaches, and indigestion. Also improves circulation; helps prevent heart attacks and strokes.

Bodily Influence: Antispasmodic, astringent, carminative, and stimulant.

THYME (Thymus vulgaris)

Therapeutic Uses: Thyme is used as a tea for bronchitis, laryngitis, and whooping cough. It is also an effective treatment for intestinal worms. Externally it is a good remedy for skin parasites such as crabs, lice, and scabies.

Bodily Influence: Antispasmodic, antiseptic, carminative, diaphoretic, expectorant, and parasiticide.

TURMERIC (Curcuma longa)

Therapeutic Uses: This spice is used to reduce fevers. It is also recommended for regulating the menstrual cycle and to cure menstrual cramps. When used externally it is effective in the healing of wounds.

Bodily Influence: Alterative, antipyretic, detergent, emollient, stimulant, and vulnerary.

AMINO ACID
SUPPLEMENTS

Amino acids are the building blocks of protein and are, for the most part, derived from egg, yeast, or animal protein. Seventy-five percent of our total body solids are made up of protein. Free form amino acids are the purest, and are taken for rapid absorption. The crystalline free form amino acids are generally extracted from a variety of grain products, although cold-pressed milk proteins are also used. Amino acids can be purchased as capsules, tablets, and powders. They are also available in combination with various protein mixtures, multivitamin combinations, and a variety of food supplements.

Nine of the known amino acids cannot be produced by the body and must be supplied through the diet. These are called, essential amino acids. All the essential amino acids must be present for the body to effectively use and synthesize protein.

ESSENTIAL AMINO ACIDS

L-Histidine   L-Isoleucine

L-Leucine   L-Lysine

L-Methionine   L-Phenylalanine

L-Threonine   L-Tryptophan

L-Valine

Amino acids compete with each other for entry to the brain. For healing purposes, always take amino acids individually and on an empty stomach to avoid competition with other amino acids for absorption. It is also wise, when taking amino acids, to also take the major vitamins that are involved in their metabolisms.

Amino Acids	Function
L-Alanine	A simple carbohydrate that aids in the metabolism of glucose that the body, in turn, uses for energy.
L-Arginine	Metabolizes body fat and tones muscle tissue, increases sperm count in males, and aids in the healing of wounds. This amino acid is also used in the retardation of tumors and cancer.
L-Asparagine	Maintains a balance in the central nervous system, preventing a person from being overly calm or overly nervous.
L-Aspartic acid	Improves stamina and endurance, increases resistance to fatigue, helps protect the central nervous system.
L-Carnitine	The amino acids' close cousin. Controls increases in body fat stored by converting nutrients into energy, enhances athletic performance, and disperses excess calories.
L-Citrulline	Stimulates the immune system, detoxifies ammonia that damages living cells, metabolizes to L-Arginine, and promotes energy.
L-Cysteine	Helps to detoxify the system, aids in protection from smoke, alcohol, and heavy metals, also helps protect the body against x-rays and nuclear radiation.
L-Cystine	This amino acid protects against copper toxicity, assists in the supply of insulin to the pancreas, strengthens white blood cells which fight disease, and is necessary for the healing of burns and wounds.
GABA	Gamma-Aminobutyric Acid is a non addictive tranquilizer. It functions as a neurotransmitter in the nervous system by decreasing neuron activity, reducing anxiety and stress.

Amino Acids   Function

Amino Acids	Function
L-Glutamic Acid	A brain fuel. The brain converts glutamic acid to a compound that regulates brain cell activity. Increases the firing of neurons in the nervous system which help correct personality disorders.
L-Glutamine	Used primarily as a brain fuel (improves intelligence). Alleviates fatigue and depression. Also used in the control of alcoholism.
L-Glutathione	A powerful antioxidant that protects against the damaging side effects of chemotherapy and x-rays. Also used in the treatment of blood disorders and as a detoxifier of metals and drugs.
L-Glycine	Needed by the immune system for the synthesis of the nonessential amino acids. Used in the treatment of gastric hyperacidity, acidema, low pituitary gland function and progressive muscular dystrophy.
L-Histidine	Important in the production of red and white blood cells and in growth and repair of tissues. Also used in the treatment of anemia, allergies, and rheumatoid arthritis.
L-Isoleucine	Taken with the correct balance of leucine and valine, it regulates and stabilizes the blood sugar and energy levels. This acid is metabolized in muscle tissues and is required in the formation of hemoglobin.
L-Leucine	Taken with the correct balance of isoleucine and valine this acid will promote the healing of bones, skin, and muscle tissue. Also lowers blood sugar levels and is recommended for people recovering from surgery.
L-Lysine	Improves concentration and mental alertness. Utilizes fatty acids required in energy production, useful in the control and prevention of herpes simplex infection.

Amino Acids	Function
L-Methionine	Not synthesized in the body, must be obtained from dietary supplements. Used in the treatment of edema and some cases of schizophrenia. It assists in the breakdown of fat and research indicates a possible link to arteriosclerosis and cholesterol deposits.
L-Ornithine	Involved in the release of human growth hormone, converts fat into energy and muscle, strengthens the immune system, and accelerates tissue repair and wound healing.
L-Phenylalanine	Controls hunger, improves memory and alertness, enhances sexual interest, and helps alleviate depression.
DL-Phenylalanine	This acid functions as a building block of all amino acids. An effective non addictive and non toxic natural pain killer, also is a very strong anti-depressant.
L- Proline	Aids in the production of collagen improving skin texture. Also strengthens joints, tendons, the heart muscle, and heals cartilage.
L-Serine	Aids in the production of antibodies and immunoglobulins. This amino acid is required for proper metabolism of fatty acids and fats, builds muscle, and a healthy immune system.
L-Taurine	This amino acid is not found in most animal proteins, so synthesis by the body is crucial. It requires vitamin B6 to be synthesized from cysteine. Aids in the control of heart disorders, arteriosclerosis, fat digestion, edema, hypoglycemia, and hypertension.
L-Threonine	L-Threonine is present in the central nervous system, heart, and skeletal muscle. Important in the formation of elastin and collagen, helps control epileptic seizures, and aids liver and lipotropic function.

Amino Acids	Function
L-Tryptophan	Anti-depressant, reduces anxiety, tension, promotes sleep, and lowers pain sensitivity. Also aids in the control of alcoholism, weight control, and is good for the heart.
L-Tyrosine	Appetite depressant, fights fatigue and depression, helps cocaine addicts kick the habit — alleviates the withdrawal symptoms (depression, fatigue, and irritability).
L-Valine	A stimulant that regulates the hydrogen and nitrogen balance in the body. Also used for better muscle metabolism and tissue repair.

HOMEOPATHY

REMEDIES AND TREATMENTS

Homeopathy - The alternative treatment that looks at an illness differently than standard medicine. Instead of dealing with physical complaints with heavy doses of medication, homeopathic medicines help realign the inner healing essence called the "vital force", stimulating the body's own healing mechanisms. Homeopathy is a safe, effective, and a relatively cheap option, for individuals who want to take responsibility for their health. Most homeopathic medicines are available from your local natural supplement store, or health food stores. Homeopathic remedies usually produce no side effects, and when used properly, offer better results than using over the counter medications.

HOMEOPATHIC

COMBINATION REMEDIES

After extensive research and experimentation, the Global Health Research Foundation would not hesitate to recommend the line of homeopathic remedies called, "Medicine From Nature" distributed by Nature's Way Products Inc. Each of the following formulas contain natural substances, that are known to be effective, in stimulating the self healing capacities of the body, and have in our opinion, demonstrated consistent high quality delivery.

ALLERGY FORMULA (Medicine from Nature)

Indications: For natural symptomatic relief of runny nose, sneezing, itchy eyes, skin rashes, and common symptoms of allergy. This formula will not cause drowsiness or impair your ability to operate a motorized vehicle.

Specifics: Allergies are commonly treated with antihistamines, which often create a host of uncomfortable side effects. Homeopathic medicines can more safely minimize symptoms of allergy and can strengthen the body to reduce the frequency and intensity of allergy symptoms.

Ingredients: The formula for allergies includes six leading homeopathic medicines, each of which contributes to its effectiveness. Allium cepa 6x, Histaminum 12x, Solidago 6x, Sabadilla 6x, Urtica sioica 3x, and Natrum 12x.

ARTHRITIS PAIN FORMULA
(Medicine from Nature)

Indications: For natural symptomatic relief of minor pain or discomfort associated with arthritis and rheumatism.

Specifics: Conventional medical treatment for arthritis usually requires long-term use of painkilling or steroidal drugs which can create serious side effects. It makes sense to first try the natural and safer alternatives that homeopathic medicines offer. If this special arthritis formula does not provide enough relief, consider seeking professional homeopathic care.

Ingredients: The formula for arthritis pain includes seven leading homeopathic medicines, each of which contributes to its effectiveness. Rhus tox 6x, Salicylicum acidum 6x, Colchicum 6x, Arnica 6x, Ruta 3x, Formica rufa, 12x, and Phytolacca 12x.

COLD and FLU FORMULA (Medicine from Nature)

Indications: For natural symptomatic relief of nasal congestion or discharge as the result of the common cold, or symptoms of influenza.

Specifics: The common cold and flu are caused by viruses which no conventional drug is known to treat effectively. On the other hand, homeopathic medicines support the body's own defenses and help the body fight infection for itself.

Ingredients: The formula for colds and flu includes six leading homeopathic medicines, each of which contributes to its effectiveness. Allium cepa 3x, Influenzinum 30x, Gelsemium 6x, Bryonia 6x, Arsenicum 9x, and Ferrum phodphorica 6x.

COLIC FORMULA (Medicine from Nature)

Indications: For natural symptomatic relief of discomfort and irritability associated with colic and gas pains.

Specifics: This homeopathic medicine is safe and gentle and will improve digestion, allay pain and discomfort, and relax the infant allowing rest and sleep. The colic formula is also effective in relieving diarrhea, gas and stomach cramps in children and adults.

Ingredients: The formula for colic includes five leading homeopathic medicines, each of which contributes to its effectiveness. Podophyllum 6x, Arsenicum 6x, Natrum sulph 3x, Camomilla 6x, and Magnesia phosphoricum 3x.

CONSTIPATION and HEMORRHOIDS FORMULA (Medicine from Nature)

Indications: For natural symptomatic relief of simple constipation, or discomfort associated with hemorrhoids.

Specifics: Conventional laxatives can be habit forming, and over time, often worsen a person's constipation. Constipation tends to cause or aggravate hemorrhoids. Homeopathic medicines are not habit forming and cause no side effects.

Ingredients: The formula for constipation and hemorrhoids includes four leading homeopathic medicines, each of which contributes to its effectiveness. Nux vomica 12x, Aesculus 3x, Hamamelis 3x, and Collinsonia 3x.

DRY COUGH FORMULA (Medicine from Nature)

Indications: For natural symptomatic relief of cough or bronchial irritation.

Specifics: Homeopathic medicines provide a gentle and more effective way to strengthen the respiratory tract so that the body can more successfully heal itself.

Ingredients: The formula for dry cough includes four leading homeopathic medicines, each of which contributes to its effectiveness. Spongia 3x, Bryonia 6x, Hepar sulfur 6x, and Phosphorus 6x.

EARACHE FORMULA (Medicine from Nature)

Indications: For natural symptomatic relief of irritability and restlessness caused by discomfort in the ear.

Specifics: This homeopathic medicine provides gentle relief of ear pain, helps reduce inflammation and speeds the healing of ear problems.

Ingredients: The formula for earache includes four leading homeopathic medicines, each of which contributes to its effectiveness. Aconitum 3x, Belladonna 6x, Chamomilla 6x, and Kali mur 3x.

FATIGUE FORMULA (Medicine from Nature)

Indications: For natural symptomatic relief of physical and/or mental fatigue.

Specifics: This homeopathic formula is an easy and effective way to begin the healing process. Since fatigue may have various causes, it may be important to consider other natural treatments concurrently to help the healing process.

Ingredients: The formula for fatigue includes seven leading homeopathic medicines, each of which contributes to its effectiveness. Alfalfa 3x, Arsenicum album 12x, Echinacea 3x, Phosphoricum acid 6x, Picuicum acid 12x, Ferrum phos 6x, Gelsemium 12x, and Scuttelaria 12x.

INDIGESTION & GAS FORMULA
(Medicine from Nature)

Indications: For natural symptomatic relief of heartburn, gas, acid indigestion, and upset stomach.

Specifics: This safe and effective homeopathic formula improves digestion and helps the body assimilate food properly. It also reduces gas, heartburn, nausea, and vomiting.

Ingredients: The formula for indigestion and gas includes seven leading homeopathic medicines, each of which contributes to its effectiveness. Nux vomica 12x, Ipecacunha 6x, Natrum phos 6x, Robinia 6x, Asafoetida 6x, Carbo veg 6x, and Antimonium crudum 12x.

INJURY and BACKACHE FORMULA
(Medicine from Nature)

Indications: For natural symptomatic relief of pain and discomfort caused by injury, including bruises, sprains, strains, and backache. This medicine is non toxic and non addictive.

Specifics: Various conventional drugs may kill the pain or alleviate the discomfort of an injury, but painkilling drugs block the person from feeling the injury and they may increase the chances of re-injury. On the other hand homeopathic medicines reduce the pain and swelling of an injury by actually speeding the healing process.

Ingredients: The formula for injury and backache includes six leading homeopathic medicines, each of which contributes to its effectiveness. Arnica 6x, Hypericum 6x, Rhus tox 6x, Bellis perennis 3x, Ruta 3x, and Phosphorus 12x.

INSOMNIA FORMULA (Medicine from Nature)

Indications: For natural symptomatic relief of simple nervous tension, restlessness, and insomnia.

Specifics: The stress of modern life makes it difficult to relax and sleep. This homeopathic remedy can effectively help you sleep whether you are using relaxation strategies or not.

Ingredients: The formula for insomnia includes six leading homeopathic medicines, each of which contributes to its effectiveness. Passiflora 3x, Scutellaria 12x, Coffea 9x, Arentum nitricum 6x, Humulus lupulus 3x, and Kali phosphoricum 3x.

MENOPAUSE FORMULA (Medicine from Nature)

Indications: For the natural relief of depression, hot flashes, insomnia, irritability, vaginal dryness, and other emotional or physical symptoms commonly associated with menopause.

Specifics: Although hormones provide some benefit, they also tend to cause various short and long-term side effects. It is safer and more prudent to use homeopathic and natural medicines that gently strengthen the woman's body.

Ingredients: The formula for menopause includes six leading homeopathic medicines, each of which contributes to its effectiveness. Lachesis 12x, Natrum mur 6x, Ignatia 12x, Belladonna 6x, Murex 12x, and Calcarea phosphorica 3x.

MIGRAINE HEADACHE FORMULA
(Medicine from Nature)

Indications: For natural symptomatic relief of occasional migraine headache pain.

Specifics: Conventional drugs may provide some relief, but they also can create aggravating side effects. Homeopathic medicines provide safer, more natural relief of head pain than do common conventional drugs.

Ingredients: The formula for migraine headache includes seven leading homeopathic medicines, each of which contributes to its effectiveness. Belladonna 6x, Iris versicolor 3x, Bryonia 6x, Natrum mur 12x, Sanguinaria 12x, Gelsemium 6x and Epiphegus 6x.

PMS FORMULA (Medicine from Nature)

Indications: For natural relief of bloating, cramps, and other discomforts associated with the menstrual cycle.

Specifics: Physical and psychological symptoms play a part in premenstrual syndrome. For two hundred years homeopathic doctors have treated both the mind and body for women suffering from this syndrome, with select homeopathic medicines.

Ingredients: The formula for PMS includes five leading homeopathic medicines, each of which contributes to its effectiveness. Pulsatilla 12x, Vibuinum opulus 3x, Aristolochia clematitis 12x, Colocynthis 6x, and Sepia 9x.

SINUSITIS FORMULA (Medicine from Nature)

Indications: For natural symptomatic relief of sinus congestion and head pain associated with sinusitis or colds.

Specifics: Sinus pain often results from a lingering cold or allergy which can block the openings from the sinuses, creating an opportunity for infection. This problem can be prevented by using the Cold and Flu, and Allergy formulas. If sinus pain has already developed, the Sinusitis formula is a good, safe and natural place to start to heal yourself.

Ingredients: The formula for sinus problems includes five leading homeopathic medicines, each of which contributes to its effectiveness. Pulsatilla 6x, Mercurius 12x, Hydrastis 6x, Kali bichromicum 6x, and Euphorbium 6x.

TEETHING FORMULA (Medicine from Nature)

Indications: For natural symptomatic relief of pain, discomfort, irritability, and restlessness associated with teething.

Specifics: Conventional medicine offers little to allay the pain and suffering that teething infants experience. On the other hand homeopathic medicine offers a safe and effective treatment for the common ailment of teething.

Ingredients: The formula for teething includes five leading homeopathic medicines, each of which contributes to its effectiveness. Chamomilla 3x, Calcarea phosphorica 3x, Belladonna 6x, Podophyllum 6x, and Caffeinum 12x.

TENSION HEADACHE FORMULA
(Medicine from Nature)

Indications: For natural symptomatic relief of occasional headache pain, resulting from tension and stress.

Specifics: Aspirin and other conventional drugs provide only temporary relief from tension headaches and can cause various side effects that can be worse than the headaches themselves. Homeopathic medicines not only can treat tension headaches without side effects but can also prevent future headaches.

Ingredients: The formula for tension headache includes five leading homeopathic medicines, each of which contributes to its effectiveness. Nux vomica 6x, Caffeinum 6x, Gelsemium 6x, Kali phosphoricum 3x, and Argentum nitricum 9x.

VAGINITIS FORMULA (Medicine from Nature)

Indications: For natural relief of minor vaginal burning and itching.

Specifics: Conventional drugs may temporarily inhibit the growth of various microorganisms that tend to cause vaginal itching and burning, but all too often these microorganisms return. Homeopathic remedies aid the body's own defenses and help the body protect and heal itself.

Ingredients: The formula for vaginitis includes six leading homeopathic medicines, each of which contributes to its effectiveness. Candida albicans 18x, Hydrastis 6x, Pulsatilla 6x, Sepia 12x, Borax 3x, and Kreosotum 6x.

HOMEOPATHIC
SINGULAR REMEDIES

ACONITUM NAPELLUS

Common Names: (Aconite) (Monkshood)

Therapeutic Uses: This remedy is given at the first sign of colds, croup, diarrhea, earache, headache, and sore throat. Also used for abdominal pain, bleeding, eye disorders, fever, measles, nausea, and vomiting.

AESCULUS

Therapeutic Uses: Recommended for the relief of constipation and hemorrhoids. This remedy also alleviates a backache that may be experienced at the same time as the constipation.

ALLIUM CEPA

Common Name: (Common Red Onion)

Therapeutic Uses: One of the most common homeopathic remedies for allergies. Also an effective treatment for hay fever and respiratory infections such as coughs, colds, and sore throats.

ANTIMONIUM CRUDUM

Therapeutic Uses: A useful treatment for the bloating and constant belching that some people with indigestion experience shortly after eating.

ANTIMONIUM TARTARICUM

Common Name: (Tartrate of Antimony and Potash)

Therapeutic Uses: Primarily used in the treatment of repertory diseases. It also heals the bluish scars of acne or chickenpox, and is an effective treatment for asthma, nausea, and vomiting.

APIS MELLIFICA

Common Name: (Apis)

Therapeutic Uses: An excellent treatment for bee stings, bites, and puncture wounds. Helps relieve allergic shock and reduce the swelling of tongue and throat passages. Also used to treat abscesses, fever, respiratory infections, and urinary problems.

ARGENTUM NITRICUM

Common Name: (Silver Nitrate)

TherapeuticUses: This remedy helps to relax the nervous system and creates a general calming influence. An effective treatment for nervousness, restlessness, and anxious anticipation of approaching deadline after extended intellectual work. Also helps control asthma, improves digestion, and is useful in the treatment of respiratory infections.

ARISTOLOCHIA CLEMATIS

TherapeuticUses: This homeopathic medicine is recommended for women who suffer from abdominal cramps and swelling of calves and feet prior to menstruation.

ARNICA MONTANA

Common Names: (Arnica) (Leopard's Bane)

TherapeuticUses: It is the first homeopathic medicine to consider giving immediately after an injury. An effective treatment for arthritic pain or backache that results from an old injury that was aggravated by overexertion. Also relieves shock, headache, bleeding, toothache, and is good for treating injuries such as bruises, burns, sprains, and strains.

ARSENICUM ALBUM

Common Names: (Arsenicum) (Arsenic Trioxide)

TherapeuticUses: A common homeopathic remedy for abdominal pain, colic, and diarrhea. Controls anxiety and anguish that is sometimes experienced at the same time as fatigue, and is also recommended for asthma, coughs, colds, fever, indigestion, nausea, respiratory infections, sore throats, toothache, and vomiting.

ASAFOETIDA

TherapeuticUses: An invaluable treatment for the relief of stomach pain caused by bloating. It also reduces excessive gas and the various stomach noises that are experienced with indigestion.

BAPTISIA

Common Name: (Wild Indigo)

TherapeuticUses: This homeopathic medicine is used to treat acute influenza, lower fever, and is recommended for respiratory infections, cough, cold, and sore throats.

BELLADONNA

Common Name: (Deadly Nightshade)

Therapeutic Uses: Relieves migraine headaches and throbbing headaches with pain that comes in waves. Useful in treating agitation, bleeding, ear problems, exhaustion, fever, hot flashes, loss of appetite, acute cramps, lower abdominal pain, and vaginal dryness. This remedy is also effective in treating colic and infant pain and discomfort during teething.

BELLIS PERENNIS

Therapeutic Uses: For natural symptomatic relief of pain and discomfort caused by injury, including bruises and sprains. Also useful in helping to heal surgical wounds after an operation.

BORAX

Common Name: (Sodium Borate)

Therapeutic Uses: An effective remedy for vaginal itching and burning, especially when it is accompanied by a white discharge. Also good for motion sickness and vaginitis.

BRYONIA ALBA

Common Names: (Bryonia) (Wild Hops)

Therapeutic Uses: One of the most common homeopathic medicines for the flu. It alleviates the irritability that may be experienced due to a splitting headache and aches in various parts of the body aggravated by motion. Also helpful if a person has stitching pains in the chest during a cough and soreness in the throat as a result of coughing.

CAFFEINUM

Common Name: (Caffeine)

Therapeutic Uses: Helps relieve the discomfort, restlessness, insomnia, and pain in infants suffering from teething. It is particularly effective in the treatment of tension headache in adults.

CALCAREA CARBONICUM

Common Names: (Calcium Carbonate) (Calcarea Ostrearum)

Therapeutic Uses: An excellent remedy for respiratory infections, coughs, colds, sinus infections, and sore throats. Also used to treat diarrhea, headache, nausea and vomiting, menstrual problems, and vaginitis.

CALCAREA PHOSPHORICA

Common Names: (Calcarea Phosphoricum) (Calcium Phosphate)

TherapeuticUses: This remedy is made from calcium phosphate so is excellent for the development of teeth during teething. Also used for asthma, colds, coughs, diarrhea, headache, menopause, menstrual problems, respiratory problems, and vaginitis.

CALENDULA OFFICINALIS

Common Names: (Marigold) (Calendula)

Therapeutic Uses: Used as ointment or lotion to promote healing and provide protection against infection for injuries such as bites, bruises, burns, and incised or lacerated wounds.

CANDIDA ALBICANS

Common Name: (Yeast)

TherapeuticUses: Candida albicans is the fungus which is known to grow during a vaginal yeast infection. Homeopathic doses relieve vaginal itching and discomfort by stimulating the body's defense systems to alleviate the condition.

CANTHARIS VESICATOR

Common Names: (Spanish fly) (Cantharis)

Therapeutic Uses: This homeopathic medicine is used for the treatment of bites, stings, puncture wounds, and burns. Also used to treat respiratory infections, bladder and kidney pain, and urinary problems.

CARBO VEGETABILIS

Common Names: (Carbo Veg) (Vegetable Charcoal)

TherapeuticUses: Recommended for natural symptomatic relief of bloating due to gas and is effective in improving digestion. Also an invaluable remedy for asthma and respiratory infections, and is a useful treatment for menstrual problems and vaginitis.

CHAMOMILLA

Common Name: (German Chamomile)

Therapeutic Uses: The premier homeopathic remedy for hyper-irritable colicky infants and to relieve the discomfort of teething. Also used for abdominal pain, asthma, throbbing earache, and urinary problems.

CINCHONA OFFICINALIS

Common Names: (Peruvian Bark) (Quinine)

Therapeutic Uses: For natural symptomatic relief of diarrhea, fever, heartburn, nausea, and vomiting.

This medicine is particularly effective if the person's condition has been aggravated by laxatives or various digestive problems which result as a side effect from taking conventional drugs.

COCCULUS INDICUS

Common Name: (Indian Cockle)

Therapeutic Uses: For natural symptomatic relief of constipation, heartburn, and upset stomach, usually caused when a person consumes a particular rich diet. Also an effective treatment for respiratory problems and motion sickness.

COFFEA CRUDA

Common Name: (Unroasted Coffee)

Therapeutic Uses: For natural relief of simple nervous tension and insomnia. This medicine is also used to treat violent throbbing toothache and is helpful to reduce the restlessness and pain in infants suffering from teething.

COLCHICUM AUTUMNALE

Common Names: (Colchicum) (Meadow Saffron)

Therapeutic Uses: Beneficial in the treatment of arthritic stiffness and gout. Also an effective remedy for diarrhea, nausea (especially in the first months of pregnancy) and vomiting.

COLLINSONIA

Therapeutic Uses: An effective remedy for obstinate constipation with protruding hemorrhoids. This treatment is particularly helpful for anyone who experiences gas with constipation and for women during pregnancy.

COLOCYNTHIS

Common Name: (Bitter Cucumber)

Therapeutic Uses: An effective remedy for abdominal pain, diarrhea, gas, headache, indigestion, menstrual problems, PMS, nausea, uterine cramping, and vomiting.

CUPRUM

Common Name: (Copper)

Therapeutic Uses: A common homeopathic medicine for abdominal pain, colic, coughs, colds, diarrhea, nausea, and vomiting. Controls anxiety and anguish that is sometimes experienced at the same time as mental and physical exhaustion.

DROSERA

Common Name: (Sundew)

TherapeuticUses: A good medicine for a dry cough or croup that is aggravated by talking and cold air. This remedy also relieves hoarseness and respiratory infections.

DULCAMARA

Common Name: (Bitter Sweet)

TherapeuticUses: Very effective in the relief of spasmodic sneezing and continuous runny nose that is commonly experienced by hay fever or allergy sufferers.

ECHINACEA ANGUSTIFOLIA

Common Name: (Echinacea)

TherapeuticUses: This homeopathic remedy helps to cleanse the blood and to invigorate a person who experiences muscular weakness felt in the arms and legs. Also effective for treating people who experience generalized fatigue.

EPIPHEGUS

TherapeuticUses: An effective homeopathic medicine that relieves headache that is primarily situated on the left side of the head. This remedy is particularly effective when the headache results from physical or mental exhaustion.

EQUISETUM HYEMALE

Common Name: (Scouring-rush)

TherapeuticUses: This remedy is used principally for urinary complaints. Relieves the burning in urethra during or after urination and controls the urge to urinate when the bladder is not full.

EUPHORBIUM PERFOLIATUM

Common Name: (Thoroughwort)

TherapeuticUses: A good treatment for many cases of influenza. Relieves the pressing and shooting pains in the head caused by sinusitis, and is helpful in healing post-nasal drip. Also reduces fever and helps eliminate respiratory infections.

EUPHRASIA OFFICINALIS

Common Name: (Eyebright)

TherapeuticUses: A useful remedy for hay fever. Recommended particularly for its action on mucus membranes of the nose and eyes.

FERRUM PHOSPHORICA

Common Names: (Iron Phosphate) (Ferrum Phos)

Therapeutic Uses: Ferrum Phosphorica is made from phosphate of iron and helps reduce the anemia that people with fatigue experience. Also a good remedy for the initial onset of the flu, and a useful treatment for abdominal pain, abscesses and inflammation, ear problems, fever, measles, mumps, respiratory infections, sties, and urinary problems.

FORMICA RUFA

Therapeutic Uses: An effective medicine for arthritic and gouty stiffness and pain, especially when the pain starts suddenly and causes great restlessness.

GELSEMIUM SEMPERVIRENS

Common Names: (Yellow Jasmine) (Gelsemium)

Therapeutic Uses: A common homeopathic remedy for the flu, extremely effective when the person experiences headache, hoarseness, diarrhea, fever, and helps alleviate the muscular weakness that fatigued people experience. Also used as a treatment for hay fever, measles, and respiratory infections.

HAMAMELIS

Common Name: (Witch Hazel)

Therapeutic Uses: This remedy is made from the common herb Witch Hazel and is an effective treatment for constipation and hemorrhoids.

HELONIAS DIOICA

Common Names: (Unicorn Plant) (Helonias)

Therapeutic Uses: A treatment for vaginitis, especially useful during pregnancy. Recommended for women who experience irritability along with minor vaginal burning and itching.

HEPAR SULPHUR

Common Names: (Sulphate of Lime) (Hepar Sulph)

Therapeutic Uses: An effective homeopathic medicine for a dry cough that is aggravated in the cold air or when any part of a person is exposed to the cold. Also used for abscesses and inflammation, croup, ear problems, respiratory infections, sore throats, and sinus infections.

HISTAMINUM

Therapeutic Uses: Small doses of this substance minimize symptoms of allergy and will help the body heal itself from allergies.

HUMULUS IUPULUS

Common Name: (Humulus)

Therapeutic Uses: This homeopathic sleep aid is made from the herb hops and is particularly useful for people who are so drowsy that they have difficulty falling asleep.

HYDRASTIS

Therapeutic Uses: A common treatment for vaginal itching and burning, especially when there is a yellow vaginal discharge. Also provides benefit to people suffering dull, pressing sinus pain after experiencing a cold. This remedy aids the body's own defenses, helping the body protect and heal itself.

HYPERICUM PERFOLIATUM

Common Names: (St. John's Wart) (Hypericum)

Therapeutic Uses: Very useful for the relief of pain caused by injuries to the nerve-rich areas of the back, toes, fingertips, and gums. Hypericum ointment may be used on infected skin wounds, where pain is associated with the injury. It is also useful in the treatment of eye disorders.

IGNATIA AMARA

Common Names: (St. Ignatius' Bean) (Ignatia)

Therapeutic Uses: An effective homeopathic remedy for emotional problems, headache, gas, indigestion, infections, menopause, menstrual problems, motion sickness, and vaginitis.

INFLUENZINUM

Common Name: (Influenza Virus)

Therapeutic Uses: Influenzinum is an exceedingly small dose of the influenza virus and it is effective in preventing the flu and in treating people who are experiencing a protracted case of the flu.

IPECACUANHA

Common Names: (Ipecac Root) (Ipecac)

Therapeutic Uses: This remedy is made from the herb Ipecac Root. It is effective in the treatment of persistent nausea not relieved by vomiting. Also used to relieve abdominal pain, asthma, indigestion, and to control bleeding.

IRIS VERSICOLOR

Common Names: (Blue Flag) (Iris)

Therapeutic Uses: This homeopathic medicine is a headache remedy. Particularly effective when constipation and/or visual symptoms are experienced at the same time that a person develops a migraine headache.

KALI BICHROMICUM

Common Name: (Potassium Bichromate)

Therapeutic Uses: A common homeopathic remedy for sinus pain when the nasal discharge is tough, stringy, and sometimes forming thick, yellow-green mucus. Also recommended for the treatment of asthma and respiratory infections.

KALI CARBONICUM

Common Name: (Potassium Carbonate)

Therapeutic Uses: For the natural symptomatic relief of abdominal pain, hemorrhoids, and menstrual problems. Also used to treat indigestion, respiratory infections, nausea, and vomiting.

KALI MURIATICUM

Common Names: (Potassium Chloride) (Kali Mur)

Therapeutic Uses: A helpful remedy for persons who experience earache along with noises in the ear. Also used for abscesses and inflammation, bleeding, chicken pox, injuries and burns, mumps, styes, and vaginal problems.

KALI PHOSPHORICUM

Common Name: (Kali Phos)

Therapeutic Uses: For natural symptomatic relief of simple nervous tension and sleeplessness. Particularly valuable for children and adults who wake in the middle of the night with fear and terror. Also a good remedy for people who are so exhausted that they have difficulty falling or staying asleep.

KREOSOTUM

Common Name: (Beechwood Kreosote)

Therapeutic Uses: A remedy for urinary problems, and vaginitis. Inhibits the growth of various microorganisms that cause vaginal itching, burning, and swelling of the labia.

LACHESIS

Common Name: (Venom of the Bushmaster Snake)

Therapeutic Uses: A common treatment to relieve the stress and tension that women experience during menopause. Also effective for asthma, back pain, coughs and colds, diarrhea, dizziness, headache, hemorrhoids, menstrual problems, sinus infections, and sore throat.

LEDUM PALUSTRE

Common Names: (Marsh Tea) (Ledum)

Therapeutic Uses: It is a good homeopathic medicine to consider giving immediately after an injury. An effective treatment for backache that results from an old injury that was aggravated by overexertion. Also useful for treating injuries such as bruises, burns, sprains, and strains.

LYCOPODIUM CLAVATUM

Common Names: (Club Moss) (Lycopodium)

Therapeutic Uses: A common homeopathic remedy for abdominal pain, colic, and diarrhea. Controls anxiety and anguish that is sometimes experienced at the same time as fatigue, and is also recommended for asthma, coughs, colds, fever, indigestion, nausea, respiratory infections, sore throats, and vomiting.

MAGNESIA PHOSPHORICUM

Common Names: (Magnesium Phosphate) (Magnesia Phos)

Therapeutic Uses: Relieves the colic in infants whose pain is reduced by the application of warmth or by bending over. Also used to relieve abdominal pain, headache, toothache, and menstrual cramps.

MANGANUM

Common Name: (Manganese)

Therapeutic Uses: One of the most common homeopathic medicines for coughs and colds. Particularly helpful if a person has stitching pains in the chest during a cough and soreness in the throat as a result of coughing.

MERCURIUS SOLUBILIS

Common Names: (Quicksilver) (Mercurius) (Merc Sol)

Therapeutic Uses: This homeopathic remedy reduces the pressure and sensation of heaviness in and behind the nose during an attack of sinusitis. Also a recommended treatment for abscesses, diarrhea, inflammation, respiratory infections, swollen glands, and urinary problems.

MUREX

Therapeutic Uses: An effective homeopathic medicine for the natural relief of acute fatigue. Also used for the relief of physical or emotional symptoms commonly associated with menopause and menstrual problems, and is recommended as a natural remedy for vaginal dryness.

NATRUM MURIATICUM

Common Names: (Sodium Chloride) (Natrum Mur)

Therapeutic Uses: Useful in treating migraine headache or throbbing headaches with pain that comes on in waves. Helps relieve both acute and chronic allergy symptoms. Also an effective treatment for colds, diarrhea, emotional trauma, gas, indigestion, menopause, menstrual problems, respiratory infections, urinary problems, vaginitis, nausea, and vomiting.

NATRUM PHOSPHORICUM

Common Names: (Sodium Phosphate) (Natrum Phos)

TherapeuticUses: A common homeopathic medicine for heartburn, indigestion, and abdominal pain caused by gas and bloating in the abdomen which cannot be relieved by passing gas. It is particularly useful for indigestion after eating milk products or rich or fatty foods.

NATRUM SULPHURICUM

Common Names: (Sodium Sulphate) (Natrum Sulph)

TherapeuticUses: An effective treatment to relieve gas and sharp pains experienced by a child due to digestive disturbances. Also used for asthma, diarrhea, and urinary problems.

NUX VOMICA

Common Name: (Poison Nut)

TherapeuticUses: For natural symptomatic relief of constipation, heartburn, and upset stomach. This medicine is particularly effective if the person's constipation has been aggravated by laxatives or various digestive problems which result as a side effect from taking conventional drugs, or when a person consumes a particular rich diet. Also an effective treatment for respiratory problems and motion sickness.

PASSIFLORA

Therapeutic Uses: An effective homeopathic sleep aid used in treating anyone who is mentally anxious or overworked. This remedy is particularly effective for infants and the elderly.

PHOSPHORUS

TherapeuticUses: A common homeopathic medicine for a dry cough that is aggravated by talking and cold air. Phosphorus is an effective treatment for reducing the bleeding that may occur after an injury and this remedy also relieves hoarseness, digestive disorders, acute respiratory infections, fever, nausea, and vomiting.

PHOSPHORICUM ACID

Common Name: (Phos Acid)

Therapeutic Uses: This homeopathic remedy is invaluable for treating fatigue that is first experienced mentally/emotionally and then developed physically. It is also effective in alleviating fatigue caused by an acute illness, or a loss of body fluids.

PHYTOLACCA

Common Name: (Poke Root)

TherapeuticUses: Helps relieve arthritic pain that is aggravated in the morning and in damp weather. Also an effective glandular remedy for many menstrual and respiratory problems.

PICRICUM ACID

Common Name: (Pic Acid)

TherapeuticUses: This homeopathic medicine helps to reduce the difficulty a fatigued person feels in getting and keeping warm. It is also known to be particularly useful in reducing the weariness felt in the arms and legs.

PODOPHYLLUM

Common Name: (May Apple)

Therapeutic Uses: The leading homeopathic remedy for acute diarrhea. Also good for abdominal pain, colic, gas, and teething problems.

PULSATILLA NIGRICANS

Common Names: (Pulsatilla) (Wood Flower)

TherapeuticUses: A recognized treatment for vaginitis, especially for women who experience emotional swings during this ailment. Pulsatilla is recommended for the relief of sinus pain and digestive disorders that may be experienced at the same time that sinus pain is felt. Also useful in the treatment of asthma, coughs, colds, ear problems, fever, headache, hemorrhoids, measles, menstrual problems, mumps, nausea, respiratory infections, PMS, and urinary problems.

PYROGENIUM
Common Name: (Pyrogen)

TherapeuticUses: One of the most common homeopathic remedies for a fever. Also an effective treatment for abscesses and inflammation, toothache, and respiratory infections such as coughs, colds, and sore throats.

RHODODENDRON
Common Name: (Dwarf Rosebag) (Snow-Rose)

TherapeuticUses: A useful remedy for pain. Particularly helpful if a person has stitching pains in the chest during a cough and soreness in the throat as a result of coughing. Also an effective medicine for toothache.

RHUS TOXICODENDRON
Common Names: (Poison Oak) (Rhus Tox)

TherapeuticUses: The most common remedy for arthritic pains, sprains, strains, and backache, especially when the pain is worse on the initial motion. Also used for chicken pox, diarrhea, motion sickness, mumps, swollen glands, and skin diseases.

ROBINIA
Therapeutic Uses: An excellent homeopathic medicine for heartburn, nausea and dull, heavy aching in the stomach, often accompanied by a headache. This remedy is often helpful when heartburn is felt at night and is worse when lying down.

RUMEX CRISPUS
Common Names: (Yellow Dock)

TherapeuticUses: For the natural symptomatic relief of abdominal pain, and diarrhea. Controls anxiety and anguish that is sometimes experienced at the same time as fatigue, and is also recommended for coughs, colds, fever, indigestion, nausea, respiratory infections, and sore throats.

RUTA GRAVEOLENS
Common Names: (Rue-Bitterwort) (Ruta)

TherapeuticUses: Relieves arthritic stiffness of the wrists and ankles, and is effective in the treatment of headaches and injuries such as bruises, sprains when the site of the injury seems to be where tendons join the bone, and strains. It is particularly effective in treating injuries to the knee, elbow, and cheekbone.

SABADILLA

Therapeutic Uses: Very effective in the relief of spasmodic sneezing and continuous runny nose that is commonly experienced by hay fever or allergy sufferers.

SALICYLICUM ACIDUM

Common Name: (Salic Acid)

Therapeutic Uses: Made from salicylic acid, the primary ingredient in aspirin. Homeopathic doses help to relieve arthritic pain and reduce swelling.

SANGUINARIA

Therapeutic Uses: This homeopathic medicine helps relieve nausea that is experienced at the same time as a migraine. It is particularly effective when the headache is on the right side, especially over the right eye.

SCUTELLARIA

Therapeutic Uses: For the natural symptomatic relief of physical and/or mental fatigue. It helps people to both relax and fall asleep. This homeopathic remedy is particularly effective in people who have difficulty concentrating, and who experience fatigue and depression after exhausting labor, or after experiencing the flu or some other infection.

SEPIA

Common Name: (Inky Juice of Cuttlefish)

Therapeutic Uses: Recommended for women who experience irritability along with minor vaginal burning and itching. Also an effective treatment for constipation, cramps, exhaustion, headache, irritability, menstrual problems, PMS, extreme nausea, and vomiting.

SILICEA

Common Names: (Silicon dioxide) (Pure Flint)

Therapeutic Uses: A helpful remedy for persons who experience earache along with noises in the ear. Also used for abscesses and inflammation, respiratory infections, sinusitis, and styes.

SOLIDAGO

Therapeutic Uses: This substance is made from the golden rod flower. When the pollen is given in homeopathic doses it helps heal hay fever symptoms.

SPONGIA TOSTA

Common Names: (Spongia) (Roasted Sponge)

Therapeutic Uses: This is one of the most common homeopathic medicines for treating anxiety due to a dry cough with hoarseness, croup, or difficult breathing. Especially effective when the person's symptoms grow worse before midnight and are aggravated by inhaling cold air.

STICTA PULMONARIA

Common Names: (Sticta) (Lungwort)

Therapeutic Uses: An excellent homeopathic medicine for respiratory infections. It alleviates the irritability that may be experienced due to head colds and aches in various parts of the body. Also helpful if a person has stitching pains in the chest during a cough and soreness in the throat as a result of coughing.

SULPHUR

Therapeutic Uses: This homeopathic remedy reduces the pressure and sensation of heaviness in and behind the nose during an attack of sinusitis. Also a recommended treatment for abscesses, diarrhea, inflammation, respiratory infections, menstrual problems, swollen glands, and vaginitis.

SYMPHYTUM

Common Name: (Comfrey Root)

Therapeutic Uses: Mainly used to heal bone injuries. Particularly musculoskeletal problems where there is disruption of the outer layer of bone causing pricking, sticking pains.

TABACUM

Common Name: (Tobacco)

Therapeutic Uses: A common homeopathic medicine for heartburn, abdominal pain caused by indigestion, nausea and vomiting. Also a good remedy for respiratory infections and motion sickness.

URTICA DIOICA or URTICA URENS

Common Name: (Dwarf Stinging Nettle)

Therapeutic Uses: This substance is made from the dwarf stinging nettle. Very effective in the treatment of hive like allergy symptoms such as prickly heat rash and small vesicles. Also used in the treatment of urinary problems.

VERATRUM ALBUM

Common Names: (White Hellebore)

TherapeuticUses: A good remedy for abdominal pain, colic, and diarrhea. This medicine is also recommended for coughs, colds, fever, and respiratory infections.

VERBASCUM

Common Names: (Mullein Flower)

TherapeuticUses: An excellent remedy for respiratory infections, coughs, colds, sinus infections, and sore throats. Also used to treat earache.

VIBURNUM OPULUS

Common Name: (Cramp Bark)

Therapeutic Uses: One of the leading homeopathic remedies in treating the physical and psychological symptoms associated with PMS. Also a valuable remedy for premenstrual and menstrual cramps, and bloating.

A WORD ABOUT TISSUE SALTS

Dr. W. H. Schuessler isolated them in the late nineteenth century. Also known as (Schuessler biochemical cell salts). Tissue salts are inorganic mineral components of your body tissues. Dr. Schuessler found that illness occurred if the body was deficient in any of these salts and the body could heal itself if the deficiency was corrected. We recommend that you use only the dosages prescribed on the manufacturer's label as there is a variant in strengths between different manufacturers.

HOMEOPATHIC

SINGULAR

TISSUE SALTS

Mineral	Actions & Uses	AffectedComponents
#1 CALC-FLUOR (Calcium Fluoride) (Fluoride of Lime)	Maintains elasticity of tissues.	Impaired circulation piles, varicose veins, muscle tendon strain, deficient enamel teeth, carbuncles, cracked skin and over-relaxed conditions.
#2 CALC-PHOS (Calcium Phosphate) (Phosphate of Lime)	Constituent of bones, teeth and gastric juices.	Impaired digestion, anemia, cold hands and feet, numbness, hydrocele, teething, sore breasts, and night sweats.
#3 CALC-SULPH (Calcium Sulfate) (Sulfate of Lime)	Blood purifier, constituent of all connective tissue in minute particles.	Acne, skin eruptions, abscesses, pimples during adolescence, sore lips, or chronic oozing ulcers.
#4 FERR-PHOS (Iron Phosphate)	The biochemic first aid oxygenates the blood.	Diarrhea, nosebleeds, coughs, colds, chills, fevers, inflammation, congestion, rheumatic pain, and excessive menses.

Mineral	Actions & Uses	AffectedComponents
#5 KALI-MUR (Potassium Chloride) (Chloride of Potash)	Blood constituent and conditioner. Found in lining under surface body cells.	Coughs, colds, respiratory ailments. also granulation of eyelids, warts, and blistering eczema.
#6 KALI-PHOS (Potassium Phosphate)	Nerve Nutrient. Found in all nerve, brain and blood cells.	Nervous exhaustion, indigestion, headaches, poor memory, anxiety, insomnia, and improper fat digestion.
#7 KALI-SULPH (Potassium Sulfate) (Sulfate of Potash)	Oxygenates the tissue salts. Constituent of skin cells and internal organ linings.	Pains in limbs, feeling of heaviness, skin eruptions with sealing or sticky exudation, falling hair, and diseased nails.
#8 MAG-PHOS (Magnesium Phosphate) (Phosphate of magnesia)	Nerve stabilizer and anti-spasmodic. Constituent of bones, teeth, brain, nerves, blood and muscle cells.	Cramps, neuralgia, shooting pains, flatulence, and colic.
#9 NAT-MUR (Sodium Chloride) (Chloride of Soda)	Water distribution. Regulates the amount of moisture in the body.	Loss of smell or taste, salt cravings, colds, watery discharges from eyes, and nose.
#10 NAT-PHOS (Sodium Phosphate) (Phosphate of Soda)	Acid-neutralizer, emulsifies fatty acids and keeps uric acid soluble in the blood.	Over acidity of the blood, jaundice, gastric disorders, heartburn, and rheumatic tendency.
#11 NAT-SULPH (Sodium Sulphate) (Sulphate of Soda)	Excess water eliminator. An irritant to tissues and functions as a stimulant for natural secretions.	Liver symptoms, gall bladder disorders, edema, depression, low fevers, bilious attacks, and watery infiltration's.
#12 SILICA (Silicic Oxide) (Silicic Acid)	Conditioner, cleanser, eliminator. Constituent of all connective tissue cells.	Lack of luster or falling hair, boils, impure blood, brittle ribbed or ingrown nails, carbuncles, and poor memory.

HOMEOPATHIC
COMBINATION TISSUE SALTS

Combination	Ingredients	Therapeutic Use
A	Ferr Phos, Kali Phos, Mag Phos.	For neuritis, neuralgia, and sciatica.
B	Calc Phos, Kali Phos, Ferr Phos.	Used during convalescence, general debility, and nervous exhaustion.
C	Mag Phos, Nat Phos, Nat Sulph, Silica.	For acidity, heartburn, and dyspepsia.
D	Kali Mur, Kali Sulph, Calc Sulph, Silica.	Acne, eczema, scalp eruptions, scaling of the skin, and all minor skin ailments.
E	Calc Phos, Mag Phos, Nat Phos, Nat Sulph.	For flatulence, colic, and indigestion.
F	Kali Phos, Mag Phos, Nat Mur, Silica.	For nervous headaches, migraine when associated with nervous weakness.
G	Calc Fluor, Calc Phos, Kali Phos, Nat Mur.	Backache, lumbago, piles, and over relaxed tissues.
H	Mag Phos, Nat Mur, Silica.	Hay fever.
I	Ferr Phos, Kali Sulph, Mag Phos.	Fibrositis, and muscular pains.
J	Ferr Phos, Kali Mur, Nat Mur.	A seasonal remedy for coughs and colds.
K	Kali Sulph, Nat Mur, Silica.	For falling hair and brittle nails.
L	Calc Fluor, Ferr Phos, Nat Mur.	Loss of elasticity of veins and arteries.
M	Nat Phos, Nat Sulph, Kali Mur, Calc Phos.	For rheumatism.
N	Calc Phos, Kali Mur, Kali Phos, Mag Phos.	For menstrual pain.
P	Calc Fluor, Calc Phos, Kali Phos, Mag Phos.	For poor circulation, chilblains, aching legs, and feet.
Q	Ferr Phos, Kali Mur, Kali Sulph, Nat Mur.	For sinus disorders.
R	Calc Fluor, Calc Phos, Ferr Phos, Mag Phos, Silica.	For infants' teething pain and to aid dentition.
S	Kali Mur, Nat Phos, Nat Sulph.	For biliousness, stomach upset, digestive and intestinal disorders, headaches.

HEALING FOODS

Food can cure. Food has been regarded as a potent medicine for thousands of years. Hypocrites was the first to say that food could be our medicine. He observed and recorded the changes that different foods brought about on the body. Different foods enable us to build up or deplete the tissues in our bodies. People who eat right, will build healthy strong bodies. A defective diet will degenerate our bodies by destroying vital tissues. Many of the worlds leading scientists and physicians are now prescribing common foods, on the bases of new understandings of the complex mechanisms of disease. Making small changes to your diet and eating foods that have a positive effect on your body can prevent or cure many acute or chronic ailments.

This section will help you to understand the healing powers and the natural active ingredients of common foods. It chronicles the latest research and the new scientific findings on the pharmacological effects and therapeutic uses of foods.

The healing foods are organized in alphabetical order for easy access.

APPLE

TherapeuticUses: Apples keep the cardiovascular system healthy by stabilizing blood sugar, lowering blood cholesterol, and lowering blood pressure. Researchers find that people who eat more apples have a higher resistance to colds and upper respiratory ailments. Apple skins are recommended to help control urinary and kidney infections. Recent studies have also shown that the chemicals in apples tend to block cancer in animals.

Beneficial Nutrients: Magnesium, Potassium, Sodium, plus Vitamins A, B1, B2, B6, Biotin, Folic Acid, Niacin, Pantothenic acid, C, and E.

APRICOT

TherapeuticUses: Scientists believe that the high concentrations of beta carotene in apricots could mitigate the latent cancerous effects of cigarette smoke and inhibit lung and smoking related cancers. This fruit is also good for anemia, catarrh, and constipation.

BeneficialNutrients: Copper, Iron, Phosphorus, Potassium, Silicon, plus Vitamins A, B1, B2, B6, Folic Acid, Niacin, Pantothenic acid, and C.

ARTICHOKE

TherapeuticUses: A general body builder. Artichokes perform as a diuretic and stimulate bile production in the liver. This vegetable also contains a constituent called cynarin, which is effective in the lowering of blood cholesterol.

Beneficial Nutrients: Iodine, Iron, Potassium, Silicon, plus Vitamins A, B1, B2, B6, Biotin, Niacin, Pantothenic acid, C, and E.

ASPARAGUS

TherapeuticUses: Asparagus is recommended in the treatment of kidney and bladder disorders.

BeneficialNutrients: Calcium, Iron, Silicon, plus Vitamins A, B1, B2, B6, Biotin, Niacin, Pantothenic acid, C, and E.

AVACADO

TherapeuticUses: Good for colitis and ulcers.

BeneficialNutrients: Chlorine, Phosphorus, Sulfur, plus Vitamins A, B1, B2, B6, Folic Acid, Niacin, Pantothenic acid, and C.

BANANA

TherapeuticUses: Bananas lower blood cholesterol and prevent and heal ulcers by strengthening the surface cells of the stomach lining, forming a barrier against noxious juices.

Beneficial Nutrients: Calcium, Chlorine, Potassium, plus Vitamins A, B1, B2, B6, Biotin, Folic Acid, Niacin, Pantothenic acid, C, and E.

BARLEY

TherapeuticUses: Recent research suggests that barley contains protease inhibitors that could suppress cancer-causing agents in the intestinal tract. This grain also lowers blood cholesterol, improves bowel function, and relieves constipation.

BeneficialNutrients: Potassium, Silicon, plus Vitamins B1, B2, Folic Acid, and Niacin.

BASS

TherapeuticUses: Bass combats early kidney disease, regulates the immune system, and is a good brain and nerve food. The omega-3 oils in fish are firmly linked to preventing heart disease. Omega-3 thins the blood, lowers blood cholesterol, lowers blood pressure, and inhibits blood clots reducing the risk of heart attack and stroke. Recent studies show that fish oils have reduced tumors in animals.

BeneficialNutrients: Chlorine, Iodine, Phosphorus, plus Vitamins A, B1, B2, B12, Niacin, Pantothenic acid.

BEANS - Lima

TherapeuticUses: Lima beans regulate functions of the colon, cure constipation, and prevent hemorrhoids and other bowel problems. Also used to reduce blood cholesterol and lower blood pressure.

Beneficial Nutrients: Calcium, Iron, Phosphorus, Potassium, plus Vitamins A, B1, B2, Niacin.

BEANS - String

TherapeuticUses: String beans contain chemicals called lignans that help fight off breast and colon cancer. This vegetable is also useful in controlling insulin and blood sugar.

BeneficialNutrients: Manganese, Nitrogen, plus Vitamins A, B1, B2, B6, Niacin, Pantothenic acid, C, and E.

BEEF

TherapeuticUses: Very high in protein. A good brain, gland, and nerve food. Beef is also recommended for the treatment of anemia.

Beneficial Nutrients: Chlorine, Phosphorus, Potassium, plus Vitamins A, B1, B2, B6, B12, Folic Acid, Niacin, and Pantothenic acid.

BEER

TherapeuticUses: Beer raises the good HDL - type blood cholesterol and helps prevent blockage of the heart arteries.

AdverseEffects: Beer drinkers have a higher rate of lung, colon, and rectal cancers. Beer is also high in purine, which the body converts into uric acid that can bring on gout.

Beneficial Nutrients: Calcium, Iron, Magnesium, Manganese, Phosphorus, Potassium, Selenium, Sodium, Zinc plus Vitamins plus Vitamins B2, B6, Folic acid, Niacin, and Pantothenic acid.

BEETS

TherapeuticUses: Beet juice combined with blackberry juice is an excellent blood builder. International surveys have found that people that consume a serving of beet leaves or spinach like vegetables every day are less likely to develop smoking related cancers. Animal tests also show that beet leaves can reduce blood cholesterol.

Beneficial Nutrients: Chlorine, Fluorine, Iron, Potassium, plus Vitamins A, B1, B2, B6, B12, Niacin, Pantothenic acid, and C.

BLACKBERRY

TherapeuticUses: Good for anemia and an effective remedy for diarrhea and dysentery.

Beneficial Nutrients: Iodine, Iron, Magnesium, Potassium, plus Vitamins A, B1, B2, B6, Biotin, Niacin, Pantothenic acid, and C.

BLUEBERRY

TherapeuticUses: A good body mineralizer and blood purifier. Recent studies show that the anthocyanosides in blueberries may protect blood vessels from destructive cholesterol deposits. They are also effective in killing infectious viruses and are used to help relieve diarrhea.

Beneficial Nutrients: Calcium, Magnesium, Potassium, plus Vitamins A, B1, B2, B6, Folic Acid, Niacin, Pantothenic acid, and C.

BREAD - Whole wheat

TherapeuticUses: Whole wheat bread is an effective laxative and will help regulate blood sugar and lowers blood cholesterol. Whole wheat is high in protease inhibitors; protease blocks the activation of cancer-causing chemicals in the intestinal tract; wheat bran is linked to lower rates of colon cancer.

Beneficial Nutrients: Calcium, Chlorine, Phosphorus, Silicon, plus Vitamins B1, B2, B6, Biotin, Folic Acid, Niacin, Pantothenic acid, and E.

BROCCOLI

TherapeuticUses: Tests show that broccoli is a versatile cancer fighter. It is rich in known cancer antidotes such as carotenoids, dithiolthiones, glucosinolates, and indoles.

Beneficial Nutrients: Chlorophyll, Potassium, plus Vitamins A, B1, B2, B6, Folic acid, Niacin, Pantothenic acid, and C.

BRUSSELS SPROUTS

TherapeuticUses: It is claimed that brussels sprouts can detoxify aflatoxin, a fungal mold linked to high rates of cancer. Eating this vegetable is a good way to boost the bodies immune system, especially for colon and stomach cancer.

BeneficialNutrients: Calcium, Potassium, Sulfur, plus Vitamins A, B1, B2, B6, Folic acid, Niacin, Pantothenic acid, and C.

BUTTER

TherapeuticUses: Butter is an easy fat to digest and an excellent source of vitamin A. Butter also helps prevent osteoporosis, peptic ulcers, chronic bronchitis, cavities, and lowers blood cholesterol and blood pressure.

BeneficialNutrients: Calcium, Chlorine, Sodium, plus Vitamins A, B1, B2, B6, B12, Folic Acid, Niacin, Pantothenic acid, C, and E.

CABBAGE

TherapeuticUses: Cabbage is rich in vitamin U. This vitamin is used to lower the risk of cancer, especially of the colon. This vegetable also kills bacteria and viruses and the juice is drank to prevent and heal ulcers.

BeneficialNutrients: Potassium, Sodium, plus Vitamins A, B1, B2, B6, Biotin, Folic acid, Niacin, Pantothenic acid, C, E, and U.

CARROTS

TherapeuticUses: Research shows that the beta carotene in carrots substantially cut down the chances of contracting cancer of the pancreas and smoking-related cancers. Carrots are good for eyes, hair, and nails and are also eaten to prevent constipation and lower blood cholesterol.

BeneficialNutrients: Calcium, Potassium, Silicon, Sulfur, plus Vitamins A, B1, B2, B6, Biotin, Folic acid, Niacin, Pantothenic acid, and C.

CASABA

TherapeuticUses: An excellent blood cleanser and cooler.

BeneficialNutrients: Chlorine, Iron, Potassium, Silicon, Sodium, plus Vitamins A, B1, B2, B6, Biotin, Niacin, Pantothenic acid, C, and E.

CAULIFLOWER

Therapeutic Uses: Tests show that cauliflower is associated with lower cancer rates of the bladder, colon, rectum, prostrate, and stomach. Cauliflower is low in carotene and chlorophyll, so is less likely to block smoking-related cancers.

Beneficial Nutrients: Calcium, Potassium, Silicon, Sulfur, plus Vitamins A, B1, B2, B6, Biotin, Folic acid, Niacin, Pantothenic acid, C, and E.

CELERY

Therapeutic Uses: Celery is a good blood cleanser. Also recommended for acidity, arthritis, rheumatism, neuritis, and high blood pressure.

Beneficial Nutrients: Chlorine, Magnesium, Potassium, Sodium, plus Vitamins A, B1, B2, B6, Biotin, Folic acid, Niacin, Pantothenic acid, C, and E.

CHEESE

Therapeutic Uses: A good source of protein, but hard to digest. Cheese also helps to prevent osteoporosis, peptic ulcers, chronic bronchitis, cavities, and lowers blood cholesterol and blood pressure.

Beneficial Nutrients: Calcium, Chlorine, Fluorine, Phosphorus, Sodium, plus Vitamins A, B1, B2, B6, B12, Folic Acid, Niacin, and Pantothenic acid.

CHERRY

Therapeutic Uses: Cherries contain a potent antibacterial agent against tooth decay and gall bladder problems. Also used in the treatment of gout, catarrh, and anemia.

Beneficial Nutrients: Iron, Magnesium, Potassium, plus Vitamins A, B1, B2, B6, Biotin, Folic Acid, Niacin, Pantothenic acid, and C.

CHERVIL

Therapeutic Uses: A good body mineralizer.

Beneficial Nutrients: Iron, Phosphorus, Potassium, Selenium, plus Vitamins A, B1, B2, B6, Biotin, Niacin, Pantothenic acid, and C.

CHICKEN

Therapeutic Uses: A good brain, gland, and nerve food. Very high in protein. Chicken is also recommended for the treatment of anemia.

Beneficial Nutrients: Chlorine, Phosphorus, Potassium, plus Vitamins A, B1, B2, B6, B12, Folic Acid, Niacin, Pantothenic acid, and C.

CHICORY

Therapeutic Uses: Chicory is an alkaline food and should be used in elimination diets. Also a good remedy for increasing peristaltic action and to strengthen liver functions.

Beneficial Nutrients: Chlorine, Iron, Potassium, Sulfur, plus Vitamins A, B1, B2, B6, Folic Acid, Niacin, Pantothenic acid, and C.

CHILI PEPPER

Therapeutic Uses: Chili peppers are an excellent medicine for the lungs, preventing and alleviating chronic bronchitis and emphysema. They also act as a decongestant, expectorant, and help to dissolve blood clots.

Adverse Effects: Hot peppers stimulate gastric acid so may aggravate stomach ulcers.

Beneficial Nutrients: Calcium, Chlorine, Copper, Iodine, Iron, Magnesium, Manganese, Phosphorus, Potassium, Selenium, Silicon, Sodium, Sulfur, Zinc plus Vitamins A, B1, B2, B6, Folic acid, Niacin, Pantothenic acid, and C.

CHIVES

Therapeutic Uses: An excellent body mineralizer. Also good for catarrh and elimination.

Beneficial Nutrients: Calcium, Potassium, Sulfur, plus Vitamins A, B1, B2, B6, Niacin, Pantothenic acid, and C.

COCONUT

Therapeutic Uses: Coconut milk is a complete protein and compares to mother's milk in its chemical balance. Recent studies show coconuts as being high on the list of possible antidotes to cancer. Coconut pulp contains high amounts of compounds called protease inhibitors. Protease inhibitors have blocked cancer in animals.

Beneficial Nutrients: Chlorine, Magnesium, Phosphorus, plus Vitamins B1, B2, B6, Folic Acid, Niacin, Pantothenic acid, C, and E.

COFFEE

TherapeuticUses: New studies in Japan and Norway suggest that drinking coffee might prevent colon cancer. Coffee boosts physical energy, elevates your mood, and improves mental performance. Also used to relieve asthma and hay fever.

Adverse Effects: People with insomnia should not drink coffee before retiring for the evening.

Beneficial Nutrients: Calcium, Copper, Iron, Magnesium, Manganese, Phosphorus, Potassium, Sodium, Zinc plus Vitamins B2, and Niacin.

CORN

TherapeuticUses: Corn lowers blood cholesterol, lowers the risk of heart disease, and is a great muscle and bone builder. It is also linked to lower rates of dental cavities.

Adverse Effects: Recent studies show that corn oil lowers the immunity in laboratory animals making them more susceptible to infections and cancer.

Beneficial Nutrients: Phosphorus, Potassium, Silicon, plus Vitamins A, B1, B2, B6, Biotin, Folic acid, Niacin, Pantothenic acid, and C.

CRANBERRY

TherapeuticUses: Cranberries help prevent urinary tract infections and inflammation of the rectal pouch. They also help prevent kidney stones, deodorize urine, and kill viruses and bacteria.

BeneficialNutrients: Calcium, Chlorine, Sulfur, plus Vitamins A, B1, B2, B6, Folic Acid, Niacin, Pantothenic acid, and C.

CREAM

Therapeutic Uses: Cream prevents osteoporosis, peptic ulcers, chronic bronchitis, cavities, and lowers blood cholesterol and blood pressure. Studies show that cream lowers the risk of colon cancer. It is believed that calcium detoxifies bile acids that can promote cancer in the intestinal tract.

Beneficial Nutrients: Calcium, Fluorine, Phosphorus, plus Vitamins A, B1, B2, B6, B12, Folic Acid, Niacin, Pantothenic acid, and C.

CUCUMBERS

TherapeuticUses: Cucumbers have a cooling effect on the body and have a purifying effect on the bowel. They are also used as a digestive aid.

Beneficial Nutrients: Calcium, Iron, Phosphorus, Potassium, Silicon, plus Vitamins A, B1, B2, B6, Biotin, Folic acid, Niacin, Pantothenic acid, C, and E.

CURRANTS

Therapeutic Uses: Recent studies using animals show that black currants help protect blood vessels against a high cholesterol diet. Currants are also recommended for colds, treating diarrhea, and soothing sore throats.

Beneficial Nutrients: Magnesium, Phosphorus, Potassium, plus Vitamins A, B1, B2, B6, Biotin, Niacin, Pantothenic acid, and C.

DATES - Dry

Therapeutic Uses: Good for ulcers. The cellulose of the date is very soft and will not irritate a sensitive bowel or stomach.

Beneficial Nutrients: Chlorine, plus Vitamins A, B1, B2, B6, Folic Acid, Niacin, and Pantothenic acid.

EGGPLANT

Therapeutic Uses: Eggplant is good for balancing diets that are heavy in starches and protein. Eggplant contains protease, this compound is believed to block certain viruses and cancer-causing agents. It also contains compounds that prevent convulsions and helps protect the arteries from cholesterol damage.

Beneficial Nutrients: Chlorine, Phosphorus, Potassium, plus Vitamins A, B1, B2, B6, Folic acid, Niacin, Pantothenic acid, C, and E.

ENDIVE

Therapeutic Uses: Very high in vitamin A. Works to rid the body of infections.

Beneficial Nutrients: Calcium, Potassium, Sulfur, plus Vitamins A, B1, B2, B6, Folic acid, Niacin, Pantothenic acid, and C.

FIGS

Therapeutic Uses: Scientists are presently testing human cancer patients with oral and injected doses of fig distillate to shrink tumors. Figs are a natural laxative, also aid digestion, and the juice kills bacteria and roundworms.

Beneficial Nutrients: Magnesium, Potassium, plus Vitamins A, B1, B2, B6, Niacin, Pantothenic acid, and C.

FISH

Therapeutic Uses: The omega-3 oils in fish are firmly linked to preventing heart disease. Omega-3 thins the blood, lowers blood cholesterol, lowers blood pressure, and inhibits blood clots reducing the risk of heart attack and stroke. Fish also combats early kidney disease, regulates the immune system, and recent studies show that fish oils have reduced tumors in animals.

Beneficial Nutrients: Calcium, Copper, Iron, Magnesium, Manganese, Phosphorus, Potassium, Sodium, Zinc plus Vitamins A, B1, B2, B6, B12, Folic Acid, Niacin, Pantothenic acid, and C.

GARLIC

Therapeutic Uses: Garlic contains potent compounds that appear to help retard cancer, heart disease, and a wide range of infections. Garlic also thins the blood and lowers blood pressure reducing the chance of strokes.

Beneficial Nutrients: Calcium, Copper, Phosphorus, Potassium, Sodium, Zinc plus Vitamins B1, Folic acid, and C.

GINGER

Therapeutic Uses: Ginger is widely used for suppressing motion induced nausea. It also thins the blood and lowers blood cholesterol.

Beneficial Nutrients: Calcium, Copper, Iron, Magnesium, Manganese, Phosphorus, Potassium, Selenium, Sodium, Zinc plus Vitamins A, B1, B2, B6, Biotin, Folic Acid, Niacin, Pantothenic acid, and C.

GRAPEFRUIT

Therapeutic Uses: Citrus fruits have definite anti cancer capabilities. In Japanese cancer tests, when grapefruit extract was injected into mice, it stopped their tumor growth and caused partial or complete remission of the malignancy. This fruit also protects the arteries from disease and lowers blood cholesterol.

Beneficial Nutrients: Calcium, Potassium, Sodium, plus Vitamins A, B1, B2, B6, Biotin, Folic Acid, Niacin, Pantothenic acid, C, and E.

GRAPES

Therapeutic Uses: A blood purifier. Grapes are especially good for catarrhal conditions.

Beneficial Nutrients: Magnesium, Potassium, plus Vitamins A, B1, B2, B6, Biotin, Folic Acid, Niacin, Pantothenic acid, and C.

HALIBUT - Smoked

TherapeuticUses: A complete protein and a good source of nerve and brain fat.

Beneficial Nutrients: Chlorine, Phosphorus, Potassium, plus Vitamins A, B1, B2, B6, B12, Biotin, Folic Acid, Niacin, and Pantothenic acid.

HONEY

TherapeuticUses: Honey is one of the best disinfectants for wounds and sores. It is also recommended for the relief of asthma, soothes sore throats, and is used to calm nerves and induce sleep.

AdverseEffects: Don't give honey to infants under one year of age. Bacterial botulism spores can germinate in a immature intestine and make a deadly toxin.

Beneficial Nutrients: Calcium, Phosphorus, Potassium, plus Vitamins A, B1, B2, B6, Biotin, Folic Acid, Niacin, Pantothenic acid, and C.

HORSERADISH

TherapeuticUses: An excellent body mineralizer and a liver and gall bladder cleanser.

BeneficialNutrients: Fluorine, Potassium, Sulfur, plus Vitamins A, B1, B2, B6, Biotin, Niacin, Pantothenic acid, and C.

KALE

TherapeuticUses: Strengthens teeth and bones. One of the richest vegetables in carotenoids, anti cancer agents. A study in Singapore showed kale as significantly diminishing the risk of lung cancer.

BeneficialNutrients: Calcium, Potassium, plus Vitamins A, B1, B2, B6, Biotin, Folic acid, Niacin, Pantothenic acid, C, and E.

KELP

TherapeuticUses: Kelp is a brown seaweed that is very rich in iodine. It heals ulcers, reduces blood cholesterol, thins the blood, lowering blood pressure, and prevents strokes. Research in Japan shows that kelp helps immunize mice against malignancies, especially breast tumors.

Beneficial Nutrients: Calcium, Iodine, Iron, Magnesium, Phosphorus, Potassium, Sodium, plus Vitamins B2, and Niacin.

KOHLRABI

TherapeuticUses: Very high in vitamin C. Good for the digestive, lymphatic, and skeletal systems.

Beneficial Nutrients: Calcium, Magnesium, Potassium, plus Vitamins A, B1, B2, B6, Folic acid, Niacin, Pantothenic acid, and C.

LAMB

Therapeutic Uses: Very high in protein. A good brain, gland, and nerve food. Lamb is also recommended for the treatment of anemia.

Beneficial Nutrients: Chlorine, Phosphorus, Potassium, plus Vitamins A, B1, B2, B6, B12, Folic Acid, Niacin, Pantothenic acid, and C.

LEEKS

TherapeuticUses: A good blood medicine. Lowers blood cholesterol, thins the blood, retards clotting, and regulates blood sugar. Also used to relieve bronchial congestion and kill bacteria. The National Cancer Institute believes that there is a link between sulfides in leeks and the bodies ability to turn off cell changes preceding cancer growth.

Beneficial Nutrients: Calcium, Sodium, plus Vitamins A, B1, B2, B6, Biotin, Folic acid, Niacin, Pantothenic acid, C, and E.

LEMON AND LIME

Therapeutic Uses: Lemon oil is effective in killing fungi and roundworms in humans. The lemon and lime peel exhibits antioxidant activity that is believed to ward off cancer and retard aging. The pectin found in the pulp of citrus fruits will lower blood cholesterol.

Beneficial Nutrients: Calcium, Magnesium, Potassium, plus Vitamins A, B1, B2, B6, Folic Acid, Niacin, Pantothenic acid, and C.

LENTILS

TherapeuticUses: Lentils regulate functions of the colon, cure constipation, and prevent hemorrhoids and other bowel problems. Also used to reduce blood cholesterol and lower blood pressure.

BeneficialNutrients: Phosphorus, Potassium, plus Vitamins A, B1, B2, and Niacin.

LETTUCE

TherapeuticUses: Lettuce is good for sleeplessness and slows the digestive effect on the intestinal tract.

BeneficialNutrients: Calcium, Chlorine, Iron, Potassium, Sodium, plus Vitamins A, B1, B2, Folic acid, Niacin, and C.

MANGOES

TherapeuticUses: Used for intestinal disorders. The mango juice will reduce excessive body heat.

Beneficial Nutrients: Calcium, Chlorine, Potassium, plus Vitamins A, B1, B2, B6, Niacin, Pantothenic acid, C, and E.

MELON

TherapeuticUses: Orange melons have been linked in numerous surveys with the lower rate of lung cancer due to their rich beta carotene content. Melons are also an effective blood thinner.

BeneficialNutrients: Potassium, Silicon, Sodium, plus Vitamins A, B1, B2, B6, Biotin, Folic Acid, Niacin, Pantothenic acid, C, and E.

MILK - Whole

TherapeuticUses: Studies show that milk lowers the risk of colon cancer. It is believed that calcium detoxifies bile acids that can promote cancer in the intestinal tract. Milk also prevents osteoporosis, peptic ulcers, chronic bronchitis, cavities, and lowers blood cholesterol and blood pressure.

Adverse Effects: People with a lactose intolerance can suffer intense stomach distress and milk has been linked to irritable bowel syndrome.

Beneficial Nutrients: Calcium, Fluorine, Phosphorus, Sodium, plus Vitamins A, B1, B2, B6, B12, Biotin, Folic Acid, Niacin, Pantothenic acid, C, and E.

MUSHROOM

TherapeuticUses: Mushrooms lower blood cholesterol, thin the blood, inactivate viruses, and stimulate the immune system. A Japanese study in 1986 shows that several mushrooms have anti tumor powers; button, shiitake, enoki, straw, and oyster mushrooms interfere with the late-stage growth of cancer.

Beneficial Nutrients: Iodine, Phosphorus, Potassium, plus Vitamins B1, B2, B6, Biotin, Folic acid, Niacin, Pantothenic acid, C, and E.

MUSTARD GREENS

TherapeuticUses: A good gall bladder and liver cleanser.

Beneficial Nutrients: Calcium, Magnesium, Potassium, Sulfur, plus Vitamins A, B1, B2, B6, Folic Acid, Niacin, and Pantothenic acid.

OATS

TherapeuticUses: This seed is high in protease inhibitors, protease blocks the activation of cancer-causing chemicals in the intestinal tract. Oats is an effective laxative and is used to combat inflammation of the skin. Also an excellent heart medicine, regulating blood sugar and lowers blood cholesterol.

Beneficial Nutrients: Iodine, Magnesium, Silicon, plus Vitamins B1, B2, B6, and Niacin.

OKRA

Therapeutic Uses: Good for ulcers and to soothe the irritated membranes of the intestinal tract.

Beneficial Nutrients: Chlorine, Sodium, plus Vitamins A, B1, B2, B6, Folic acid, Niacin, Pantothenic acid, and C.

OLIVE OIL

TherapeuticUses: An infallible treatment for heart diseases. Olive oil thins the blood lowering blood pressure, reduces LDL cholesterol, and raises HDL cholesterol. Tests show that olive oil inserted into human cells makes them less susceptible to destruction by cancer agents "free radicals".

AdverseEffects: High consumption of olive oil has a mild laxative effect and can cause diarrhea.

BeneficialNutrients: Phosphorus, Potassium, plus Vitamin E.

ONION

Therapeutic Uses: A good blood medicine. Lowers blood cholesterol, thins the blood, retards clotting, and regulates blood sugar. Also used to relieve bronchial congestion and kill bacteria. The National Cancer Institute believes that there is a link between sulfides in onions and the bodies ability to turn off cell changes preceding cancer growth.

BeneficialNutrients: Potassium, Sulfur, plus Vitamins B1, B2, B6, Biotin, Folic acid, Niacin, Pantothenic acid, C, and E.

ORANGE

Therapeutic Uses: This fruit protects the arteries from disease, fights arterial plaque, and lowers blood cholesterol. Citrus fruits have definite anti cancer capabilities. In Japanese cancer tests, when citrus extract was injected into mice, it stopped their tumor growth and caused partial or complete remission of the malignancy.

Beneficial Nutrients: Calcium, Magnesium, Potassium, Sodium, plus Vitamins A, B1, B2, B6, Biotin, Folic Acid, Niacin, Pantothenic acid, C, and E.

PAPAYA

Therapeutic Uses: Papaya is high in digestive properties and has a tonic effect on the stomach. Used to treat ulcers, intestinal disorders, and fevers.

Beneficial Nutrients: Chlorine, Magnesium, Sodium, Sulfur, plus Vitamins A, B1, B2, B6, Niacin, Pantothenic acid, and C.

PARSLEY

Therapeutic Uses: Parsley is a good blood purifier and is used to cleanse the kidneys and stimulate the bowel.

Beneficial Nutrients: Calcium, Iron, Potassium, Sulfur, plus Vitamins A, B1, B2, B6, Biotin, Niacin, Pantothenic acid, and C.

PARSNIPS

Therapeutic Uses: Parsnips strengthen the liver and improve bowel action.

Beneficial Nutrients: Calcium, Potassium, Silicon, plus Vitamins A, B1, B2, B6, Biotin, Folic Acid, Niacin, Pantothenic acid, and C.

PEACHES

Therapeutic Uses: Scientists believe that the high concentrations of beta carotene in peaches could mitigate the latent cancerous effects of cigarette smoke and inhibit lung and smoking related cancers.

Beneficial Nutrients: Calcium, Phosphorus, Potassium, plus Vitamins A, B1, B2, B6, Biotin, Folic Acid, Niacin, Pantothenic acid, and C.

PEANUTS

Therapeutic Uses: Peanuts contain high amounts of compounds called protease inhibitors. Protease inhibitors have blocked cancer in animals. Peanut oils also lower blood cholesterol and regulate blood sugar.

Beneficial Nutrients: Phosphorus, Potassium, Silicon, plus Vitamins B1, B2, B6, Folic Acid, Niacin, and Pantothenic acid.

PEARS

TherapeuticUses: A good intestinal and bowel regulator.

Beneficial Nutrients: Phosphorus, Sodium, plus Vitamins A, B1, B2, B6, Biotin, Folic Acid, Niacin, Pantothenic acid, and C.

PEAS

Therapeutic Uses: Peas can prevent appendicitis, lower blood cholesterol, and are high in contraceptive agents. Studies show that this seed is high in protease inhibitors: Peas have been linked to lower rates of intestinal and prostrate cancers.

Beneficial Nutrients: Calcium, Chlorine, Magnesium, plus Vitamins A, B1, B2, B6, Folic Acid, Niacin, Pantothenic acid, C, and E.

PECANS

TherapeuticUses: Recent studies show pecans as being high on the list of possible antidotes to cancer. Pecans contain high amounts of compounds called protease inhibitors. Protease inhibitors have blocked cancer in animals. Nut oils also lower blood cholesterol and regulate blood sugar.

Beneficial Nutrients: Calcium, Phosphorus, Potassium, plus Vitamins B1, B2, B6, Folic Acid, Niacin, and Pantothenic acid.

PERSIMMONS

TherapeuticUses: A rich source of fruit sugars and a good remedy for an irritable intestinal tract.

Beneficial Nutrients: Calcium, Phosphorus, plus Vitamins A, B1, B2, B6, Niacin, Pantothenic acid, and C.

PINEAPPLE

TherapeuticUses: Pineapple is an excellent blood builder. Used to aid digestion and catarrhal conditions.

Beneficial Nutrients: Calcium, Iodine, Magnesium, Sodium, plus Vitamins A, B1, B2, B6, Folic Acid, Niacin, Pantothenic acid, and C.

PLUMS

TherapeuticUses: A bowel regulator and a good laxative.

Beneficial Nutrients: Magnesium, plus Vitamins A, B1, B2, B6, Biotin, Folic Acid, Niacin, Pantothenic acid, and C.

POMEGRANATE

Therapeutic Uses: Pomegranate juice is used for bladder and kidney disorders.

Beneficial Nutrients: Magnesium, Sodium, plus Vitamins B1, B2, B6, Niacin, Pantothenic acid, and C.

POPCORN

TherapeuticUses: A good source of intestinal roughage.

Beneficial Nutrients: Phosphorus, plus Vitamins A, B1, B2, B6, Biotin, Niacin, Pantothenic acid, and C.

POTATO

Therapeutic Uses: Raw potatoes have protease inhibitors that neutralize certain viruses and carcinogens. Potato peels are rich in chlorogenic acid, this chemical can prevent cell mutations that lead to cancer.

Adverse Effects: Potatoes could be detrimental to diabetics as they raise insulin and blood sugar levels quickly.

Beneficial Nutrients: Magnesium, Phosphorus, Potassium, Silicon, plus Vitamins B1, B2, Folic Acid, Niacin, Pantothenic acid, and C.

PRUNES

TherapeuticUses: Prunes act as a powerful laxative due to the high content of magnesium ammonium phosphate. They are also a good source of nerve salts.

Beneficial Nutrients: Magnesium, Phosphorus, Potassium, plus Vitamins A, B1, B2, B6, Folic Acid, Niacin, Pantothenic acid, and C.

PUMPKIN

Therapeutic Uses: Pumpkins have been linked in numerous surveys with the lower rate of lung cancer due to their rich beta carotene content. Smokers and people who are around smokers should eat more deep-orange vegetables like pumpkin and winter squash.

Beneficial Nutrients: Iron, Phosphorus, Sodium, plus Vitamins A, B1, B2, B6, Folic Acid, Niacin, Pantothenic acid, and C.

RADISHES

Therapeutic Uses: Helpful in catarrhal conditions and aid in cleansing the liver and gall bladder.

Beneficial Nutrients: Magnesium, Phosphorus, Potassium, plus Vitamins A, B1, B2, B6, Folic Acid, Niacin, Pantothenic acid, and C.

RAISINS

Therapeutic Uses: A high energy food and a good body builder.

Beneficial Nutrients: Chlorine, Phosphorus, Potassium, plus Vitamins B1, B2, B6, Biotin, Folic Acid, Niacin, and C.

RASPBERRIES

Therapeutic Uses: A cleanser for mucus and toxins.

Beneficial Nutrients: Iron, Sodium, plus Vitamins A, B1, B2, B6, Biotin, Niacin, Pantothenic acid, and C.

RICE

Therapeutic Uses: Rice is known to clear up psoriasis, prevent kidney stones, regulate blood sugar, lower blood pressure, and control diarrhea. Rice contains protease inhibitors. Lab experiments on animals slashed the risk of bowel cancer and anti tumor substances isolated from rice bran suppressed solid tumors in mice.

Beneficial Nutrients: Phosphorus, Sodium, plus Vitamins B1, B2, B6, Folic Acid, Niacin, Pantothenic acid.

RYE

Therapeutic Uses: This seed is high in protease inhibitors, protease blocks the activation of cancer-causing chemicals in the intestinal tract. Rye is an effective laxative and is used to combat inflammation of the skin. Also an excellent heart medicine, regulating blood sugar and lowers blood cholesterol.

Beneficial Nutrients: Magnesium, Phosphorus, Silicon, plus Vitamins B1, B2, B6, Folic Acid, Niacin, Pantothenic acid.

SEAWEED - Laminaria species

TherapeuticUses: Research in Japan shows that Laminaria helps immunize mice against malignancies; especially breast tumors. Laminaria is a brown seaweed that is very rich iodine. It heals ulcers, reduces blood cholesterol, thins the blood, lowering blood pressure, and prevents strokes.

Beneficial Nutrients: Calcium, Iodine, Iron, Magnesium, Phosphorus, Potassium, Sodium, plus Vitamins B2, and Niacin.

SHELLFISH

Therapeutic Uses: Oysters and clams have been used as an aphrodisiac for many centuries. Shellfish lower blood cholesterol, and stimulate brain cells boosting mental energy.

Beneficial Nutrients: Calcium, Copper, Iodine, Iron, Magnesium, Manganese, Phosphorus, Potassium, Selenium, Sodium, Zinc plus Vitamins A, B1, B2, B6, B12, Folic Acid, Niacin, and Pantothenic acid.

SOYBEAN

TherapeuticUses: Soybeans regulate functions of the colon, cure constipation, and prevent hemorrhoids and other bowel problems. Also used to reduce blood cholesterol, regulate blood sugar, and lower blood pressure. Soybeans also contain chemicals called, lignans that help fight off breast and colon cancer. This vegetable is also useful in controlling insulin and blood sugar.

Beneficial Nutrients: Calcium, Chlorine, Iodine, Iron, Phosphorus, Potassium, Sodium, plus Vitamins A, B1, B2, Niacin, and C.

SPINACH

TherapeuticUses: International surveys have found that people who consume a serving of spinach like vegetables every day are less likely to develop smoking related cancers. Animal tests also show that spinach can reduce blood cholesterol.

Beneficial Nutrients: Potassium, Silicon, plus Vitamins A, B1, B2, B6, Biotin, Folic Acid, Niacin, Pantothenic acid, C, and E.

SQUASH

TherapeuticUses: This vegetable is an effective blood thinner and hubbards and butternut squash have been linked in numerous surveys with the lower rate of lung cancer due to their rich beta carotene content.

Beneficial Nutrients: Magnesium, Sodium, plus Vitamins A, B1, B2, B6, Niacin, Pantothenic acid, and C.

STRAWBERRIES

Therapeutic Uses: These berries are very high in pectin, the fiber that is found to substantially reduce blood cholesterol. In a recent cancer research study in New Jersey, strawberries capped a list of foods linked to lower rates of cancer deaths in the elderly.

Beneficial Nutrients: Calcium, Sodium, plus Vitamins A, B1, B2, B6, Biotin, Folic Acid, Niacin, Pantothenic acid, and C.

SWISS CHARD

Therapeutic Uses: Contains the vitamins and minerals essential for proper digestive action.

Beneficial Nutrients: Calcium, Iron, Magnesium, Sodium, plus Vitamins A, B1, B2, B6, Biotin, Folic Acid, Niacin, Pantothenic acid, and C.

TEA

Therapeutic Uses: Black and green teas have been used as medicines for 4000 years in china. Tea fights infections, kills bacteria and viruses, lowers blood pressure, slows arteriosclerosis and strengthens capillaries. In a Japanese study green tea drinkers had lower rates of stomach cancer.

Adverse Effects: Tea stimulates gastric acid in the stomach, so is not recommended for people with ulcers.

Beneficial Nutrients: Calcium, Copper, Iron, Magnesium, Manganese, Phosphorus, Potassium, Selenium, Sodium, Zinc.

TOMATO

Therapeutic Uses: Tomatoes are highly praised as a protector against acute appendicitis and supply both beta carotene and lycopene; anti cancer agents.

Beneficial Nutrients: Chlorine, Potassium, Sodium, plus Vitamins A, B1, B2, B6, Niacin, Pantothenic acid, and C.

TURNIPS

Therapeutic Uses: Turnips have been used for many years as a treatment for tuberculosis of the bones and lungs. They also contain compounds that block the development of cancer in laboratory animals.

Beneficial Nutrients: Calcium, Potassium, plus Vitamins B1, B2, B6, Biotin, Folic Acid, Niacin, Pantothenic acid, C, and E.

TURNIP LEAVES

Therapeutic Uses: Turnip greens are rich in carotenoids, so are among the top foods eaten by people with lower than average rates of cancer, in particular lung cancer.

Beneficial Nutrients: Calcium, Magnesium, plus Vitamins A, B1, B2, B6, Folic Acid, Niacin, Pantothenic acid, C, and E.

WALNUTS

Therapeutic Uses: Recent studies show walnuts as being high on the list of possible antidotes to cancer. Walnuts contain high amounts of compounds called protease inhibitors. protease inhibitors have blocked cancer in animals. Nuts also lower blood cholesterol and regulate blood sugar.

Beneficial Nutrients: Magnesium, Manganese, Phosphorus, plus Vitamins A, B1, B2, B6, and Niacin.

WATERCRESS

Therapeutic Uses: A good blood purifier.

Beneficial Nutrients: Calcium, Chlorine, Sulfur, plus Vitamins A, B1, B2, B6, Biotin, Folic Acid, Niacin, Pantothenic acid, and C.

WATERMELON

Therapeutic Uses: A blood cooler.

Beneficial Nutrients: Calcium, Silicon, Sodium, plus Vitamins A, B1, B2, B6, Niacin, Pantothenic acid, and C.

WHEAT BRAN

Therapeutic Uses: Wheat bran is an effective laxative and is used to combat inflammation of the skin. Also an excellent heart medicine, regulating blood sugar and lowers blood cholesterol. This seed is high in protease inhibitors, protease blocks the activation of cancer-causing chemicals in the intestinal tract; wheat bran is linked to lower rates of colon cancer.

Adverse Effects: Wheat bran is not advised for those with Crohn's disease.

Beneficial Nutrients: Phosphorus, Silicon, plus Vitamins B1, B2, B6, Folic Acid, Niacin, Pantothenic acid, and C.

WHEY

TherapeuticUses: A blood builder.

BeneficialNutrients: Calcium, Chlorine, Sodium, plus Vitamins A, B1, B2, B6, B12, Folic Acid, Niacin, Pantothenic acid, and C.

WINE

TherapeuticUses: One glass of wine a day will boost the beneficial HDL blood cholesterol by up to seven percent. Wine is also good for killing bacteria and viruses and is rich in chemicals that prevent cancer in animals.

Adverse Effects: People susceptible to migraine headaches should not drink red wine and wine is also a hazard to people with a tendency toward gout.

Beneficial Nutrients: Calcium, Copper, Iron, Magnesium, Phosphorus, Potassium, Sodium, Zinc plus Vitamins A, B1, B2, B6, Folic Acid, Niacin, Pantothenic acid, and C.

YAM

TherapeuticUses: Several studies have shown that yams and sweet potatoes as being particularly effective in thwarting the long-stage progress of lung cancer and other smoking related cancers.

Beneficial Nutrients: Calcium, Copper, Iron, Magnesium, Phosphorus, Potassium, Sodium, Zinc plus Vitamins B1, B2, B6, Folic Acid, Niacin, Pantothenic acid, and C.

YOGURT

Therapeutic Uses: Yogurt is a natural antibiotic; it treats and prevents intestinal infections, controls diarrhea, contains chemicals that prevent ulcers, improves bowel functions, lowers blood cholesterol, and strengthens the immune system. Scientists have found several cancer fighting properties in yogurt that may help to block colon cancer.

Beneficial Nutrients: Calcium, Iron, Magnesium, Phosphorus, Potassium, Sodium, Sulfur, Zinc plus Vitamins A, B1, B2, B6, B12, Folic Acid, Niacin, Pantothenic acid, and C.

GLOSSARY

Term

Definition

Absorption --- The process by which nutrients are absorbed into the bloodstream.

Acetate --- A derivative of acetic acid.

Aceticacid --- An inorganic acid used as a synthetic flavoring agent. Vinegar is made from 5% Acetic acid and water.

Acetone --- A colorless solvent for oils, fat, and waxes. Taken in large amounts it can have a narcotic effect.

Acute --- Disorders or symptoms that occur abruptly and run a short course. The opposite of chronic.

Adaptogen --- Balances and restores tone to a particular area.

Addiction --- Emotional or Physical dependence on a substance, usually requiring increased amounts.

Adrenal Gland --- Endocrine glands that produce corticosteroid, epinephrine, and norepinephrine hormones.

Albumin --- A protein found widely in plant and animal tissues. Its presence in the urine is one sign of kidney disease.

Allergen --- A substance that produces an allergic response in the body.

Allergy --- A reaction caused by a specific substance anywhere in the body's tissue.

Alterative --- Blood purifier, promotes cleansing and detoxification of blood.

Term		Definition
Amino Acid	---	An organic acid that contains nitrogen building blocks. Aids in the production of protein in the body.
Anabolic compounds	---	Conversion of nutritive material into complex living matter in the constructive metabolism.
Analgestic	---	Taken to relieve pain without causing loss of consciousness.
Anaphylaxis	---	An immediate and sometimes life threatening allergic hypersensitivity reaction.
Androgen	---	A hormone such as andosterone and testosterone responsible for the development of male characteristics.
Aneurysm	---	The local swelling or bulging of a blood vessel, to form a sac.
Anodyne	---	Herb used to ease or relieve pain.
Anorexia	---	Loss of appetite.
Antacid	---	Helps regulate acid conditions in the stomach.
Anthelmintic	---	Used to expel intestinal worms.
Antiabortive	—	Help to inhibit abortive tendencies.
Antiasthmatic	—	Relieves the symptoms of asthma.
Antibilious	---	Acts on the bile, relieving biliousness.
Antibiotic	---	Inhibits the growth of, or eradicates viruses and bacteria.
Antibody	---	A protein molecule that counteracts the effects of invading organisms and other foreign substances.
Anticatarrhal	---	Eliminate or counteract the formation of mucus.
Antiemetic	---	Stops vomiting.
		produce antibodies.
Antileptic	---	Relieves fits.

Term		Definition
Antihistamine	---	Any drug that reduces the effect associated with histamine production in colds and allergies.
Antioxidant	---	A substance that slows oxidation.
Antiperiodic	---	Arrests morbid periodic movements.
Antipyretic	---	Cools system reducing fevers.
Antirheumatic	---	Relieves or cures rheumatism.
Antiscorbutic	---	Cures or prevents scurvy.
Antiseptic	---	Helps prevent putrification.
Antispasmodic	---	Relieves or prevents spasms.
Antisyphilitic	---	Having effect or curing venereal diseases.
Aorta	---	The artery that carries blood from the heart's left ventricle and distributes it throughout the entire body.
Aphrodisiaca	---	Improve sexual potency and power.
Ascorbicacid	---	An organic acid (vitamin C). Used as an antioxidant.
Astringent	---	Constricting or binding effect, checks hemorrhages and secretions.
Ataxia	---	The loss of coordinated movement caused by a disease of the nervous system.
Autoimmune disease	---	When the body's immune system reacts to and damages its own tissues and organs.
Autologous transfusion	---	Using one's own blood that has been preserved for later use.
Avidin	---	A protein found in egg whites capable of inactivating biotin.
Bacteria	---	Harmful and friendly microscopic germs.
Bacteriophage	---	A virus that infects bacteria.
Bariatrician	---	A weight control doctor.

Term		Definition
B-Cells	---	White blood cells, made in the bone marrow that produce antibodies upon instructions from the white blood cells manufactured in the thymus.
Benign	---	Refers to cells that are not cancerous (non malignant).
Bile	---	Substance released by the liver into the intestines for the digestion of fat.
Bioflavonoid	---	Crystalline compounds (Vitamin P) needed to maintain healthy blood vessel walls and essential for the stability and absorption of ascorbic acid.
Biopsy	---	Excision of tissue from a living being for diagnosis.
Bloodcount	---	Number of red and white blood cells and platelets in a sample of blood.
Bronchi	---	The two main breathing tubes leading from the trachea to the lungs.
Carcinogen	---	Any agent that can cause cancer.
Cardiac	---	Pertaining to, or affecting the heart.
Cardiacarrest	---	Sudden stopping of circulation by cessation of the heart.
Cardiovascular	---	Pertaining to the heart and blood vessels.
Carminative	---	Expels gas from the bowels.
Carotidartery	---	Principal artery of the neck; carries blood to the head and brain.
Cathartic	---	Cause evacuating from the bowels.
Cell	---	All living tissue is composed of cells; very small complex units consisting of a nucleus, cytoplasm, and a cell membrane.
Cellulose	---	A nondigestable carbohydrate found in the peel or skin of fruits and vegetables.
Cephalic	---	Remedies used in diseases of the head.

Term		Definition
Cerebellum	---	The portion of the brain responsible for balance and coordinating movements.
Cerebrovascular	---	Pertaining to the blood vessels of the brain.
Chelation	---	A process by which mineral substances are changed into a digestible form.
Chemotherapy	---	A chemical treatment used to treat cancer.
Chronic	---	Constant, continuing, and of long duration.
Cholagogue	---	Increases the flow of bile.
Chyme	---	Mixture of partly digested food and digestive secretions found in the stomach.
Coagulate	---	To change from a liquid to a semisolid, as when blood clots.
Cobalt60	---	A radioactive isotope of the element cobalt.
Collagen	---	The primary organic constituent of bone, cartilage, and connective tissue.
Colon	---	The large intestine running from the small intestine to the anus.
Condiment	---	Improves the flavor of food.
Congenital	---	Not hereditary, condition existing at birth.
Congestion	---	The presence of excessive blood or fluid, such as mucus, in an organ or tissue.
Constipation	---	The difficult passage of hard or dry stools.
Contraceptive	---	A product used to prevent pregnancy.
Contusion	---	An injury in which the skin is not broken.
Convulsion	---	Contractions of the voluntary muscles that results from abnormal cerebral stimulation.
Coronary	---	Related to arteries that supply blood to the heart.
Cranium	---	Portion of the skull that houses the brain.
Cyst	---	A closed sac or cavity filled with a fluid , semisolid substance, or gas.

Term   ## Definition

Term		Definition
Cystoscope	---	The instrument used to examine the urinary bladder.
Debility	---	A state of physical weakness.
Dehydration	---	Excessive loss of water from the body.
Delirium	---	A state of mental confusion sometimes characterized by disordered speech and hallucinations.
Demulcent	---	Soothing, relieves internal inflammation.
Deobstruent	---	Removes obstructions.
Depression	---	A feeling of extreme sadness and discourage ment. Symptoms include lack of energy and disruption of eating and sleeping patterns.
Depurative	---	Purifies the blood.
Dermis	---	The layer of skin beneath the epidermis.
Detergent	---	Cleansing boils, ulcers, wounds, etc.
Detoxification	---	Reducing the body's toxic build-up of poisonous substances.
Dialysis	---	A technique used in the removal of toxins and waste from the blood.
Diaphoretic	---	Produces and increases perspiration.
Diaphragm	---	The muscle that separates the abdomen from the chest.
Discutient	---	Dissolves and heals tumors and abnormal growths.
Diuretic	---	Increases the secretion and flow of urine.
DNA	---	The substance that genetically codes and determines the type of life form into which a cell will develop.
Duodenum	---	The part of the small intestine closest to the stomach.
EDTA	---	Organic molecule used in chelation therapy.

Term		Definition
EEG	---	A test that measures brain wave activity.
Effusion	---	Accumulation of fluid in the body cavities or between tissues.
Essentialfatty acids	---	Substances that cannot be manufactured in the body, so must be supplied in the diet.
Emetic	---	Substance that induces vomiting.
Emmenagogue	---	Promotes and stimulates menstrual flow.
Emollient	---	Softens and soothes inflamed tissue.
Endocardium	---	The inner membrane that lines the heart muscle.
Enzyme	---	A protein found in living cells that brings about chemical changes necessary for the digestion of food.
Epicardium	---	The exterior membrane that protects the heart muscle.
Epidermis	---	Outer layer of skin.
Erythema	---	Area of reddened skin due to dilatation of capillaries beneath the skin.
Esculent	---	Edible as a food.
Exanthematous	---	Remedy for skin eruptions and diseases.
Expectorant	---	Expulsion of phlegm from mucus membrane.
Febrifuge	---	Abates and reduces fevers.
Fetus	---	A child in the uterus from the second month of pregnancy to delivery.
Fibrillation	---	Uncontrollable contraction or quivering of heart muscles, causing irregular heart beat.
Fibroid	---	A benign tumor of connective and muscular tissue.
Flatulence	---	Excessive gas in the stomach and intestine.
Fracture	---	A break or a crack in a bone.

Term   ## Definition

Free radical --- An atom or group of atoms that has at least one impaired electron.

Fructose --- A natural fruit sugar.

Fungus --- A one-celled organism belonging to the plant kingdom.

Galactagogue --- Promotes secretion of breast milk.

Gallbladder --- A sac located under the liver that stores the bile secreted from the liver and releases it into the small intestine.

Gamma globulin -- A protein found in the blood that helps fight infection.

Gastrointestinal--- The stomach and intestines.

Genetic --- Characteristics that are inherited.

Gestation --- Period of time from conception to birth.

Globulin --- A category of blood proteins of which anti-bodies are formed.

Glucose --- A blood sugar that is the product of the body's assimilation of carbohydrates.

Gluten --- The combination of two proteins (gliadin and glutenin) present in barley, oats, rye, and wheat.

Granulocytes --- White blood cells that contain granules, manufactured in the bone marrow.

Hamstrings --- Muscles at the back of the thigh.

Hemangioma --- A benign tumor of dilated blood vessels.

Hematuria --- Blood in the urine.

Hemicellulose --- An indigestible carbohydrate resembling cellulose.

Hemoglobin --- A molecule in which the essential component is iron. Required by the red blood cells to transport oxygen.

Hemorrhage --- Profuse bleeding due to damage to a blood vessel.

Term		Definition
Hemostatic	---	Agent that arrests internal bleeding.
Hepatic	---	For liver diseases, stimulates secretive functions.
Herpatic	---	A remedy for skin diseases of all types.
Histamine	---	A chemical that constricts bronchial tube muscles, increases secretion of stomach acid, and dilates small blood vessels.
Hormone	---	A substance secreted by the endocrine gland that regulates the various body functions.
Host	---	An organism in which another micro-organism lives and obtains nourishment.
Hydrolyzed	---	Put into water-soluble form.
Hymen	---	A membrane that partially covers the opening to the vagina.
Hyperglycemia	---	An excess of sugar in the bloodstream.
Hypertension	---	Abnormally high blood pressure.
Hypoglycemia	---	Abnormally low blood sugar count in the bloodstream.
Immunity	---	A condition that enables a living organism to resist disease and infection.
Incontence	---	Inability to control the release of feces or urine.
Indigestion	---	Abnormal or incomplete digestion.
Infection	---	The invasion of a body by organisms such as bacteria, fungi, protozoa, or virus.
Inflammation	---	Body tissue's reaction to injury from irritation, infection, or a physical blow.
Intestines	---	The portion of the digestive tract extending from the stomach to anus.
Insulin	---	The hormone secreted by the pancreas that controls the metabolism of sugar in the body.
IU	---	International unit.

Term   ## Definition

IV --- A needle placed in a vein to assist the giving of medication or fluid replacement.

Jejunum --- The portion of the small intestine between the ileum and duodenum.

Jugularveins --- The two veins on the sides of the neck that carry blood from the brain to the heart.

Keratin --- Protein found in the outer layers of skin, hair, and nails.

Kyphosis --- Excessive curvature of the spine resulting in rounding of the shoulders or hunchback.

Laser --- An instrument used in surgical procedures.

Laxative --- Promotes bowel action.

Leukocytes --- White blood cells that fight infection.

Lipid --- A fatty substance.

Lipotropic --- Preventing excessive accumulation of fat in the liver.

Lithontryptic --- Dissolves and discharges calculi in urinary organs.

Lumbar --- The lower back .

Lymphatic --- Used to stimulate and cleanse lymphatic system.

Malabsorption --- Inadequate absorption of nutrients from the small intestine.

Malignant --- A term used to describe a cancerous growth that is predisposed to spreading.

Mammary gland - A compound gland of the breast that secretes milk.

Maturating --- Ripens or brings boils to a head.

Membrane --- A thin soft layer of tissue that separates, covers, or lines structures or organs.

Meninges --- The three membranes that cover the brain and spinal cord.

<u>Term</u>	<u>Definition</u>
Metabolize	--- Undergoing change by physical and chemical process.
Microbes	--- One-celled organisms.
Mucilaginous	--- Soothing to all inflammation.
Muscle	--- Tissue with the ability to contract producing movement.
Nauseant	--- Produces vomiting.
Nerve	--- Fibers through which impulses pass connecting the spinal cord and brain with the other parts of the body.
Nervine	--- Acts on nervous system, stops nervous excitement.
Nutritive	--- Supplies nutrients, aids building and toning body.
Oncology	--- The study of cancer.
Oncologist	--- A cancer specialist
Opticnerve	--- The nerve that carries light impulses from the retina to the brain.
Opthalmicum	--- A remedy for the healing of eye diseases.
Oxidation	--- A chemical reaction occurring when oxygen is added, resulting in a chemical transformation.
Oxytocin	--- Pituitary hormone that acts to stimulate the breasts to release milk.
Pancreas	--- The gland that produces enzymes essential to the digestion of food.
Paptest	--- Examining the cells collected from the vagina and cervix to test for uterine cancer.
Parasite	--- An organism that lives off other organisms.
Parasiticide	--- Kills and expels parasites from the skin or digestive tract.
Paroxysm	--- A sudden attack such as a recurrence of symptoms of a disease, a spasm, or a convulsion.

Term

Definition

Term		Definition
Parturient	---	Induces and promotes labor at childbirth.
Pectoral	---	A remedy for chest affections.
Pepsin	---	The main enzyme of the digestive juices of the stomach.
Pericardium	---	Membranous sac enclosing the heart.
Peroxides	---	By-products of free radicals formed in our bodies when molecules of fat react with oxygen.
Phlegm	---	Thick mucus usually found in the sinuses or respiratory tract.
Pinealbody	---	A cone-shaped gland at the back of the brain.
Pituitary gland	---	An endocrine gland that produces hormones that control growth, reproductive capabilities, and day to day functioning.
Placebo	---	A pharmacological inactive substance used to compare the effects of pharmacologically active substances.
Precursor	---	Starts a chain reaction which accelerates growth.
Prolactin	---	Pituitary hormone responsible for stimulating the breasts to produce milk.
Protein	---	Essential for the body's growth and repair. A complex compound formed from nitrogen and found in all animal and vegetable tissues.
Prostategland	---	Located at the base of the bladder in men.
Provitamin	---	Precursor; a chemical necessary to produce a vitamin.
Pumonary	---	Pertaining to the lungs.
Purgative	---	Causes copious excretions from the bowels.
Purlent	---	Forming or containing pus.
Pylorus	---	The lower opening of the stomach.

Term		Definition
Radiation	---	The release of energy by unstable particles, not unlike the emission and transmission of energy referred to as actual radiation.
Refrigerant	---	Cooling.
Renal	---	Pertaining to the kidneys.
Resolvent	---	Dissolves boils and tumors.
RDA	---	Recommended daily allowance of vitamins or other nutrients as determined by the FDA.
Remission	---	Abatement of disease.
Retrovirus	---	A virus with its core being nucleic acid. This group is the causative agent of AIDS and viruses that cause immune deficiency.
RNA	---	Ribonucleic acid found in plant and animal cells.
Rubifacient	---	Increases circulation and produces red skin.
Saturates	---	Solid animal fats.
Sciaticnerve	---	The largest nerve in the body. It emerges from the base of the spinal cord as a number of roots and passes through the pelvis and down the back of the thigh.
Sedative	---	Nerve tonic, relieves excitement, promotes sleep.
Serum	---	A cell-free fluid of the blood stream, as reveiled in a test tube after a blood clot.
Sialogogue	---	Increases the secretion of saliva.
Spasm	---	A muscular contraction that causes an involuntary movement.
Spinalcolumn	---	The bony assemblage of vertebrae that enclose the spinal cord.
Spinalcord	---	A cord like bundle of nerves that link nerves of the trunk and extremities to the brain.
Stimulant	---	Increases energy, assists functional activity.

Term	Definition
Stomachic	Strengthens and tones stomach. Relieves indigestion.
Stroke	A medical emergency produced by a blood clot that lodges in an artery blocking the flow of blood to a portion of the brain.
Styptic	Contracts tissues, blood vessels, arrests bleeding.
Sudorific	Produces profuse perspiration.
Suppuration	The formation and discharge of pus from an injury or infection.
Symptom	Reaction to a bodily disorder.
Syncope	Fainting; A short loss of consciousness.
Syndrome	A combination of signs and symptoms that are presumed to characterize a disease.
Synergism	Interaction between two or more nutrients.
Synthetic	Artificial.
Tartar	Plaque deposits on the teeth.
T-Cell	A lymphocyte involved in the direct attack on invading organisms, crucial to the immune system.
Tendon	Cord-like tissue that connects muscles to bones.
Teratological	Abnormal formations in plants or animals.
Thrombin	An enzyme that is part of the process of blood coagulation.
Tissue	A collection of similar cells that, taken together, form a body structure
Tonic	A remedy which is invigorating and strengthening.
Toxin	A poison that impairs bodily functions.
Trauma	An injury such as a burn, broken bone, or wound.

Term		Definition
Tremor	---	Involuntary trembling.
Triglycerides	---	Fatty substances in the blood.
Tumor	---	An abnormal growth or tissue that resembles normal tissue but has no function.
Uterus	---	The female organ that contains the embryo and fetus. Sometimes called the womb.
Vaccine	---	A substance administered to induce immunity against specific agents.
Vagina	---	A tube of muscle and membrane connecting the external female genitalia with the uterus.
Vermifuge	---	Destroys and expels worms from the system.
Virus	---	A group of single celled structures composed of a protein coat and a core of DNA or RNA.
Vital Signs	---	Temperature, blood pressure, breathing, and pulse.
Vulnerary	---	Promotes healing by stimulating cell growth.
Vulva	---	External female genitalia, including the clitoris and labia.
Wen	---	A cyst that develops in a sebaceous gland.
Western Blot	---	The test designed to find the AIDS virus exposure by assessing the presence of the AIDS virus antibody.
Withdrawal	---	Detoxification, termination of a habit forming drug.
Xerosis	---	A condition of dryness.
Yeast	---	A single celled organism that can cause infection on any and all body parts.
Zein	---	Protein from corn.
Zyme	---	Fermenting.

BIBLIOGRAPHY

Adams, Ruth. - *Vitamin E, Wonder Worker of the 70's.* New York, U.S.A: Larchmont books 1972.

Adams, Ruth. - *Body, Mind, & B Vitamins.* New York, U.S.A: Larchmont books 1972.

Airola, Paavo. - *How to Get Well.* Ariz. U.S.A: Health Plus, 1974.

Alexeev, U.E. - *Herbal Plants of the U.S.S.R.* Moscow, U.S.S.R: MISL, 1971.

Allshorn, George, E. - *Domestic Homeopathic Practice.* London, England: Houston and Write, 1871.

Ancowitz, Aurthur. - *Strokes and Their Prevention.* New York, U.S.A: Jove Publications, 1982.

Andrews, Ralph W. - *Indian Primitive.* New York, U.S.A: Bonanza Books, 1962.

Atkins, Robert C. - *Dr. Atkins' Nutrition Breakthrough.* New York, U.S.A: Bantom Books 1981.

Bakuleff, A. N. and Petroff, F.N. - *Popular Medical Encyclopedia.* Moscow, U.S.A: Bolshaya Soviet Encyclopedia, 1965.

Bailey, Herbert. - *Vitamin E: Your Key to a Healthy Heart.* New York, U.S.A: Ark Books, 1970.

Basu, T.K. - *About Mothers, Children and Their Nutrition.* London, England: Thorsons Publishing, 1981.

Bender, George, A. - *Great Moments in Medicine.* Michigan, U.S.A: Park Davis, 1961.

Bodman, Frank. - *Insights into Homeotherapeutics.* London, England: Beakonsfield Publisher, 1990.

Bogorad, B.B. - *Dictionary of Biological Terms.* Moscow, U.S.S.R. Ministry of Education, 1963.

Borsaak, Henry. - *Vitamins: What they are and How They Can Effect You.* New York, U.S.A: Pyramid Books, 1971.

Brennan, R.O. - *Nutrigenetics.* New York, U.S.A: New American Library, 1977.

Brewster, Dorothy Patricia. - *You Can Breastfeed Your Baby.* PA U.S.A: Rodale Press, 1979.

Chopra, R. N. *Glossary of Indian Medicinal Plants.* New Delhi, India: Scientific & Industrial Research, 1956.

Clarke, J. H. - *The Prescriber.* Rustington, England: Health Science Press, 1968.

Clymer, R. - *Nature's Healing Agents.* PA, U.S.A; Dorrance Co., 1963.

Daraban, E. V. *Medical Preparations.* Zsoeovie, Kiev: Medication Ukrainian, 1966.

Davis, Adelle. - *Let's Get Well.* New York, U.S.A: New American Library, 1972.

Dastur, J.F. - *Medicinal Plants of India and Pakistan.* Bombay, India: Taraporevala Sons and Co., 1962.

De-Vries, Arnold. - *Primitive Man and His Food.* Chicago, U.S.A: Chandler Book Co., 1952.

Dewey, W.A. - *Practical Homeopathic Therapeutics.* New Delhi, India: Jain Publishing Co., No Date.

Doole, Louise E. - *Herbs and Garden Ideas.* New York, U.S.A: Sterling Publishing Co., 1964.

Dunne, Lavon J. - *Nutrition Almanac.* New York, U.S.A: McGraw-Hill Book Co., 1979.

Farrandez, V. L. - *Guia de Medicina Vegetal.* Celoni, Spain: J. Impentor, 1967.

Farrington, E.A. - *Clinical Materia Medica.* New Delhi, India: Jain Publishers, 1981.

Feingold, Ben W. - *Why Your Child is Hyperactive.* New York, U.S.A: Random House, 1975.

Fortisevn, Zeke. - *Global Herb Manual.* Alberta, Canada: Global Health Ltd., 1992.

Fox, William. - *Family Botanic Guide.* California, U.S.A: Health Research, 1963.

Gibbons, Euell. - *Stalking The Healthful Herbs.* New York, U.S.A: David Mckay Co. Inc. 1966.

Graham, Judy. - *Multiple Sclerosis.* Wellingborough, England: Thorsons Publishers, 1982.

Harper, Shove. - *Prescriber and Clinical Repertory of Medicinal Herbs.* Sussex, England: Health Science Press, 1938.

Hauschka, Rudolf. - *The Nature of Substance.* London, England: Stuart & Watkins, 1966.

Hutchens, Alma R. - *Indian Herbalogy of North America.* Michigan, U.S.A: Ann Arbor, 1982

Hunter, Kathleen. - *Health Foods and Herbs.* Glasgow, U.K: Collins, 1962.

James, Claudia V. - *Herbs and the Fountain of Youth.* Alberta, Canada: Armita Books, 1963.

Jolliffe, Norman. - *ClinicalNutrition.* 2d ed. New York, U.S.A: Harper & Brothers, 1962.

Jouanny, Jacques. - *TheEssentialsofHomeopathicMateria Medica.* Lyon, France: Laboratoires Boiron, 1984.

Kareev, F. I. - *Plants for Daily Use.* Moscow, U.S.S.R: Moscow University, 1963.

Katz, Marcella. - *Vitamins, Food, and Your Health.* U.S.A: Public Affairs Committee, 1975.

Korth, Leslie O. - *Some Unusual Healing Methods.* Surrey, England: Health Science Press, 1960.

Kushi, Michio. - *The Book of Macrobiotics.* Tokyo, Japan: Japan Publications, 1977.

Kushi, Michio. - *The Book of Oriental Diagnosis..* Tokyo, Japan: Japan Publications, 1980.

Locke, David M. - *Enzymes-The Agents of Life.* New York, U.S.A: Crown Press, 1971.

Mindell, Earl. - *Mindell's Vitamin Bible.* New York, U.S.A: Warner Books, 1980.

Mindell, Earl. - *Mindell's Herb Bible.* New York, U.S.A: Simon & Schuster, 1992.

Meshkovsky, M. D. - *LedaretvennyeSredstva.* Moscow, U.S.S.R: Medicina, 1967.

Meyer, Joseph E. - *TheHerbalist.* Illinois, U.S.A: Meyerbooks, 1991.

Newbold, H.L. - *Mega-Nutrients for Your Nerves.* New York, U.S.A: Berkley Publishing, 1981.

Nyholt, David H. - *The Athlete's Bible.* Alberta, Canada: Global Health Ltd., 1989.

Nyholt, David H. - *The Vitamin & Herb Guide.* Alberta, Canada: Global Health Ltd., 1992.

Oliver, J. H. - *Proven Remedies.* London, England: Thorsons Publishers Ltd., 1962.

Passwater, Ritchard A. - *Selenium as Food and Medicine.* Conn., U.S.A: Keats Publishing Co., 1980.

Pearson, Durk, and Sandy Shaw - *Life Extension.* New York, U.S.A: Warner Books, 1982.

Phillips, Charles D. - *Materia Medica and Therapeutics.* New York, U.S.A: William Wood and Co., 1897.

Pollack, Edward. - *New, Old and Forgotten Remedies.* Calcutta, India: Roy publishing House, 1966.

Rodale, J.I. - *Be a Healthy Mother, Have a Healthy Baby.* PA, U.S.A: Rodale Books, 1973.

Rodenberg, Harold. and Feldzaman, A.N. - *Doctors Book of Vitamin Therapy: Megavitamins for Health.* New York, U.S.A: Putnam's, 1974.

Shepherd, Dorothy. - *Homeopathy for the First Aider.* Sussex, England: Health Science Press, 1953.

Sokol, Steve. - *The Fitness Formula.* Alberta, Canada: Global Health Ltd., 1992.

Sweet, Muriel. - *Common Edible and Useful Plants of the West.* California, U.S.A: Naturegraph Co., 1962.

Thomas, Clayton L. - *Taber's Cyclopedia Medical Dictionary* 12th ed. PA, U.S.A: Davis Co., 1973

Tobe, John H. - *Proven Herbal Remedies.* Ontario, Canada. Provoker, 1969.

Vogel, Virgil J. - *American Indian Medicine.* Oklahoma, U.S.A: University of Oklahoma, 1970.

Wade, Carlson. - *Helping Your Health with Enzymes.* New York, U.S.A: Universal-Award House, 1971.

Wheatly, Michael. - *About Nutrition.* London, England: Thorsons, 1971.

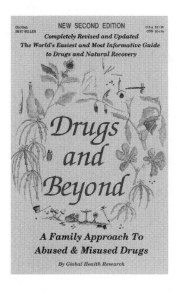
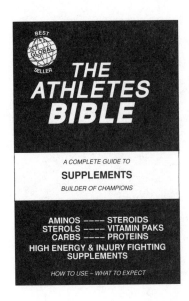

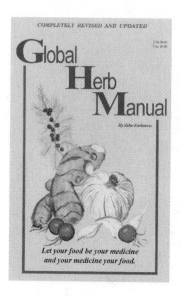

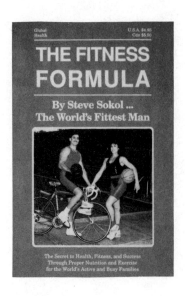

Global Herb Manual

New Sixth Edition
The Latest in Herbal Science
by Zeke Fortisevn
$4.95 U.S.A./ $5.95 Cdn.

This manual is a vast storehouse of knowledge on herbs. Discover the amazing healing and preventative properties of ancient and modern herbs. Plants are mankind's chief method of healing and main source of medicine. This simplified book contains all of the common herbs and characteristics, the effective herbal combinations, extracts, oils and syrups, and their specific functions. Proven herbal cleansing diets, over 50 herbal treatments for the world's most common ailments, plus a comprehensive index and glossary.

The Fitness Formula

A Must For The World's Active and Busy Families
by Steve Sokol
$4.95 U.S.A./ $5.95 Cdn.

The Secret to Health, Fitness, and Success. Steve Sokol is not only a talented writer and spokesman for numerous health related associations, but also holds over twenty world fitness records. In this book Steve shares with you his proven techniques designed for people of all skill levels, to increase energy levels, mental alertness, health, and fitness. A sensible plan to feel and look your personal best. Building confidence and success through proper nutrition and exercise.